RENAL DIET COOKBOOK FOR BEGINNERS

600+ Healthy, Easy and Delicious Recipes-

28-Day Handpicked Diet Meal Plan –
5 Proven Tips for Success-
Lose Up to 20 Pounds in Just 3-Weeks

CHRISTOPHER S. MULLINS

TABLE OF CONTENTS

INTRODUCTION **1**
BREAKFAST **2**
01. Berry Chia with Yogurt 2
02. Arugula Eggs with Chili Peppers 2
03. Breakfast Skillet 2
04. Eggs in Tomato Rings 3
05. Eggplant Chicken Sandwich 3
06. Eggplant Caprese 3
07. Chorizo Bowl with Corn 4
08. Panzanella Salad 4
09. Shrimp Bruschetta 4
10. Strawberry Muesli 5
11. Yogurt Bulgur 5
12. Chia Pudding 5
13. Goat Cheese Omelet 5
14. Vanilla Scones 6
15. Olive Bread 6
16. Yufka Pies 6
17. Breakfast Potato Latkes with Spinach 7
18. Cherry Tomatoes and Feta Fritatta 7
19. Egg White Scramble 7
20. Beet Smoothie 8
21. Chia Bars 8
22. Green Eggs Mix 8
23. Chia Pudding 9
24. Pineapple Smoothie 9
25. Anti-Inflammatory Porridge 9
26. Cucumber and Pineapple Smoothie 9
27. Quinoa Porridge 10
28. Raspberry Smoothie 10
29. Gingerbread Oatmeal 10
30. Rhubarb Muffins 11
31. Winter Fruit Salad 11
32. Buckwheat Granola 11
33. Mushroom Frittata 12
34. Breakfast Crepes 12
35. Millet Muffins 12
36. Kale Smoothie 12
37. Apple Muesli 13
38. Veggie and Onion Mix 13
39. Coconut Flour Naan Bread with Paprika Mushrooms 13
40. Zucchini Noodles 14
41. Kohlrabi with a Creamy Mushroom Sauce 14
42. Spinach and Strawberry Salad 14
43. Japanese Enoki Mushrooms with Oyster Sauce and Sesame Seeds 15
44. Creamy Cauliflower Soup 15
45. Invigorating Nutty Spring Salad 15
46. Cremini Mushroom Casserole with a Kick 16
47. Sautéed Broccoflower with Blue Cheese Sauce 16
48. Roasted Cherry Tomatoes with Parmesan Cheese. 16
49. Buttery Savoy Cabbage 17
50. Broccoli and Vegetable "Rice" Delight 17
51. Shrimp Bok Choy 18
52. Cheesy Cauliflower and Mushroom Casserole 18
53. Cheddar and Spinach Muffins 18
54. Muffins with Kale and Gruyère Cheese 19
55. Family Vegetable Pizza 19
MAINS **20**
56. Dolmas Wrap 20
57. Salad al Tonno 20
58. Arlecchino Rice Salad 20
59. Greek Salad 21
60. Sauteed Chickpea and Lentil Mix 21
61. Baked Vegetables Soup 21
62. Pesto Chicken Salad 22
63. Falafel 22
64. Israeli Pasta Salad 22
65. Artichoke Matzo Mina 23
66. Stuffed Zucchini Boats with Goat Cheese 23
67. Greek Style Quesadillas 24
68. Creamy Penne 24
69. Light Paprika Moussaka 24
70. Cucumber Bowl with Spices and Greek Yogurt 25
71. tuffed Bell Peppers with Quinoa 25
72. Mediterranean Burrito 25
73. Sweet Potato Bacon Mash 26
74. Prosciutto Wrapped Mozzarella Balls 26
75. Garlic Chicken Balls 26
76. Stuffed Tomatoes with Cheese and Meat 27
77. Stuffed Meatballs with Eggs 27
SIDES **28**
78. Dill Orzo 28
79. Quinoa Tabbouleh 28
Baked Grapes with Feta 28
81. 4-Ingredients Spinach Salad 28
82. Celeriac Tortilla 29
83. Caraway Mushroom Caps 29
84. Stuffed Sweet Potato 29
85. Garlic Grated Beets 29
86. Mujadara n 30
87. Olives Quinoa with Jalapeno 30
88. Cauliflower Puree with Bacon 30
89. Citrus Salad 31
90. Spanakorizo Spinach Rice 31
91. Walnut Salad 31
92. Baked Olives 32
93. Sliced Figs Salad 32
94. Lemon Cucumbers with Dill 32

95. Honey Apple Bites 32
96. Cucumber Salad 33
97. Sesame Seeds Escarole 33
98. Yogurt Eggplants 33
SEAFOOD 34
99. Fish Packets 34
100. Salmon Baked in Foil with Fresh Thyme 34
101. Poached Halibut in Orange Sauce 34
102. Fish en Papillote 35
103. Tuna Casserole 35
104. Oregano Salmon with Crunchy Crust 35
105. Sardine Fish Cakes 35
106. Cajun Catfish 36
107. Poached Gennaro/Seabass with Red Peppers 36
108. 4-Ingredients Salmon Fillet 36
109. Spanish Cod in Sauce 37
110. Fish Shakshuka 37
111. Mackerel Skillet with Greens 37
112. Salmon Balls with Cream Cheese 38
113. Fish Chili with Lentils 38
114. Chili Mussels 38
115. Fried Scallops in Heavy Cream 39
116. Lettuce Seafood Wraps 39
117. Mango Tilapia Fillets 39
118. Seafood Gratin 39
119. Ginger Seabass Stir-Fry 40
120. Teriyaki Tuna 40
121. Shrimp Korma 40
122. Tandoori Salmon Skewers 41
123. Prawns Kebabs 41
124. Lime Lobsters 41
125. Asian Sesame and Miso Salmon 42
126. Orange Herbed Sauced White Bass 42
127. Grilled Salmon Teriyaki 42
128. Pecan Crusted Trout 43
129. Oysters on the Shell 43
130. Breaded and Spiced Halibut 43
131. Baked Salmon with Greens 44
132. Oysters Rockefeller 44
133. Smoked Herring Sandwich 45
134. Roasted Salmon Garden Salad 45
135. Tuna Caprese Open-Faced Flatbread 45
136. Tuna-Hummus on Flatbread 46
137. Tuna & Sun-Dried Tomato-Wich 46
138. Tuna-Avo Boat Salad 47
139. Grilled Salmon-Lettuce Wraps 47
140. Black Bean 'n Salmon Salad 47
141. Easy 'n Healthy Tuna Salad 48
142. Fresh Tomato 'n Tuna Salad Sandwich 48
143. Baked Salmon Burger Patty 49
144. Baked Halibut with Avocado-Blueberry Salsa 49
145. Rice 'n Tuna Casserole 49
146. Sardine Salad Pickled Pepper Boats 50
147. Asian-Inspired Tilapia Chowder 50
148. Smoked Salmon and Cheese Stuffed Tomatoes 50
149. Chilean Sea Bass with Cauliflower and Chutney 51
150. Grilled Halloumi and Tuna Salad 51
151. Colorful Tuna Salad with Bocconcini 52
152. Tuna Fillets with Greens 52
153. One-Pot Seafood Stew 52
154. Seafood and Andouille Medley 53
155. Quatre Épices Salmon Fillets with Cheese 53
156. Easy Parmesan Crusted Tilapia 54
157. Creamy Anchovy Salad 54
158. Moms' Aromatic Fish Curry 54
159. Pan-Seared Trout Fillets with Chimichurri 55
160. Sunday Amber jack Fillets with Parmesan Sauce 55
161. Crab meat, Prosciutto and Vegetable Delight 56
162. Fish with Cremini Mushrooms and Sour Cream Sauce 56
163. Spring Salad with Harissa Crab Mayo 56
164. Grilled Clams with Tomato Sauce 57
165. Prawn and Avocado Cocktail Salad 57
166. Chinese-Style Milk fish with Mushroom-Pepper Coulis 57
167. Tuna and Vegetable Kebabs 58
168. Mackerel Steak Casserole with Cheese and Veggies 58
169. Classic Seafood Chowder 59
170. Smoky Cholula Seafood Dip 59
171. Smoked Creamy Fish Fat Bombs 59
172. Steamed Bream with Fennel 60
173. Egg and Fish Fry 60
174. Tuna Salad with Avocado, Sesame and Mint 61
175. Almond Breaded Crayfish with Herbs 61
176. Aromatic Cuttlefish with Spinach 61
177. Baked Shrimp Saganaki with Feta 62
178. Breaded Catfish Fillets 62
179. Calamari and Shrimp Stew 62
180. Catalonian Shrimp Stew 63
181. Cuttlefish with Green Olives and Fennel 63
182. Delicious Shrimp with Broccoli 63
183. Fried Mussels with Mustard and Lemon 64
184. Fried Wine Octopus Patties 64
185. Grilled King Prawns with Parsley Sauce 64
186. Cajun Lime Grilled Shrimp 65
187. Iberian Shrimp Fritters 65
188. Mussels with Herbed Butter on Grill 65
189. Mussels with Saffron 66
190. Mussels with Spinach Stir-fry 66
191. Shrimp and Octopus Soup 66
192. Shrimp with Curry and Coconut Milk 67
193. Spicy Razor Clams 67

194. Squid with Homemade Pesto Sauce........................67
195. Traditional Hungarian Halászlé..............................68
196. Salmon Fillets in Marsala Sauce..............................68
197. Old Bay Prawns with Sour Cream...........................68
198. Dad's Fish Jambalaya...69
199. Mediterranean Haddock with Cheese Sauce..........69
200. Fish Cakes with Classic Horseradish Sauce...........69
201. Classic Fish Curry...69
202. 34Sea Bass with Dill Sauce......................................70
203. Salmon Lettuce Tacos..70
204. Traditional Mahi Mahi Ceviche..............................70
205. Fried Cod Fillets...71
206. Shrimp and Ham Jambalaya...................................71
207. Herring and Spinach Salad.......................................71
208. Haddock and Parmesan Fish Burgers....................71
209. Greek-Style Halibut Fillets.......................................72
210. Cod Fish à La Nage..72
211. Tilapia in Garlic Butter Sauce.................................72
212. Chinese Fish Salad..72
213. 36Indian Fish Fry...73
214. 36Tilapia and Shrimp Soup.....................................73
215. 36Provençal Fish and Prawn Stew.........................73
216.36Mexican-Style Grilled Salmon..............................74
217. 36Portuguese Caldeirada De Peixe.........................74
218. 36Sea Bass with Peppers..74
219. 36Cod Fish Salad (Insalata di Baccalà)....................74
POULTRY 76
220. Ground Chicken & Peas Curry...............................76
221. Chicken Meatballs Curry..76
222. Ground Chicken with Basil......................................77
223. Chicken &Veggie Casserole....................................77
224. Chicken & Cauliflower Rice Casserole..................78
225. Chicken Meatloaf with Veggies..............................78
226. Roasted Spatchcock Chicken..................................79
227. Roasted Chicken with Veggies & Orange.............80
228. Roasted Chicken Breast...80
229. Roasted Chicken Drumsticks..................................80
230. Grilled Chicken...81
231. Grilled Chicken Breast...81
232. Grilled Chicken with Pineapple & Veggies............82
233. Ground Turkey with Veggies..................................82
234. Ground Turkey with Asparagus..............................83
235. Ground Turkey with Peas & Potato.......................83
236. Turkey & Pumpkin Chili...84
237. Turkey & Veggies Chili..84
238. Ground Turkey with Lentils....................................85
239. Roasted Whole Turkey...85
240. Grilled Turkey Breast...86
241. Duck with Bok Choy...86
242. Grilled Duck Breast & Peach..................................86
243. Slow Cooker Turkey Legs.......................................87
244. Turkey and Cauliflower Soup like Grandma Used to Make... 87
245. Chicken Leftovers Chowder 88
246. Amazing Turkey Kebabs 88
247. Healthy Chicken Salad 88
248. Spicy Chicken and Hemp Seeds 89
249. Chicken with a Mustard and Cream Sauce........... 89
250. Delicious and Easy Chicken Drumettes............... 90
251. Salsa Chicken Sausage 90
252. Simple Turkey and Herb Drumsticks 91
253. Chicken Drumsticks Mediterranean-Style with Aioli 91
254. Cheesy Chicken with Peppers............................... 91
255. The Tastiest Chicken Tacos Ever.......................... 92
256. Turkey and Baby Bok Choy Soup 92
257. Turkey Soup like Mom Used to Make.................. 93
258. Duck Fillets with Vodka and Sour Cream............ 93
259. Chicken with Spices and Brussels Sprouts........... 93
260. Chicken Salad with Tarragon 93
261. Her by Chorizo and Asiago Cheese 94
262. Chicken and Cauliflower Creamy Soup................ 94
263. Turkey and Cheese Dip with Fresno Chiles......... 95
264. Turkey Bacon and Habanero Balls........................ 95
265. Crispy Chicken in the Oven 95
266. Prosciutto Wrapped Holiday Turkey 96
267. Chicken Thighs with a Rum Glaze........................ 96
268. Oven Baked Creamy Chicken Thighs.................. 96
269. Roasted Turkey Mushroom Loaf 97
270. Chicken Artichoke Casserole 97
271. Chicken Liver and Pancetta Casserole.................. 98
272. Chicken Casserole... 98
273. Chicken with Curry and Coriander Casserole....... 98
274. Instant Pot Asiago Chicken Wings........................ 99
275. Instant Pot Chicken Cilantro Wraps..................... 99
276. Instant Pot Perfect Braised Turkey Breast.......... 100
277. Instant Pot Roasted Whole Chicken................... 100
278. Instant Pot Serrano Chicken Stir Fry.................. 100
279. Instant Pot Tasty Chicken Curry 101
280. Slow cooker Chicken Thighs in Coconut Sauce. 101
281. Delicious Chicken Breast with Turmeric............ 102
282. Chicken Cutlets with Spinach Stir-Fry................ 102
283. Chicken and Zoodle Stir Fry............................... 102
284. Hungarian Chicken Fillet Stir-fry........................ 103
285. Spicy Chicken Stir-Fry.. 103
286. Shredded Turkey with Asparagus Stir-fry........... 103
287. Squash Spaghetti and Ground Chicken Stir-fry.. 104
288. Ground Turkey and Green Beans Stir-fry.......... 104
289. Turkey Chili with Monterey Jack Cheese 105
290. Swiss Turkey and Pepper Timbale 105
291. Chicken and Vegetable Souvlaki.......................... 105
292. 10Hungarian Chicken Paprikash 105
293. Sri Lankan Curry... 106

294. Traditional Japanese Ramen....106
295. Summer Turkey Drumstick....106
296. Greek-Style Roasted Chicken with Herbs....107
297. Garlicky Roasted Chicken Drumsticks....107
298. Chicken Breasts in Creamy Mushroom Sauce....107
299. Easy Cocktail Party Meatballs....108
300. Chinese Duck with Onion....108
301. Chicken Drumstick Soup....108
302. Oven-Roasted Buffalo Chicken....108
303. Chicken Drumsticks with Tomato....109
304. Creamed Chicken Salad....109
305. Rustic Italian Stuffed Turkey....109
306. Chicken with Tomato and Romano Cheese....110
307. Indian Chicken Masala....110
308. Authentic Italian Puttanesca....110
309. Chicken with Wine-Mushroom Sauce....110
310. 12Gourmet Italian Turkey Fillets....111
311. Mediterranean Chicken with Thyme and Olives.111
312. Duck with Zucchini and Marinara Sauce....111
MEAT....112
313. Grilled Skirt Steak....112
314. Spicy Lamb Curry....112
315. Lamb with Prunes....113
316. Lamb with Zucchini & Couscous....113
317. Baked Lamb with Spinach....114
318. Ground Lamb with Harissa....114
319. Ground Lamb with Peas....115
320. Roasted Leg of Lamb....115
321. Broiled Lamb Shoulder....116
322. Pan-Seared Lamb Chops....116
323. Roasted Lamb Chops with Relish....117
324. Grilled Lamb Chops....117
325. Lamb Burgers with Avocado Dip....118
326. Lamb & Pineapple Kebabs....118
327. Baked Meatballs & Scallions....119
328. Pork with Bell Pepper....119
329. Pork with Pineapple....120
330. Spiced Pork....120
331. Pork Chili....121
332. Ground Pork with Water Chestnuts....121
333. Glazed Pork chops with Peach....122
334. Pork chops in Creamy Sauce....122
335. Baked Pork & Mushroom Meatballs....123
336. Butternut Squash, Kale and Ground Beef Breakfast Bowl....123
337. Light Beef Soup....124
338. Beef Noodle Soup....124
339. Spanish Rice Casserole with Beef....124
340. Kefta Styled Beef Patties with Cucumber Salad..125
341. Broiled Lamb Chops....125
342. Mustard Chops with Apricot-Basil Relish....126
343. Sirloin Rolls with Brussels Sprouts & Fennel....126
344. Stone Fruit Slaw Topped Grilled Chops....127
345. Lamb Stew....127
346. Lamb with Spinach Sauce....128
347. Pepper Steak Taco....128
348. Tenderloin Steaks with Caramelized Onions....129
349. Lamb Burger on Arugula....129
350. Roasted Leg of Lamb....130
351. Cashew Beef Stir Fry....130
352. Lamb Curry Stew with Artichoke Hearts....131
353. Beefy Cabbage Bowls....131
354. Mexican Pork Carnitas....132
355. Slow Cooked Beef Pot Roast....132
356. Beef Ragu....132
357. Asian-Inspired Porkchops....133
358. Asian Beef Short Ribs....133
359. Stir-Fried Ground Beef....134
360. Traditional Scotch Eggs Recipe....134
361. Burrito Breakfast Bowl....134
362. Stir-Fried Mushrooms and Beef....135
363. Malaysian Beef Stew....135
364. Homemade Meatballs....135
365. Goat Curry....136
366. Pork Breakfast Muffins....136
367. Pork Gumbo for Entertaining....136
368. Pork Meatloaf with Tomato Sauce....137
369. Pork Shoulder a Cheesy Sauce....137
370. Meatloaf Muffins....138
371. A Mug of Breakfast Pork....138
372. Spicy and Creamy Pork Soup....138
373. Lettuce Wraps with Pork....139
374. Pork Steaks....139
375. Pork and Veggie Skewers....139
376. Pork with Bamboo Shoots and Cauliflower....140
377. Easy Fragrant Pork Chops....140
378. Crispy Pork Shoulder....141
379. Frittata with Spicy Sausage....141
380. Pork Stir-Fry Chinese-Style with Muenster Cheese....141
381. Slow Cooker Hungarian Goulash....142
382. Pork and Bell Pepper Quiche....142
383. Grilled Summer Baby Back Ribs....143
384. Skillet of Pork and Swiss chard....143
385. Roasted Peppers with Pork Ribs....143
386. Meatloaf for the Holidays....144
387. Pork Gumbo For a Special Dinner....144
388. Meatloaf with Gruyere....144
389. Roasted Fillet Mignon in Foil....145
390. Stewed Beef with Green Beans....145
391. Beef and Chicken Meatballs with Curry Sauce....146
392. Creamy and Peppery Beef Fillets....146

393. Perfect Oven Roasted Spareribs 147
394. Baked Ground Beef and Eggplant Casserole...... 147
395. Festive Rosemary Beef Fillet 147
396. Grilled Fillet Mignon with Black Peppercorn..... 148
397. Keto Beef Satay 148
398. Keto Beef Stroganoff 148
399. Tasty Veal Roast with Herb Crust 149
400. Beef Prosciutto Casserole 149
401. Ground Beef and Baby Spinach Casserole 150
402. Instant Pot Tangy Beef Chuck Roast 150
403. Beef Roast with Herbs and Mustard 150
404. Ground Beef with Swiss Chard Stir-fry 151
405. Ground Beef Kale Stew with Almonds 151
406. Perfect Keto Beef and Broccoli Stir-Fry 151
407. Grilled Lamb Skewers 152
408. Grilled Lamb Patties 152
409. Roasted Lamb Loin with Yogurt Sauce 153
410. Grilled Lamb Chops 153
411. Grilled Lamb Chops with Sweet Marinade 153
412. Instant Pot Lamb Chops with Greens 154
VEGETABLES 155
413. Collard Green Wrap 155
414. Zucchini Garlic Fries 155
415. Mashed Cauliflower 155
416. Stir-Fried Eggplant 156
417. Sautéed Garlic Mushrooms 156
418. Stir Fried Asparagus and Bell Pepper 156
419. Stir fried Brussels Sprouts And Pecans............... 157
420. Stir Fried Kale 157
421. Stir Fried Bok Choy 157
422. Vegetable Curry.. 158
423. Braised Carrots 'n Kale 158
424. Butternut Squash Hummus 158
425. Stir Fried Gingery Veggies.................................... 159
426. Cauliflower Fritters 159
427. Stir-Fried Squash.. 159
428. Cauliflower Hash Brown 160
429. Sweet Potato Puree 160
430. Curried Okra 160
431. Zucchini Pasta with Mango-Kiwi Sauce 161
432. Ratatouille 161
433. Roasted Eggplant with Feta Dip 161
434. Vegetable Potpie 162
435. Marsala Roasted Carrots 162
436. Cajun Asparagus 163
SOUPS AND STEWS 164
437. Beef Stroganoff Soup 164
438. Buffalo Ranch Chicken Soup 164
439. Chicken Stew 165
440. Chicken Fajita Soup 165
441. Italian Wedding Soup 166
442. Cream of Chicken Soup 166
443. Coffee and Wine Beef Stew 167
444. Green chicken enchilada soup 167
445. Beef Stew 167
446. Bacon Cheeseburger Soup 168
447. Roasted Garlic Soup 168
448. Fat Bomb Hamburger Soup 169
449. Mulligatawny 169
450. Chicken "Noodle" Soup 170
451. Broccoli Cheddar Soup 170
452. French Onion Soup 170
453. Curried Beef Stew 171
454. Green Chile Pork Stew 171
455. Wonderful Multi-Veggie Soup 172
456. Healthy Kale Soup 172
457. Delicious Carrot Soup 172
458. Mind Blowing Pumpkin Soup 172
459. Healthy Cabbage Soup 172
460. Broccoli Delight Soup 173
461. Chicken & Egg Drop Soup 173
462.Beef & Egg Drop Delight...................................... 173
463. Super-Crafted Egg & Vegetable Soup 174
464. Bacon Master Blaster 174
465. Basic Quinoa Soup 174
466. Marvellous Beans Soup 174
467. Tasty Shrimp Soup 174
468. Roasted Pepper Soup 175
469. Herb Flavored Potato Soup 175
470. Creamy Carrot Soup 175
471. Roasted Pork Soup 175
SAUCE RECIPES 177
472. Easy Garlicky Cherry Tomato Sauce 177
473. Avocado Cilantro Detox Dressing 177
474. Golden Turmeric Sauce 177
475. Creamy Turmeric Dressing 178
476. Dijon Mustard Vinaigrette 178
477. Anti-Inflammatory Caesar Dressing 178
478. Fresh Tomato Vinaigrette 178
479. Ginger Sesame Sauce 179
480. Golden Turmeric Tahini Sauce 179
481. Healthy Teriyaki Sauce 179
482. Yogurt Garlic Sauce 180
483. Chunky Tomato Sauce 180
484. Sweet Balsamic Dressing 180
485. Citrus Salad Sauce 180
486. Anti-Inflammatory Applesauce 181
487. Healthy Pizza Sauce 181
488. Green Goddess Sauce 181
489. Chimichurri Sauce 182
490. Raspberry Vinaigrette Sauce 182
491. Clean BBQ Sauce 182

EGGS AND DAIRY 183
492. Cheese Stuffed Peppers 183
493. Italian Zucchini Sandwiches 183
494.Creamy Dilled Egg Salad 183
495. Eggs with Goat Cheese 183
496. Dukkah Frittata with Cheese 184
497. Classic Italian Omelet 184
498. Egg Salad with Anchovies 184
499. Classic Keto Muffins 184
500. Authentic Spanish Migas 185
501. Double Cheese Fondue 185
502. Savory Rolls with Bacon and Cheese 185
503. Broccoli Cheese Pie 185
504. Herbed Cheese Ball 186
505. Mexican Eggs with Vegetables 186
506. Masala Eggs with Brown Mushrooms 186
507. Easy Keto Quesadillas 186
508. Ham and Cheese Muffins 187
509. Aleppo Pepper Deviled Eggs 187
510. Skinny Eggs with Spinach 187
511. Oven-Baked Eggs with Ham 188
512. Famous Double-Cheese Chips 188
513. Fast and Simple Spicy Eggs 188
514. Favorite Breakfast Tabbouleh 188
515. Egg Cups with Ham 189
516. Seasoned Egg Porridge for Breakfast. 189
517. Savory Feta Spinach Egg Cups. 189
518. Tasty and Soft-Boiled Egg. 190
519. Poached Tomatoes with Eggs. 190
520. Tasty and Simple French Toast. 190
521. Hard Boiled Large Eggs Recipe. 191
522. Spinach, Sliced Bacon with Eggs 191
523. Breakfast Jar with Bacon. 191
524. Tasty Scrambled Eggs & Bacon. 192
525. Tomato Spinach Quiche with Parmesan Cheese.192
526. Seasoned Cheesy Hash Brown. 193
527. Seasoned Creamy Sausage Frittata. 193
528. Seasoned Egg Side Dish Recipe. 193
529. Bacon and Egg with Cheese Muffins. 194
SNACKS 195
530. Cheesy Spicy Sausage Stuffed Mushrooms 195
531. Buffalo Cauliflower Bites with Dairy Free Ranch Dressing 195
532. Mini Zucchini Pizza Bites 195
533. Sugar Free Sweet & Spicy Bacon Chicken Bites .196
534. Baked Cream Cheese Crab Dip 196
535. Philly Cheesesteak Stuffed Mushrooms 196
536. Cheddar Cheese Straws and the Cabot Fit Team 197
537. Crispy Parmesan Tomato Chips 197
538. Parmesan Zucchini Rounds 197
539. Cheddar Cauliflower Bacon Bites 198
540. Jalapeno Popper Dip 198
541. Cream Cheese Stuffed Meatballs 198
542. Cucumber Cream Cheese Sandwiches 199
543. Salt and Vinegar Zucchini Chips 199
544. Chicken Salad Cucumber Bites 199
545. Ham and Dill Pickle Bites 200
546. Smoked Salmon & Cucumber 200
SMOOTHIES & JUICE 201
547. Almonds & Blueberries Smoothie 201
548. Almonds and Zucchini Smoothie 201
549. Avocado with Walnut Butter Smoothie 201
550. Baby Spinach and Dill Smoothie 201
551. Blueberries and Coconut Smoothie 202
552. Collard Greens and Cucumber Smoothie 202
553. Creamy Dandelion Greens and Celery Smoothie202
554. Dark Turnip Greens Smoothie 202
555. Butter Pecan and Coconut Smoothie 203
556. Fresh Cucumber, Kale and Raspberry Smoothie 203
557. Fresh Lettuce and Cucumber-Lemon Smoothie.203
558. Green Coconut Smoothie 204
559. Instant Coffee Smoothie 204
560. Keto Blood Sugar Adjuster Smoothie 204
561. Lime Spinach Smoothie 204
562. Protein Coconut Smoothie 205
563. Strong Spinach and Hemp Smoothie 205
564. Total Almond Smoothie 205
565. Ultimate Green Mix Smoothie 205
DESSERTS 207
566. Fruit Trifle 207
567. Berry Crumble 207
568. Greek Cheesecake 207
569. Lemon Pie 208
570. Galaktoboureko 208
571. Honey Cake 209
572. Portokalopita 209
573. Finikia 210
574. Vasilopita 210
575. Vanilla Biscuits 210
576. Semolina Pudding 211
577. Watermelon Jelly 211
578. Greek Cookies 211
579. Baked Figs with Honey 212
580. Cream Strawberry Pies 212
581. Banana Muffins 212
582. Grilled Pineapple 213
583. Coconut-Mint Bars 213
584. Hummingbird Cake 213
585. Cool Mango Mousse 214
586. Sweet Potato Brownies 214
587. Pumpkin Cookies 214
588. Baked Plums 214

589. Classic Parfait 215
590. Melon Popsicles 215
591. Watermelon Salad with Shaved Chocolate 215
592. No-Bake Strawberry Cheesecake 215
593. Raw Lime, Avocado & Coconut Pie 216
594. Blackberry & Apple Skillet Cake 216
595. Pudding Muffins 217
596. Black Forest Pudding 218
597. Pineapple Sticks 218
598. Fried Pineapple Slices 218
599. Grilled Peaches 218
600. Baked Apples 219
601. Stuffed Apples 219
602. Rhubarb & Blueberry Granita 219
603. Citrus Strawberry Granita 220
604. Pumpkin Ice-Cream 220
605. Chocolaty Cherry Ice-Cream 220
606. Pineapple & Banana Ice-Cream 221
607. Chocolate Sorbet 221
608. Lemon Sorbet 221
609. Zesty Mousse 221
610. Chocolate & Coffee Mousse 222
611. Chocolaty Avocado Mousse 222
612. Chocolaty Chia Pudding 222
613. Carrot Chia Pudding 223
614. Apple Chia Pudding 223
28 DAY MEAL PLAN 224
5 TIPS 225
CONCLUSION 225

DESCRIPTION

Our kidneys make an essential organ that is responsible for filtering our blood on a daily basis. However, when our kidneys start mal functioning, different organs can get affected and our body becomes unable to get rid of the excess of fluids and the toxic wastes of our body. Therefore, keeping our kidneys healthy is the cornerstone of our well-being, long and healthy life.

Thus, when living with a chronic kidney disease, controlling what you eat and what you drink makes an important step that can help prevent your health condition from deteriorating. And this is where this book stems from. In fact, this "Cope with your kidney disease and say good bye to dialysis" has proven its efficiency in controlling all types of kidney diseases that can endanger your life and that can change your basic lifestyle forever.

This book offers 600+ easy to make, delicious and succulent low phosphorus, low sodium and low potassium recipes that will help reduce any strain on your kidneys and will help you achieve better results.

And to make this book easier to read for you, I have made sure to categorize the recipes under certain subcategories like breakfast, mains, sides, seafood, poultry, meat, vegetables, soups, stews, smoothies and desserts **... AND MORE!!!**

The 28 day meal plan I have included in this book will help you decide what you eat every day without thinking too much about what you should and what you should not eat and with each recipe, you will find the recipe's nutritional information with specific Calories, protein, potassium, sodium and phosphorus. It is also recommended that you consult a renal dietician. And remember that as a kidney disease keeps progressing throughout time, your diet needs to be adjusted to the new condition. Try this book, you never know; it can save your life.

What are you waiting for? **Click buy now!!!!!**

INTRODUCTION

When you are recovering from acute renal failure or when you are on a renal failure diet, then your doctor or dietician would recommend a particular diet that would help you in limiting the stress on your kidneys. Your dietician would analyze and then depending upon your current situation would suggest a diet that would reduce the pressure on your kidneys. Here are certain lifestyle changes that would help you in the recovery process and also help you to have healthy kidneys.

You should opt for foods that have a low level of potassium or no potassium at all. Foods that are rich in potassium are bananas, spinach, tomatoes, oranges and even potatoes. You can instead consume foods that have a low level of potassium in them like apples, cabbage, grapes, strawberries and green beans as well. You should avoid products that have added salt in them. You should cut down on the amount of sodium that you consume on a daily basis and this can be done by simply avoiding packed and canned foods, even frozen foods, you should also avoid processed meats as well as cheeses. Phosphorus is generally found in dairy products like milk, cheese and butter, also in beans and nuts. You will need to reduce the amount of phosphorus that you consume because this weakens your bones and also cause skin irritation. Once your kidneys start recovering, your diet would change but that doesn't mean that you should stop eating healthy foods.

Renal failure is more often than not, difficult to predict or even prevent. But you can certainly lower your risk of renal failure by taking good care of your kidneys. Here are the things that you can keep in mind for taking good care of your kidneys. Whenever you are buying any over the counter medication, you should pay close attention to the labels. You should always follow the instructions that are given on these over-the-counter medicines like aspirin, ibuprofen and acetaminophen. Taking excess of the pain medication would increase the risk of renal failure and this is more likely when you already have any pre-existing kidney disease or any other problem like diabetes or high blood pressure. You should work along with your doctor for managing your kidney problems. Like mentioned earlier, if you have any preexisting condition or any other disease, then the risk of kidney failure increases. Especially when you have diabetes, high blood pressure or any other kidney related problem. Therefore, you should stay on track with your treatment and follow the doctor's recommendations for managing your condition. You should make living healthy as your lifestyle choice and priority. Keep yourself active, stay fit by exercising regularly and eat a balanced diet and consume alcohol in moderation, if you drink.

BREAKFAST

01. BERRY CHIA WITH YOGURT

Preparation Time: 35 minutes
Cooking time: 5 minutes
Servings:4

Ingredients:

- ½ cup chia seeds, dried
- 2 cup Plain yogurt
- 1/3 cup strawberries, chopped
- ¼ cup blackberries
- ¼ cup raspberries
- 4 teaspoons Splenda

Directions:

1. Mix up together Plain yogurt with Splenda, and chia seeds.
2. Transfer the mixture into the serving ramekins (jars) and leave for 35 minutes.
3. After this, add blackberries, raspberries, and strawberries. Mix up the meal well.
4. Serve it immediately or store in the fridge up to 2 days.

Nutrition: calories 257, fat 10.3, fiber 11, carbs 27.2, protein 12

02. ARUGULA EGGS WITH CHILI PEPPERS

Preparation Time: 7 minutes
Cooking time: 10 minutes
Servings: 4

Ingredients:

- 2 cups arugula, chopped
- 3 eggs, beaten
- ½ chili pepper, chopped
- 1 tablespoon butter
- 1 oz Parmesan, grated

Directions:

1. Toss butter in the skillet and melt it.
2. Add arugula and saute it over the medium heat for 5 minutes. Stir it from time to time.
3. Meanwhile, mix up together Parmesan, chili pepper, and eggs.
4. Pour the egg mixture over the arugula and scramble well.
5. Cook the breakfast for 5 minutes more over the medium heat.

Nutrition: calories 98, fat 7.8, fiber 0.2, carbs 0.9, protein 6.7

03. BREAKFAST SKILLET

Preparation Time: 7 minutes
Cooking time: 25 minutes
Servings: 5

Ingredients:

- 1 cup cauliflower, chopped
- 1 tablespoon olive oil
- ½ red onion, diced
- 1 tablespoon Plain yogurt
- ½ teaspoon ground black pepper
- 1 teaspoon dried cilantro
- 1 teaspoon dried oregano
- 1 bell pepper, chopped
- 1/3 cup milk
- ½ teaspoon Za'atar
- 1 tablespoon lemon juice
- 1 russet potato, chopped

Directions:

1. Pour olive oil in the skillet and preheat it.
2. Add chopped russet potato and roast it for 5 minutes.
3. After this, add cauliflower, ground black pepper, cilantro, oregano, and bell pepper.
4. Roast the mixture for 10 minutes over the medium heat.
5. Then add milk, Za'atar, and Plain Yogurt. Stir it well.
6. Saute the mixture 10 minutes.
7. Top the cooked meal with diced red onion and sprinkle with lemon juice.
8. It is recommended to serve the breakfast hot.

Nutrition: calories 112, fat 3.4, fiber 2.6, carbs 18.1, protein 3.1

04. EGGS IN TOMATO RINGS

Preparation Time: 8 minutes
Cooking time: 5 minutes
Servings: 2

Ingredients:

- 1 tomato
- 2 eggs
- ¼ teaspoon chili flakes
- ¾ teaspoon salt
- ½ teaspoon butter

Directions:

1. Trim the tomato and slice it into 2 rings.
2. Remove the tomato flesh.
3. Toss butter in the skillet and melt it.
4. Then arrange the tomato rings.
5. Crack the eggs in the tomato rings. Sprinkle them with salt and chili flakes.
6. Cook the eggs for 4 minutes over the medium heat with the closed lid.
7. Transfer the cooked eggs into the serving plates with the help of the spatula.

Nutrition: calories 77, fat 5.4, fiber 0.4, carbs 1.6, protein 5.8

05. EGGPLANT CHICKEN SANDWICH

Preparation Time: 10 minutes
Cooking time: 15 minutes
Servings: 2

Ingredients:

- 1 eggplant, trimmed
- 10 oz chicken fillet
- 1 teaspoon Plain yogurt
- ½ teaspoon minced garlic
- 1 tablespoon fresh cilantro, chopped
- 2 lettuce leaves
- 1 teaspoon olive oil
- ½ teaspoon salt
- ½ teaspoon chili pepper
- 1 teaspoon butter

Directions:

1. Slice the eggplant lengthwise into 4 slices.
2. Rub the eggplant slices with minced garlic and brush with olive oil.
3. Grill the eggplant slices on the preheated to 375F grill for 3 minutes from each side.
4. Meanwhile, rub the chicken fillet with salt and chili pepper.
5. Place it in the skillet and add butter.
6. Roast the chicken for 6 minutes from each side over the medium-high heat.
7. Cool the cooked eggplants gently and spread one side of them with Plain yogurt.
8. Add lettuce leaves and chopped fresh cilantro.
9. After this, slice the cooked chicken fillet and add over the lettuce.
10. Cover it with the remaining sliced eggplant to get the sandwich shape. Pin the sandwich with the toothpick if needed.

Nutrition: calories 368, fat 15.2, fiber 8.2, carbs 14.2, protein 43.5

06. EGGPLANT CAPRESE

Preparation Time: 15 minutes
Cooking time: 13 minutes
Servings: 3

Ingredients:

- 1 eggplant, trimmed, sliced
- ½ teaspoon dried basil
- 1 teaspoon salt
- ½ teaspoon ground black pepper
- 2 tomatoes, sliced
- 7 oz Mozzarella, sliced
- 1 teaspoon lemon juice
- 2 tablespoons olive oil

Directions:

1. Sprinkle the sliced eggplant with salt and leave for 10 minutes or until they give juice.
2. Then sprinkle the sliced eggplants with ground black pepper, lemon juice, and dried basil.
3. Arrange the eggplant, tomato, and sliced Mozzarella one-by-one in the casserole mold.
4. Drizzle it with olive oil and cover with foil.
5. Bake the caprese for 13 minutes.

Nutrition: calories 321, fat 21.5, fiber 6.5, carbs 14.8, protein 20.9

07. CHORIZO BOWL WITH CORN

Preparation Time: 10 minutes
Cooking time: 15 minutes
Servings: 4

Ingredients:

- 9 oz chorizo
- 1 tablespoon almond butter
- ½ cup corn kernels
- 1 tomato, chopped
- ¾ cup heavy cream
- 1 teaspoon butter
- ¼ teaspoon chili pepper
- 1 tablespoon dill, chopped

Directions:

1. Chop the chorizo and place in the skillet.
2. Add almond butter and chili pepper.
3. Roast the chorizo for 3 minutes.
4. After this, add tomato and corn kernels.
5. Add butter and chopped the dill. Mix up the mixture well. Cook for 2 minutes.
6. Close the lid and simmer the meal for 10 minutes over the low heat.
7. Transfer the cooked meal into the serving bowls.

Nutrition: calories 422, fat 36.2, fiber 1.2, carbs 7.3, protein 17.6

08. PANZANELLA SALAD

Preparation Time: 10 minutes
Cooking time: 5 minutes
Servings: 4

Ingredients:

- 3 tomatoes, chopped
- 2 cucumbers, chopped
- 1 red onion, sliced
- 2 red bell peppers, chopped
- ¼ cup fresh cilantro, chopped
- 1 tablespoon capers
- 1 oz whole-grain bread, chopped
- 1 tablespoon canola oil
- ½ teaspoon minced garlic
- 1 tablespoon Dijon mustard
- 1 teaspoon olive oil
- 1 teaspoon lime juice

Directions:

Pour canola oil in the skillet and bring it to boil.
Add chopped bread and roast it until crunchy (3-5 minutes).
Meanwhile, in the salad bowl combine together sliced red onion, cucumbers, tomatoes, bell peppers, cilantro, capers, and mix up gently.
Make the dressing: mix up together lime juice, olive oil, Dijon mustard, and minced garlic.
Pour the dressing over the salad and stir it directly before serving.

Nutrition: calories 136, fat 5.7, fiber 4.1, carbs 20.2, protein 4.1

09. SHRIMP BRUSCHETTA

Preparation Time: 15 minutes
Cooking time: 10 minutes
Servings: 4

Ingredients:

- 13 oz shrimps, peeled
- 1 tablespoon tomato sauce
- ½ teaspoon Splenda
- ¼ teaspoon garlic powder
- 1 teaspoon fresh parsley, chopped
- ½ teaspoon olive oil
- 1 teaspoon lemon juice
- 4 whole-grain bread slices
- 1 cup water, for cooking

Directions:

1. Pour water in the saucepan and bring it to boil.
2. Add shrimps and boil them over the high heat for 5 minutes.
3. After this, drain shrimps and chill them to the room temperature.
4. Mix up together shrimps with Splenda, garlic powder, tomato sauce, and fresh parsley.
5. Add lemon juice and stir gently.
6. Preheat the oven to 360F.
7. Brush the bread slices with olive oil and bake for 3 minutes.
8. Then place the shrimp mixture on the bread. Bruschetta is cooked.

Nutrition: calories 199, fat 3.7, fiber 2.1, carbs 15.3, protein 24.1

10. STRAWBERRY MUESLI

Preparation Time: 10 minutes
Cooking time: 30 minutes
Servings: 4

Ingredients:

- 2 cups Greek yogurt
- 1 ½ cup strawberries, sliced
- 1 ½ cup Muesli
- 4 teaspoon maple syrup
- ¾ teaspoon ground cinnamon

Directions:

1. Put Greek yogurt in the food processor.
2. Add 1 cup of strawberries, maple syrup, and ground cinnamon.
3. Blend the ingredients until you get smooth mass.
4. Transfer the yogurt mass in the serving bowls.
5. Add Muesli and stir well.
6. Leave the meal for 30 minutes in the fridge.
7. After this, decorate it with remaining sliced strawberries.

Nutrition: calories 149, fat 2.6, fiber 3.6, carbs 21.6, protein 12

11. YOGURT BULGUR

Preparation Time: 10 minutes
Cooking time: 15 minutes
Servings: 3

Ingredients:

- 1 cup bulgur
- 2 cups Greek yogurt
- 1 ½ cup water
- ½ teaspoon salt
- 1 teaspoon olive oil

Directions:

1. Pour olive oil in the saucepan and add bulgur.
2. Roast it over the medium heat for 2-3 minutes. Stir it from time to time.
3. After this, add salt and water.
4. Close the lid and cook bulgur for 15 minutes over the medium heat.
5. Then chill the cooked bulgur well and combine it with Greek yogurt. Stir it carefully.
6. Transfer the cooked meal into the serving plates. The yogurt bulgur tastes the best when it is cold.

Nutrition: calories 274, fat 4.9, fiber 8.5, carbs 40.8, protein 19.2

12. CHIA PUDDING

Preparation Time: 10 minutes
Cooking time: 30 minutes
Servings: 2

Ingredients:

- ½ cup raspberries
- 2 teaspoons maple syrup
- 1 ½ cup Plain yogurt
- ¼ teaspoon ground cardamom
- 1/3 cup Chia seeds, dried

Directions:

1. Mix up together Plain yogurt with maple syrup and ground cardamom.
2. Add Chia seeds. Stir it gently.
3. Put the yogurt in the serving glasses and top with the raspberries.
4. Refrigerate the breakfast for at least 30 minutes or overnight.

Nutrition: calories 303, fat 11.2, fiber 11.8, carbs 33.2, protein 15.5

13. GOAT CHEESE OMELET

Preparation Time: 10 minutes
Cooking time: 25 minutes
Servings: 8

Ingredients:

- 8 eggs, beaten
- 6 oz Goat cheese, crumbled
- ½ teaspoon salt
- 3 tablespoons sour cream
- 1 teaspoon butter
- ½ teaspoon canola oil
- ¼ teaspoon sage
- ¼ teaspoon dried oregano
- 1 teaspoon chives, chopped

Directions:

1. Put butter in the skillet. Add canola oil and preheat the mixture until it is homogenous.
2. Meanwhile, in the mixing bowl combine together salt, sour cream, sage, dried oregano, and chives. Add eggs and stir the mixture carefully with the help of the spoon/fork.
3. Pour the egg mixture in the skillet with butter-oil liquid.
4. Sprinkle the omelet with goat cheese and close the lid.
5. Cook the breakfast for 20 minutes over the low heat. The cooked omelet should be solid.
6. Slice it into the and transfer in the plates.

Nutrition: calories 176, fat 13.7, fiber 0, carbs 0, protein 12.2

14. VANILLA SCONES

Preparation Time: 20 minutes
Cooking time: 10 minutes
Servings: 4

Ingredients:

- ½ cup wheat flour, whole grain
- 1 teaspoon baking powder
- 1 tablespoon butter, melted
- 1 teaspoon vanilla extract
- 1 egg, beaten
- ¾ teaspoon salt
- 3 tablespoons milk
- 1 teaspoon vanilla sugar

Directions:

1. In the mixing bowl combine together wheat flour, baking powder, butter, vanilla extract, and egg. Add salt and knead the soft and non-sticky dough. Add more flour if needed.
2. Then make the log from the dough and cut it into the triangles.
3. Line the tray with baking paper.
4. Arrange the dough triangles on the baking paper and transfer in the preheat to the 360F oven.
5. Cook the scones for 10 minutes or until they are light brown.
6. After this, chill the scones and brush with milk and sprinkle with vanilla sugar.

Nutrition: calories 112, fat 4.4, fiber 0.5, carbs 14.3, protein 3.4

15. OLIVE BREAD

Preparation Time: 20 minutes
Cooking time: 50 minutes
Servings: 6

Ingredients:

- 1 cup black olives, pitted, chopped
- 1 tablespoon olive oil
- ½ teaspoon fresh yeast
- ½ cup milk, preheated
- ½ teaspoon salt
- 1 teaspoon baking powder
- 2 cup wheat flour, whole grain
- 2 eggs, beaten
- 1 teaspoon butter, melted
- 1 teaspoon sugar

Directions:

1. In the big bowl combine together fresh yeast, sugar, and milk. Stir it until yeast is dissolved.
2. Then add salt, baking powder, butter, and eggs. Stir the dough mixture until homogenous and add 1 cup of wheat flour. Mix it up until smooth.
3. Add olives and remaining flour. Knead the non-sticky dough.
4. Transfer the dough into the non-sticky dough mold.
5. Bake the bread for 50 minutes at 350 F.
6. Check if the bread is cooked with the help of the toothpick. Is it is dry, the bread is cooked.
7. Remove the bread from the oven and let it chill for 10-15 minutes.
8. Remove it from the loaf mold and slice.

Nutrition: calories 238, fat 7.7, fiber 1.9, carbs 35.5, protein 7.2

16. YUFKA PIES

Preparation Time: 15 minutes
Cooking time: 20 minutes
Servings: 6

Ingredients:

- 7 oz yufka dough/phyllo dough
- 1 cup Cheddar cheese, shredded
- 1 cup fresh cilantro, chopped
- 2 eggs, beaten
- 1 teaspoon paprika
- ¼ teaspoon chili flakes
- ½ teaspoon salt
- 2 tablespoons sour cream
- 1 teaspoon olive oil

Directions:

1. In the mixing bowl, combine together sour cream, salt, chili flakes, paprika, and beaten eggs.
2. Brush the springform pan with olive oil.
3. Place ¼ part of all yufka dough in the pan and sprinkle it with ¼ part of the egg mixture.
4. Add a ¼ cup of cheese and ¼ cup of cilantro.
5. Cover the mixture with 1/3 part of remaining yufka dough and repeat the all the steps again. You should get 4 layers.
6. Cut the yufka mixture into 6 pies and bake at 360F for 20 minutes. The cooked pies should have a golden brown color.

Nutrition: calories 213, fat 11.4, fiber 0.8, carbs 18.2, protein 9.1

17. BREAKFAST POTATO LATKES WITH SPINACH

Preparation Time: 10 minutes
Cooking time: 6 minutes
Servings: 4

Ingredients:

- 2 potatoes, peeled
- ½ onion, diced
- ½ cup spinach, chopped
- 2 eggs, beaten
- ½ teaspoon salt
- ½ teaspoon ground black pepper
- 1 teaspoon olive oil

Directions:

1. Grate the potato and mix it with chopped spinach, diced onion, salt, and ground black pepper.
2. Add eggs and stir until homogenous.
3. Then pour olive oil in the skillet and preheat it well.
4. Make the medium latkes with the help of 2 spoons and transfer them in the preheated oil.
5. Roast the latkes for 3 minutes from each side or until they are golden brown.
6. Dry the cooked latkes with the help of the paper towel if needed.

Nutrition: calories 122, fat 3.5, fiber 3, carbs 18.5, protein 4.9

18. CHERRY TOMATOES AND FETA FRITATTA

Preparation Time: 10 minutes
Cooking time: 25 minutes
Servings: 4

Ingredients:

- 4 eggs, beaten
- 1/3 cup cherry tomatoes
- 2 oz Feta cheese, crumbled
- 1 teaspoon butter
- 1 teaspoon fresh parsley, chopped
- ½ teaspoon salt
- ½ teaspoon dried oregano

Directions:

1. Cut the cherry tomatoes into the halves.
2. Then spread the round springform pan with butter.
3. Arrange the cherry tomatoes halves in the pan in one layer.
4. Then add the layer of Feta cheese.
5. In the mixing bowl mix up together beaten eggs, dried oregano, salt, and parsley.
6. Pour the egg mixture over the cheese.
7. Preheat the oven to 360F.
8. Put the pan with frittata in the oven and cook it for 25 minutes at 355F.

Nutrition: calories 112, fat 8.4, fiber 0.3, carbs 1.6, protein 7.7

19. EGG WHITE SCRAMBLE

Preparation Time: 10 minutes
Cooking time: 6 hours

Servings: 4

Ingredients:

- 1 teaspoon almond butter
- 4 egg whites
- ¼ teaspoon salt
- ½ teaspoon paprika
- 2 tablespoons heavy cream

Directions:

1. Whisk the egg whites gently and add heavy cream.
2. Put the almond butter in the skillet and melt it.
3. Then add egg white mixture.
4. Sprinkle it with salt and cook for 2 minutes over the medium heat.
5. After this, scramble the egg whites with the help of the fork or spatula and sprinkle with paprika.
6. Cook the scrambled egg whites for 3 minutes more.
7. Transfer the meal into the serving plates.

Nutrition: calories 68, fat 5.1, fiber 0.5, carbs 1.3, protein 4.6

20. BEET SMOOTHIE

Preparation time: 10 minutes
Cooking time: 0 minutes
Servings: 2

Ingredients:

- 10 ounces almond milk, unsweetened
- 2 beets, peeled and quartered
- ½ banana, peeled and frozen
- ½ cup cherries, pitted
- 1 tablespoon almond butter

Directions:

1. In your blender, mix the milk with the beets, banana, cherries and butter. Pulse well, pour into glasses and serve.
2. Enjoy!

Nutrition: calories 165, fat 5, fiber 6, carbs 22, protein 5

21. CHIA BARS

Preparation time: 4 hours
Cooking time: 0 minutes
Servings: 4

Ingredients:

- 1½ cups dates, pitted and chopped
- ½ cup chia seeds
- 1/3 cup cocoa powder
- ½ cup shredded coconut, unsweetened
- 1 cup chopped walnuts
- ½ cup oats
- ½ cup dark chocolate, chopped
- 1 teaspoon vanilla extract

Directions:

1. In your food processor, mix the dates with the chia seeds, cocoa, coconut, walnuts, oats, chocolate and vanilla. Pulse well then press into a lined baking dish. Keep in the freezer for 4 hours, cut into 12 bars and serve for breakfast.
2. Enjoy!

Nutrition: calories 125, fat 5, fiber 4, carbs 12, protein 5

22. GREEN EGGS MIX

Preparation time: 10 minutes
Cooking time: 30 minutes
Servings: 4

Ingredients:

- 2 garlic cloves, minced
- 1 pound spinach, torn
- 2 tablespoons olive oil
- 1 yellow onion, chopped
- 1 jalapeno, chopped
- 1 teaspoon cumin, dried
- A pinch of salt and black pepper
- 1 teaspoon coriander, ground
- 2 tablespoons harissa
- ½ cup veggie stock
- 8 eggs
- 1 tablespoon cilantro, chopped
- 1 tablespoon parsley, chopped

Directions:

1. Heat up a pan with the oil over medium heat, add the onion, stir and cook for 4 minutes. Add the jalapeno and the garlic, stir and cook for a few more seconds. Add

the spinach, stir and cook for 4 minutes. Add salt, pepper, harissa, coriander and cumin. Cook for 1 minute, transfer to your food processor, add the stock then pulse well, return the mix to the pan and spread it well. Make 8 holes in this mix and crack an egg in each hole. Place the dish in the oven, bake at 350 degrees F for 20 minutes, divide between plates, sprinkle cilantro and parsley on top and serve.
2. Enjoy!

Nutrition: calories 251, fat 12, fiber 4, carbs 12, protein 14

23. CHIA PUDDING

Preparation time: 4 hours
Cooking time: 0 minutes
Servings: 3

Ingredients:

- 2 cups coconut milk, unsweetened
- 1 banana, peeled and sliced
- ½ cup chia seeds
- ½ teaspoon vanilla extract
- 2 tablespoon raw honey
- 1 tablespoon cocoa powder
- 2 tablespoon cocoa nibs

Directions:

1. In a bowl, mix the banana with the chia seeds, and mash using a fork. Add the milk, the vanilla extract, honey, cocoa powder and cocoa nibs, mix and keep in the fridge for 4 hours before serving.
2. Enjoy!

Nutrition: calories 313, fat 14, fiber 17, carbs 36, protein 10

24. PINEAPPLE SMOOTHIE

Preparation time: 10 minutes
Cooking time: 0 minutes
Servings: 1

Ingredients:

- 1 cup coconut water
- 1 orange, peeled and cut into quarters
- 1½ cups pineapple chunks
- 1 tablespoon fresh grated ginger
- 1 teaspoon chia seeds
- 1 teaspoon turmeric powder
- A pinch of black pepper

Directions:

1. In your blender, mix the coconut water with the orange, pineapple, ginger, chia seeds, turmeric and black pepper. Pulse well, pour into a glass and serve for breakfast.
2. Enjoy!

Nutrition: calories 151, fat 2, fiber 6, carbs 12, protein 4

25. ANTI-INFLAMMATORY PORRIDGE

Preparation time: 10 minutes
Cooking time: 5 minutes
Servings: 2

Ingredients:

- ¼ cup walnuts, chopped and toasted
- 2 tablespoons hemp seeds, toasted
- 2 tablespoons chia seeds
- 1 cup almond milk, unsweetened
- ¼ cup coconut milk, unsweetened
- ¼ cup coconut, shredded and toasted
- ¼ cup almond butter
- 1 tablespoon coconut oil, melted
- ½ teaspoon turmeric powder
- 1 teaspoon bee pollen
- A pinch of black pepper

Directions:

1. Heat up a pot with the almond and coconut milk over medium heat, add the walnuts, hemp seeds, chia seeds, coconut, turmeric, black pepper and the bee pollen, stir, cook for 5 minutes. Take off heat, add the coconut oil and the almond butter, stir and let sit for 10 minutes then divide into 2 bowls and serve.
2. Enjoy!

Nutrition: calories 152, fat 11, fiber 6, carbs 15, protein 11

26. CUCUMBER AND PINEAPPLE

SMOOTHIE

Preparation time: 10 minutes
Cooking time: 0 minutes
Servings: 2

Ingredients:

- 2 cups kale, torn
- 1 cup brewed green tea
- 1 cup pineapple chunks
- 1 cup cucumber, peeled and chopped
- ½ cup mango chunks, frozen
- ½ banana, peeled
- 1 teaspoon ground ginger
- ¼ teaspoon ground turmeric
- 3 mint leaves, chopped
- 1 tablespoon chia seeds
- 4 ice cubes
- 1 scoop protein powder

Directions:

1. In your blender, mix the kale with the green tea, pineapple, cucumber, mango, banana, ginger, turmeric, mint, protein powder and ice. Pulse well then add the chia seeds. Stir, divide into 2 glasses and serve.
2. Enjoy!

Nutrition: calories 161, fat 2, fiber 6, carbs 11, protein 5

27. QUINOA PORRIDGE

Preparation time: 10 minutes
Cooking time: 0 minutes
Servings: 2

Ingredients:

- 1 cup cashew milk, warm
- 1 cup blueberries
- 2 cups quinoa, cooked
- ¼ cup chopped walnuts, toasted
- 2 teaspoons raw honey
- ½ teaspoon ground cinnamon
- 1 tablespoon chia seeds

Directions:

1. In a bowl, mix the cashew milk with the blueberries, quinoa, walnuts, honey, cinnamon and chia seeds. Stir well, divide into 2 small bowls and serve.
2. Enjoy!

Nutrition: calories 151, fat 2, fiber 11, carbs 14, protein 13

28. RASPBERRY SMOOTHIE

Preparation time: 10 minutes
Cooking time: 0 minutes
Servings: 2

Ingredients:

- 1 avocado, pitted and peeled
- ¾ cup raspberry juice
- ¾ cup orange juice
- ½ cup raspberries

Directions:

1. In your blender, mix the avocado with the raspberry juice, orange juice and raspberries. Pulse well, divide into 2 glasses and serve.
2. Enjoy!

Nutrition: calories 125, fat 11, fiber 7, carbs 9, protein 3

29. GINGERBREAD OATMEAL

Preparation time: 10 minutes
Cooking time: 15 minutes
Servings: 4

Ingredients:

- 1 cup steel cut oats
- 4 cups water
- ¼ teaspoon ground coriander
- 1½ tablespoons ground cinnamon
- ¼ teaspoon ground cloves
- ¼ teaspoon fresh grated ginger
- ¼ teaspoon ground allspice
- ¼ teaspoon ground cardamom
- A pinch of ground nutmeg

Directions:

1. Heat up a pan with the water over medium-high heat, add the oats and stir. Add the coriander, cinnamon, cloves, ginger, allspice, cardamom and nutmeg, stir, cook for 15 minutes, divide into bowls and serve.

2. Enjoy!

Nutrition: calories 188, fat 3, fiber 6, carbs 13, protein 6

30. RHUBARB MUFFINS

Preparation time: 10 minutes
Cooking time: 25 minutes
Servings: 8

Ingredients:

- ½ cup almond meal
- 2 tablespoons crystallized ginger
- ¼ cup coconut sugar
- 1 tablespoon linseed meal
- ½ cup buckwheat flour
- ¼ cup brown rice flour
- 2 tablespoons powdered arrowroot
- 2 teaspoon gluten-free baking powder
- ½ teaspoon fresh grated ginger
- ½ teaspoon ground cinnamon
- 1 cup rhubarb, sliced
- 1 apple, cored, peeled and chopped
- 1/3 cup almond milk, unsweetened
- ¼ cup olive oil
- 1 free-range egg
- 1 teaspoon vanilla extract

Directions:

1. In a bowl, mix the almond meal with the crystallized ginger, sugar, linseed meal, buckwheat flour, rice flour, arrowroot powder, grated ginger, baking powder and cinnamon and stir. In another bowl, mix the rhubarb with the apple, almond milk, oil, egg and vanilla and stir well. Combine the 2 mixtures, stir well, and divide into a lined muffin tray. Place in the oven at 350 degrees F and bake for 25 minutes. Serve the muffins for breakfast.
2. Enjoy!

Nutrition: calories 200, fat 4, fiber 6, carbs 13, protein 8

31. WINTER FRUIT SALAD

Preparation time: 10 minutes
Cooking time: 0 minutes
Servings: 6

Ingredients:

- 4 persimmons, cubed
- 4 pears, cubed
- 1 cup grapes, halved
- 1 cup apples, peeled, cored and cubed
- ¾ cup pecans, halved
- 1 tablespoon olive oil
- 1 tablespoon peanut oil
- 1 tablespoon pomegranate flavored vinegar
- 2 tablespoons agave nectar

Directions:

1. In a salad bowl, mix the persimmons with the pears, grapes, apples and pecans. In another bowl, mix the olive oil with the peanut oil, vinegar and agave nectar. Whisk well then pour over the salad, toss and serve for breakfast.
2. Enjoy!

Nutrition: calories 125, fat 3, fiber 6, carbs 14, protein 8

32. BUCKWHEAT GRANOLA

Preparation time: 10 minutes
Cooking time: 45 minutes
Servings: 6

Ingredients:

- 2 cups oats
- 1 cup buckwheat
- 1 cup sunflower seeds
- 1 cup pumpkin seeds
- 1½ cups dates, pitted and chopped
- 1 cup apple puree
- 6 tablespoons coconut oil
- 5 tablespoons cocoa powder
- 1 teaspoon fresh grated ginger

Directions:

1. In a large bowl, mix the oats with the buckwheat, sunflower seeds, pumpkin seeds, dates, apple puree, oil, cocoa powder and ginger then stir really well. Spread on a lined baking sheet, press well and place in the oven at 360 degrees F for 45 minutes. Leave the granola to cool down, slice and serve for breakfast.

2. Enjoy!

Nutrition: calories 161, fat 3, fiber 5, carbs 11, protein 7

33. MUSHROOM FRITTATA

Preparation time: 10 minutes
Cooking time: 30 minutes
Servings: 4

Ingredients:

- ¼ cup coconut milk, unsweetened
- 6 eggs
- 1 yellow onion, chopped
- 4 ounces white mushrooms, sliced
- 2 tablespoons olive oil
- 2 cups baby spinach
- A pinch of salt and black pepper

Directions:

1. Heat up a pan with the oil over medium-high heat, add the onion, stir and cook for 2-3 minutes. Add the mushrooms, salt and pepper, stir and cook for 2 minutes more. In a bowl, mix the eggs with salt and pepper, stir well and pour over the mushrooms. Add the spinach, mix a bit, place in the oven and bake at 360 degrees F for 25 minutes. Slice the frittata and serve it for breakfast.
2. Enjoy!

Nutrition: calories 200, fat 3, fiber 6, carbs 14, protein 6

34. BREAKFAST CREPES

Preparation time: 10 minutes
Cooking time: 10 minutes
Servings: 4

Ingredients:

- 2 eggs
- 1 teaspoon vanilla extract
- ½ cup almond milk, unsweetened
- ½ cup water
- 2 tablespoons agave nectar
- 1 cup coconut flour
- 3 tablespoons coconut oil, melted

Directions:

1. In a bowl, whisk the eggs with the vanilla extract, almond milk, water and agave nectar. Add the flour and 2 tablespoons oil gradually and stir until you obtain a smooth batter. Heat up a pan with the rest of the oil over medium heat, add some of the batter, spread into the pan and cook the crepe until it's golden on both sides then transfer to a plate. Repeat with the rest of the batter and serve the crepes for breakfast.
2. Enjoy!

Nutrition: calories 121, fat 3, fiber 6, carbs 14, protein 6

35. MILLET MUFFINS

Preparation time: 10 minutes
Cooking time: 15 minutes
Servings: 12

Ingredients:

- ¼ cup coconut oil, melted
- 1 egg
- ½ teaspoon vanilla extract
- 1 teaspoon baking powder
- 1½ cups organic millet, cooked
- ½ cup coconut sugar
- Cooking spray

Directions:

1. In a blender, blend the melted coconut oil with the egg, vanilla extract, baking powder, millet and sugar. Grease a muffin tray with cooking spray and divide the millet mix into each cup. Place the muffins in the oven and bake at 350 degrees F for 30 minutes. Let the muffins cool and then serve!
2. Enjoy!

Nutrition: calories 167, fat 4, fiber 7, carbs 15, protein 6

36. KALE SMOOTHIE

Preparation time: 10 minutes
Cooking time: 0 minutes
Servings: 5

Ingredients:

- 10 kale leaves

- 5 bananas, peeled and cut into chunks
- 2 pears, chopped
- 5 tablespoons almond butter
- 5 cups almond milk

Directions:

1. In your blender, mix the kale with the bananas, pears, almond butter and almond milk, pulse well, divide into glasses and serve for breakfast.
2. Enjoy!

Nutrition: calories 267, fat 11, fiber 7, carbs 15, protein 7

37. APPLE MUESLI

Preparation time: 10 minutes
Cooking time: 0 minutes
Servings: 4

Ingredients:

- 2 apples, peeled, cored and grated
- 1 cup rolled oats
- 3 tablespoons flax seeds
- 1¼ cups coconut cream
- 1¼ cups coconut water
- ½ cup goji berries
- 2 tablespoons chopped mint
- 3 tablespoons raw honey

Directions:

1. In a bowl, mix the apples with the oats, flax seeds, coconut cream, coconut water, goji berries, mint and honey. Stir well, divide into smaller bowls and serve for breakfast.
2. Enjoy!

Nutrition: calories 171, fat 2, fiber 6, carbs 14, protein 5

38. VEGGIE AND ONION MIX

Preparation time: 10 minutes
Cooking time: 10 minutes
Servings: 2

Ingredients:

- ½ cup chopped yellow onions
- ½ cup chopped red bell pepper
- A pinch of garlic powder
- A pinch of salt and black pepper
- 1 tablespoon olive oil
- 2 eggs

Directions:

1. Heat up a pan with the oil over medium-high heat, add the onions, stir and cook for 1-2 minutes. Add the bell pepper, garlic powder, salt and pepper then stir and cook for 3 minutes more. Add the eggs, stir and cook until the eggs are done, about 1-2 minutes. Divide everything between plates and serve.
2. Enjoy!

Nutrition: calories 221, fat 6, fiber 6, carbs 14, protein 11

39. COCONUT FLOUR NAAN BREAD WITH PAPRIKA MUSHROOMS

Servings 6
Preparation Time: 20 minutes

Ingredients

- 2 tablespoons psyllium powder
- A pinch of salt
- 3/4 cup coconut flour
- 1/2 teaspoon baking powder
- 1 beaten egg plus 1 egg yolk
- 8 tablespoons melted coconut oil
- 1/8 cup hot water
- 1 pound thinly sliced Cremini mushrooms
- 1 teaspoon smoked paprika
- 1 teaspoon kosher salt

Directions

1. Mix together psyllium powder, salt, coconut flour and baking powder in a mixing bowl.
2. Put in the egg and egg yolk in with 6 tablespoons of coconut oil and add some hot water to form a dough. Let it rest at room temperature for 10 minutes.
3. Make 6 balls out of the dough and then flatten them so that they look like naan bread. Now, divide the dough into 6 balls; and flatten them on a working surface.
4. Put 1 tablespoon coconut oil in a pan and

preheat on a moderate heat. Fry the naan bread until they are a golden color.

5. Heat the last tablespoon of coconut oil in a frying pan and sauté the mushrooms until soft and aromatic. Season with the smoked paprika and the kosher salt.
6. Serve with the naan bread and enjoy!

Nutrition: Calories281 ,Protein 6.4g ,Fat 21.4g Carbs, 6.1g ,Sugar 0.1g

40. ZUCCHINI NOODLES

Servings 4
Preparation Time: 15 minutes

Ingredients

- 2 zucchinis
- 1 teaspoon minced garlic
- 1 tablespoon minced shallots
- 2 tablespoons avocado oil
- 1 pound chopped mushrooms,
- 1 cup chicken stock
- 2 ripe chopped tomatoes
- 1/4 teaspoon chili powder
- 1 teaspoon dried basil
- 1/2 teaspoon dried oregano

Directions

1. Cut the end of the ends of the zucchini. Make noodles out of them by using a mandolin, a spiralizer or a julienne peeler.
2. Bring to the boil a pan of salted water and boil the zucchini noodles for a minute. Drain the noodles.
3. Heat the avocado oil over moderate heat. Sauté the garlic and the shallots for 2 minutes. Then put the mushrooms in and cook for 3 minutes.
4. Stir in the chicken stock, chopped tomatoes, chili powder, basil and oregano. Simmer over a moderate-low heat until everything is hot.
5. Put the noodles on plates and top with the mushroom sauce. Enjoy!

Nutrition: Calories 85, Protein 5.8g, Fat 3.5g, Carbs 6.4g, Sugar 2.5g

41. KOHLRABI WITH A CREAMY MUSHROOM SAUCE

Servings 4
Preparation Time: 25 minutes

Ingredients

- 3/4 pound trimmed and thinly sliced kohlrabi
- 3 tablespoons butter
- 1 minced garlic clove
- 1/2 cup chopped scallions
- 1/2 pound sliced mushrooms
- 1/4 teaspoon red pepper flakes
- 1/2 teaspoon ground black pepper
- 1 teaspoon sea salt
- 1 1/2 cups double cream

Directions

1. Bring to the boil a large pot of salted water. Add the kohlrabi and parboil for 7 – 9 minutes. Drain.
2. Heat the butter over a moderate-low heat and sauté the garlic, scallions and mushrooms until soft and aromatic.
3. Put in the red pepper flakes, the black pepper and salt.
4. Pour in the cream slowly, whisking all the time until the sauce thickens. This takes about 8 – 12 minutes.
5. Put the kohlrabi on separate plates and pour the creamy mushroom sauce on top.

Nutrition: Calories220 ,Protein 4g ,Fat 20g ,Carbs 5.3 ,Sugar 3.1g

42. SPINACH AND STRAWBERRY SALAD

Servings 4
Preparation Time: 10 minutes

Ingredients

- 4 cups baby spinach
- 1 cup pitted, peeled and sliced avocado
- 1/2 cup hulled and sliced strawberries
- 1/2 freshly squeezed lime
- 1/2 teaspoon kosher salt
- 2 tablespoons olive oil
- White pepper, to taste
- 1/3 cup crumbled brie cheese
- 2 tablespoons chopped fresh basil leaves,

Directions

1. Dry the spinach leaves and put them in a bowl.
2. Add the slices of avocado and strawberries.
3. Make the dressing by whisking together the lime juice, salt, pepper and olive oil. Pour this over the salad and crumble the cheese on top.
4. Garnish with the basil leaves. Bon appétit!

Nutrition: Calories190 ,Protein 4.3g ,Fat 17.6g ,Carbs 4.6 ,Sugar 1.4g

43. JAPANESE ENOKI MUSHROOMS WITH OYSTER SAUCE AND SESAME SEEDS

Servings 3
Preparation Time: 15 minutes

Ingredients

- 1 1/2 tablespoons ghee at room temperature
- 2 minced cloves garlic
- 1 cup scallions
- 7-ounce pack Enoki mushrooms, trimmed away about 1-inch of the root section
- 1/2 teaspoon Sansho Japanese pepper
- 1/2 teaspoon salt
- 2 teaspoons oyster sauce
- 1/2 teaspoon wasabi powder
- 1 tablespoon black sesame seeds

Directions

1. Turn on the heat to medium and melt the ghee in a wok. Sauté the garlic and scallions until they are tender. This should take about 5 minutes.
2. Put in the mushrooms and cook for 4 minutes. Remove from the heat and add the wasabi powder, salt and pepper.
3. Add the oyster sauce and stir. Toast the sesame seeds and put them on top of the mushrooms.

Nutrition: Calories 103 ,Protein 2.7g ,Fat 6.7g ,Carbs 5.9g ,Sugar 1g

44. CREAMY CAULIFLOWER SOUP

Servings 4
Preparation Time: 20 minutes

Ingredients

- 3 cups cauliflower florets
- 3 cups chicken broth
- 1 cup pitted and chopped avocado
- 1 cup unsweetened almond milk
- 1/4 teaspoon freshly cracked mixed peppercorns
- 1/4 teaspoon Himalayan rock salt
- 1 bay leaf

Directions

1. Put the chicken broth on to simmer over medium heat. Put in the cauliflower florets and cook for 10 minutes.
2. Turn down the heat and add the avocado, almond milk, peppercorns, salt and the bay leaf. Cook for another 5 minutes.
3. Take the bay leaf out and then process the mixture in a blender. Bon appétit!

Nutrition: Calories 260 ,Protein 7.2g ,Fat 22.5g ,Carbs 4.1g ,Sugar 1.5g

45. INVIGORATING NUTTY SPRING SALAD

Servings 4
Preparation Time: 5 minutes

Ingredients

- 1 medium-sized head lettuce, torn into small pieces
- 1 cup thinly sliced radishes
- 2 sliced spring onions
- 1/2 pound thinly sliced cucumber
- 1 ounce chopped macadamia nuts
- Coarse salt to taste
- 1/2 teaspoon red pepper flakes
- 1/2 freshly squeezed lime
- 3 tablespoons olive oil
- 1 teaspoon sugar-free chili sauce
- 1 tablespoon lightly toasted sesame seeds

Directions

1. Toss the lettuce, radishes, spring onions,

cucumber together with the macadamia nuts.
2. Whisk together the salt, pepper, lime, olive oil and chili sauce.
3. Pour the dressing over the salad. Toast the sesame seeds and put them on top of the salad.

Nutrition: Calories184 ,Protein 2.1g ,Fat 16.8g ,Carbs 4g ,Sugar 1.4g

46. CREMINI MUSHROOM CASSEROLE WITH A KICK

Servings 4
Preparation Time: 30 minutes

Ingredients

- 1 tablespoon olive oil
- 1/2 pound chopped Cremini mushrooms
- 1 chopped celery
- 1 cup chopped shallots
- 1 teaspoon finely minced chili pepper
- 1 teaspoon minced garlic
- 2 1/2 cups low-sodium bone broth
- 1/2 cup water
- 1/4 cup dry white wine
- 2 crushed ripe tomatoes
- Salt and ground black pepper, to taste
- 1/4 teaspoon ground cinnamon
- 1/2 teaspoon ground allspice
- 1/4 teaspoon ground ginger
- 2 bay leaves
- 1/2 cup chopped fresh basil

Directions

1. Preheat a pot on a medium flame and heat the olive oil. Then cook the mushrooms, celery, shallots, chili pepper and garlic for 8 minutes.
2. Add the broth, wine, tomatoes, salt, pepper, cinnamon, allspice, ginger and bay leaves and bring to the boil. Then simmer for 18 minutes stirring now and again.
3. Put into individual bowls and garnish with fresh basil leaves. Bon appétit!

Nutrition: Calories 133 ,Protein 14g ,Fat 3.7g ,Carbs 5.7g ,Sugar 2.4g

47. SAUTÉED BROCCOFLOWER WITH BLUE CHEESE SAUCE

Servings 6
Preparation Time: 30 minutes

Ingredients

- 2 pounds broccoflower florets
- 1 1/2 tablespoons olive oil
- 2 smashed garlic cloves
- 2 chopped green onions
- 1/2 teaspoon minced fresh ginger root
- 1/4 teaspoon curry powder
- Freshly ground black pepper and flaky sea salt to taste
- 1 tablespoon chopped fresh cilantro
- For the Blue Cheese Sauce:
- 1 1/2 tablespoons ghee
- 1/3 cup double cream
- 1/4 teaspoon freshly cracked mixed peppercorns
- 1 cup crumbled blue cheese

Directions

1. Parboil the broccoflower for 2 – 3 minutes. Drain.
2. Heat a pan over medium heat and add the oil. Cook the onions for 2 minutes and then add the garlic. Cook until it is aromatic. This should take 1 – 2 minutes.
3. Add the broccoflower, florets ginger, curry powder, salt and pepper and sauté for 3 minutes while stirring.
4. Add a little water and cover. Cook for another 6 minutes until everything has softened.
5. Warm the ghee over medium heat and stir in the cream. Make sure that it's hot and then add the blue cheese and peppercorns.
6. Keep stirring until the cheese has melted. If the mixture is too thick, add a little water.
7. Put the broccoflower on individual plates and sprinkle over the fresh cilantro. Put the blue cheese on the side. Bon appétit!

Nutrition: Calories159 ,Protein 5.7g ,Fat 12.3g ,Carbs 7.2g ,Sugar 2.2g

48. ROASTED CHERRY

TOMATOES WITH PARMESAN CHEESE

Servings 4
Preparation Time: 25 minutes

Ingredients

- 1 1/2 pounds halved cherry tomatoes
- 1/4 cup olive oil
- 1 tablespoon white wine vinegar
- 1 tablespoon Worcestershire sauce
- 1 teaspoon minced garlic
- Sea salt and freshly ground black pepper to taste
- 2 sprigs of chopped fresh thyme
- 2 sprigs of f chopped fresh rosemary
- 1 cup freshly grated Parmesan cheese

Directions

1. Put the oven on at 4000F.
2. Put the tomatoes in a ceramic baking dish which is broiler-proof and pour over the Worcestershire sauce, vinegar and olive oil.
3. Add the garlic, rosemary, thyme, salt and pepper to the tomatoes and put the Parmesan on top.
4. Roast the tomatoes for 20 minutes until the tomatoes begin to caramelize. Bon appétit!

Nutrition: Calories247 ,Protein 11g ,Fat 19.8g ,Carbs 5.3g ,Sugar 2.2

49. BUTTERY SAVOY CABBAGE

Servings 4
Preparation Time: 20 minutes

Ingredients

- 1/2 stick melted butter
- 1 minced garlic clove
- 1 bunch chopped scallions
- 1 pound cored and shredded Savoy cabbage, without outer leaves
- 1/2 teaspoon sea salt
- 1/2 teaspoon freshly cracked mixed peppercorn
- 1/4 teaspoon fresh grated ginger
- 1 tablespoon dry white wine
- 1/4 cup chicken stock
- 1/3 teaspoon mustard seeds
- A pinch of nutmeg

Directions

1. Put a pan on a moderate flame and melt the butter. Sauté the garlic and scallions until soft and aromatic.
2. Mix in the cabbage and ginger. Cook for 10 minutes, stirring every now and then.
3. Add the salt, pepper, wine, chicken stock, mustard seeds and nutmeg and cook for another 5 minutes. Check to see that the Savoy cabbage has cooked to your liking. Enjoy!

Nutrition: Calories 142 ,Protein 2g ,Fat 11.6 g; Carbs 5.7g, Sugar2g

50. BROCCOLI AND VEGETABLE "RICE" DELIGHT

Servings 4
Preparation Time: 20 minutes

Ingredients

- 1 head broccoli florets
- 1/2 stick butter
- 1 minced garlic clove
- 1/2 chopped yellow onion
- 1/2 chopped celery stalk
- 1 chopped red pepper
- 1 Aji Fantasy minced chili pepper
- Salt and ground black pepper, to taste

Directions

1. Put the broccoli in your food processor and blitz. Stop when it reaches a rice-like texture.
2. On medium heat, melt the butter in a pan. Cook the onion for 2 – 3 minutes and then add the garlic. Cook until it is aromatic and slightly browned.
3. Add the celery, the red pepper and the Aji Fantasy chill pepper and cook for 4 minutes when they should all be tender. Mix in the broccoli "rice" and season to taste with pepper and salt.
4. Cook for another 5 minutes stirring every now and then. Serve warm and if you want it as a main meal with a curry. Serve

warm and enjoy!

Nutrition: Calories 126 ,Protein 1.3g ,Fat 11.6g ,Carbs 5.4g ,Sugar 2.5g

51. SHRIMP BOK CHOY

Servings 4
Preparation Time: 15 minutes

Ingredients

- 2 tablespoons coconut oil
- 2 crushed garlic cloves
- 1 1/2 inch piece of freshly grated ginger
- 1/2 pound trimmed and thinly sliced Bok Choy
- 1 teaspoon cayenne pepper
- 1 tablespoon oyster sauce
- Ground black pepper and salt to taste
- 10 ounces peeled and deveined shrimp

Directions

1. Put a pan on medium heat and warm up the coconut oil. Cook the garlic until it is slightly brown.
2. Mix in the ginger and the Bok Choy. Then put in the cayenne pepper, oyster sauce, pepper and salt. Stir while cooking for another 5 minutes. Put on a serving plate.
3. Heat the other tablespoon of coconut oil in the pan and cook the shrimp, while stirring every now and then. It should take around 3 minutes for the shrimp to turn pink and opaque.
4. Put the shrimp on top of the Bok Choy and serve with lemon wedges.

Nutrition: Calories 171 ,Protein 18.9g ,Fat 8.4g ,Carbs 5.8g ,Sugar 2.1g

52. CHEESY CAULIFLOWER AND MUSHROOM CASSEROLE

Servings 4
Preparation Time: 35 minutes

Ingredients

- 2 tablespoons lard
- 1 teaspoon yellow mustard
- 1 tablespoon Piri Piri sauce
- 1 cup aged goat cheese
- 1 cup chicken stock
- 4 lightly beaten eggs
- 1/2 Cup of sour cream
- Cup chive & onion cream cheese
- 1/2 pound thinly sliced brown Cremini mushrooms
- 1 teaspoon fresh or dry rosemary, minced
- 1/3 teaspoon freshly ground pepper
- 1/2teaspoon salt
- 1 large head cauliflower florets

Directions

1. Preheat the oven to 3000F. Spray a casserole dish with nonstick cooking spray.
2. Preheat a pan over medium heat and then melt the lard. Put in the mustard, Piri Piri sauce, goat cheese, cream cheese, sour cream, chicken stock and eggs. Cook these until they're hot.
3. In the baking dish layer the cauliflower with the mushrooms. Season with pepper, salt and rosemary.
4. Put the other mixture on top of the vegetables and cook for 25 – 30 minutes. Best served hot.

Nutrition: Calories 275 ,Protein 14g ,Fat 21.3g Carbs, 5.3g ,Sugar 2.6g

53. CHEDDAR AND SPINACH MUFFINS

Servings 6
Preparation Time: 30 minutes

Ingredients

- 8 eggs
- 1 cup full-fat milk
- 2 tablespoons olive oil
- 1/4 teaspoon ground black pepper
- 1/3 teaspoon salt
- 1 cup chopped spinach
- 1 ½ cups grated cheddar cheese

Directions

1. Put your oven on to 3500F.
2. Mix together the oil, eggs and milk. Add the pepper and salt, the spinach and the cheese. Combine well.
3. Put the mixture into a greased muffin tin.

4. Put in the oven and bake for 25 minutes. The muffins should spring back when touched.

Nutrition: Calories 252 ,Protein 16.1g ,Fat 19.7g ,Carbs 3g ,Sugar 1.6g

54. MUFFINS WITH KALE AND GRUYÈRE CHEESE

Servings 6
Preparation Time: 25 minutes

Ingredients

- 1/2 cup full-fat milk
- 1/2 teaspoon dried basil
- 1 1/2 cup grated Gruyere cheese
- Sea salt to taste
- 5 eggs
- 1/2 pound chopped prosciutto
- 10 ounces cooked and drained kale

Directions

1. Preheat your oven to 3600F. Spray a muffin tin with a nonstick cooking spray.
2. Whisk together the eggs, milk, basil, Gruyere cheese and salt. Then put in the prosciutto and the kale. Put the mixture in the muffin tin, making sure that each muffin cup is filled 3/4 full.
3. Bake for around 25 minutes. They are good served with sour cream.

Nutrition: Calories 275 Protein 21.6 ,Fat 15.8g ,Carbs 2.2g ,Sugar 0.4g

55. FAMILY VEGETABLE PIZZA

Servings 4
Preparation Time: 25 minutes

Ingredients

- For the Crust:
- A spray coating
- 1 pound cauliflower
- 1 tablespoon olive oil
- 1/2 cup Edam cheese
- 1⁄4 cup heavy cream
- 4 medium-sized eggs
- Salt, to taste
- For the Topping:
- 1 cup spring mix
- 2 tablespoons finely chopped chives
- 1 tablespoon fresh sage
- 3/4 cup sugar-free tomato sauce
- 1/4 cup pitted and sliced Kalamata olives
- 1 cup mozzarella cheese

Directions

1. Cut the cauliflower into florets and cook in a large pot of salted water until soft. Add the basil-infused oil, Edam cheese, heavy cream, 4 eggs and salt.
2. Preheat your oven to 3800F. Grease a baking tin with non-stick spray.
3. Put the crust mixture in the baking tin and bake for 15 minutes in the middle of the oven.
4. Take out of the oven and put on the spring mix, the chives, sage, tomato sauce and the olives. End up sprinkling the mozzarella cheese on top of the pizza. Put back in the oven until the cheese has melted,
5. Add some grinds of black pepper if desired or parmesan cheese.

Nutrition: Calories 234 ,Protein 16.1g ,Fat 6.3g ,Carbs 13.6g , Sugar 3.5g

56. DOLMAS WRAP

Preparation Time: 10 minutes
Servings: 2

Ingredients:

- 2 whole wheat wrap
- 6 dolmas (stuffed grape leaves)
- 1 tomato, chopped
- 1 cucumber, chopped
- 2 oz Greek yogurt
- ½ teaspoon minced garlic
- ¼ cup lettuce, chopped
- 2 oz Feta, crumbled

Directions:

1. In the mixing bowl combine together chopped tomato, cucumber, Greek yogurt, minced garlic, lettuce, and Feta.
2. When the mixture is homogenous transfer it in the center of every wheat wrap.
3. Arrange dolma over the vegetable mixture.
4. Carefully wrap the wheat wraps.

Nutrition: calories 341, fat 12.9, fiber 9.2, carbs 52.4, protein 13.2

57. SALAD AL TONNO

Preparation Time: 15 minutes
Servings: 2

Ingredients:

- 1/3 cup stuffed green olives
- 1 ½ cup lettuce leaves, teared
- ½ cup cherry tomatoes, halved
- ½ teaspoon garlic powder
- ½ teaspoon salt
- ½ teaspoon ground black pepper
- 1 tablespoon lemon juice
- 1 teaspoon olive oil
- 6 oz tuna, canned, drained

Directions:

1. Chop the tuna roughly and put it in the salad bowl.
2. Add cherry tomatoes, lettuce leaves, salt, garlic powder, ground black pepper. Lemon juice, and olive oil.
3. Then slice the stuffed olives and add them in the salad too.
4. Give a good shake to the salad.
5. Salad can be stored in the fridge for up to 3 hours.

Nutrition: calories 235, fat 12, fiber 1, carbs 6.5, protein 23.4

58. ARLECCHINO RICE SALAD

Preparation Time: 10 minutes
Cooking time: 15 minutes
Servings: 3

Ingredients:

- ½ cup white rice, dried
- 1 cup chicken stock
- 1 zucchini, shredded
- 2 tablespoons capers
- 1 carrot, shredded
- 1 tomato, chopped
- 1 tablespoon apple cider vinegar
- ½ teaspoon salt
- 2 tablespoons fresh parsley, chopped
- 1 tablespoon canola oil

Directions:

1. Put rice in the pan.
2. Add chicken stock and boil it with the closed lid for 15-20 minutes or until rice absorbs all water.
3. Meanwhile, in the mixing bowl combine together shredded zucchini, capers, carrot, and tomato.
4. Add fresh parsley.
5. Make the dressing: mix up together canola oil, salt, and apple cider vinegar.
6. Chill the cooked rice little and add it in the salad bowl to the vegetables.
7. Add dressing and mix up salad well.

Nutrition: calories 183, fat 5.3, fiber 2.1, carbs 30.4, protein 3.8

59. GREEK SALAD

Preparation Time: 10 minutes
Servings: 2

Ingredients:

- 2 cups lettuce leaves
- 4 oz black olives
- 2 tomatoes
- 2 cucumbers
- 1 tablespoon lemon juice
- 1 teaspoon olive oil
- ¼ teaspoon dried oregano
- ½ teaspoon salt
- ¼ teaspoon chili flakes
- 4 oz Feta cheese

Directions:

1. Chop Feta cheese into the small cubes.
2. Chop the lettuce leaves roughly put them in the salad bowl.
3. Slice black olives and add them in the lettuce.
4. Then chop tomatoes and cucumbers into the cubes. Add them in the lettuce bowl.
5. For the dressing: whisk together chili flakes, salt, dried oregano, olive oil, and lemon juice.
6. Pour the dressing over the lettuce mixture and mix up well.
7. Sprinkle the salad with Feta cubes and shake gently.

Nutrition: calories 312, fat 21.2, fiber 5.3, carbs 23.5, protein 11.9

60. SAUTEED CHICKPEA AND LENTIL MIX

Preparation Time: 10 minutes
Cooking time: 50 minutes
Servings: 4

Ingredients:

- 1 cup chickpeas, half-cooked
- 1 cup lentils
- 5 cups chicken stock
- ½ cup fresh cilantro, chopped
- 1 teaspoon salt
- ½ teaspoon chili flakes
- ¼ cup onion, diced
- 1 tablespoon tomato paste

Directions:

1. Place chickpeas in the pan.
2. Add water, salt, and chili flakes.
3. Boil the chickpeas for 30 minutes over the medium heat.
4. Then add diced onion, lentils, and tomato paste. Stir well.
5. Close the lid and cook the mix for 15 minutes.
6. After this, add chopped cilantro, stir the meal well and cook it for 5 minutes more.
7. Let the cooked lunch chill little before serving.

Nutrition: calories 370, fat 4.3, fiber 23.7, carbs 61.6, protein 23.2

61. BAKED VEGETABLES SOUP

Preparation Time: 15 minutes
Cooking time: 5 hours
Servings: 2

Ingredients:

- 1 carrot, peeled
- 1 onion, peeled
- 1 eggplant, peeled
- 2 oz asparagus, peeled
- 2 tablespoons sour cream
- 1 teaspoon salt
- ½ teaspoon ground black pepper
- 1 tablespoon dried dill
- 2 cups of water

Directions:

1. Place all vegetables in the tray and bake them for 30 minutes at 360F.
2. When the vegetables are tender, chop them roughly and put in the pan.
3. Add water, dried dill, ground black pepper, salt, and close the lid.
4. Simmer the soup for 10 minutes.
5. After this, gently blend the soup. It should have a soft but not smooth texture.
6. Simmer the soup for 2-3 minutes and remove from the heat.
7. Add more salt if needed.

Nutrition: calories 128, fat 3.1, fiber 11, carbs

24.4, protein 4.5

62. PESTO CHICKEN SALAD

Preparation Time: 15 minutes
Cooking time: 15 minutes
Servings: 4

Ingredients:

- 1-pound chicken breast, skinless, boneless
- 1 teaspoon salt
- 1 teaspoon ground black pepper
- 1 teaspoon olive oil
- 1 cup cherry tomatoes, halved
- 2 cucumbers, chopped
- 1 cup lettuce, chopped
- 1 red onion, sliced
- 3 tablespoons fresh basil
- 2 oz Parmesan, grated
- 1 tablespoon walnut
- ½ teaspoon minced garlic
- 4 tablespoons avocado oil
- 1 tablespoon canola oil
- 1 tablespoon lemon juice

Directions:

1. Preheat the grill to 360F.
2. Rub the chicken breast with salt, ground black pepper, and olive oil.
3. Grill the chicken for 7 minutes from each side. The cooked chicken breast should have a crunchy crust.
4. Meanwhile, mix up together tomatoes, cucumbers, lettuce, red onion, and mix up the mixture well. Add lemon juice and canola oil. Mix up the salad well again.
5. Make pesto sauce: blend in the blender avocado oil, minced garlic, walnuts, Parmesan, and basil.
6. Chop the cooked grilled chicken breast roughly and put over salad.
7. Drizzle the salad with pesto sauce.

Nutrition: calories 293, fat 13.9, fiber 2.9, carbs 12.3, protein 31.1

63. FALAFEL

Preparation Time: 10 minutes
Cooking time: 6 minutes
Servings: 4

Ingredients:

- 1 cup chickpeas, soaked, cooked
- 1/3 cup white onion, diced
- 3 garlic cloves, chopped
- 3 tablespoons fresh parsley, chopped
- 1 tablespoon chickpea flour
- ½ teaspoon salt
- ½ teaspoon ground cumin
- ¾ teaspoon ground coriander
- ½ teaspoon chili flakes
- ½ teaspoon cayenne pepper
- ½ teaspoon ground cardamom
- 3 tablespoons olive oil

Directions:

1. Blend together chickpeas, onion, garlic cloves, parsley, chickpea flour, salt, ground cumin, ground coriander, chili flakes, cayenne pepper, and ground cardamom.
2. When the chickpea mixture is homogenous and smooth transfer it in the mixing bowl.
3. Make the medium balls from the chickpea mixture.
4. Pour olive oil in the skillet and heat it up.
5. Fry the chickpea balls for 2 minutes from each side over the medium heat.
6. The cooked falafel should have a light brown color.
7. Dry the falafel with a paper towel if needed.

Nutrition: calories 283, fat 13.7, fiber 9.2, carbs 32.6, protein 10.1

64. ISRAELI PASTA SALAD

Preparation Time: 10 minutes
Cooking time: 15 minutes
Servings: 2

Ingredients:

- 2 bell peppers, chopped
- 3 oz Feta cheese, chopped
- 1/3 cup black olives, chopped
- 1 red onion, chopped
- 1 tomato, chopped
- 1 cucumber, chopped
- ½ cup elbow macaroni, dried

- 1 teaspoon dried oregano
- 1 tablespoon lemon juice
- 1 teaspoon olive oil
- 1 cup water for macaroni

Directions:

1. Pour water in the pan, add macaroni and boil them according to the
2. Directions of the manufacturer (appx. 15 minutes).
3. Then drain water and chill the macaroni little.
4. Meanwhile, in the salad bowl mix up together Feta cheese, bell peppers, olives, onion, tomato, and cucumber.
5. Make the dressing for the salad: combine together dried oregano, lemon juice, and olive oil.
6. Add cooked macaroni in the salad bowl and mix up well.
7. Drizzle the salad with dressing and shake gently.

Nutrition: calories 328, fat 14.8, fiber 5.6, carbs 40.3, protein 12.2

65. ARTICHOKE MATZO MINA

Preparation Time: 10 minutes
Cooking time: 45 minutes
Servings: 6

Ingredients:

- 4 sheets matzo
- ½ cup artichoke hearts, canned
- 1 cup cream cheese
- 1 cup spinach, chopped
- ½ teaspoon salt
- 1 teaspoon ground black pepper
- 3 tablespoons fresh dill, chopped
- 3 eggs, beaten
- 1 teaspoon canola oil
- ½ cup cottage cheese

Directions:

1. In the bowl combine together cream cheese, spinach, salt, ground black pepper, dill, and cottage cheese.
2. Pour canola oil in the skillet, add artichoke hearts and roast them for 2-3 minutes over the medium heat. Stir them from time to time.
3. Then add roasted artichoke hearts in the cheese mixture.
4. Add eggs and stir until homogenous.
5. Place one sheet of matzo in the casserole mold.
6. Then spread it with cheese mixture generously.
7. Cover the cheese layer with the second sheet of matzo.
8. Repeat the steps till you use all ingredients.
9. Then preheat oven to 360F.
10. Bake matzo mina for 40 minutes.
11. Cut the cooked meal into the.

Nutrition: calories 272, fat 17.3, fiber 4.3, carbs 20.2, protein 11.8

66. STUFFED ZUCCHINI BOATS WITH GOAT CHEESE

Preparation Time: 15 minutes
Cooking time: 30 minutes
Servings: 4

Ingredients:

- 1 cup ground chicken
- 3 oz goat cheese, crumbled
- 2 zucchini, trimmed
- 1 tablespoon sour cream
- ½ teaspoon salt
- ½ teaspoon chili flakes
- ½ teaspoon dried oregano
- 1 tablespoon tomato sauce
- 4 teaspoons butter

Directions:

1. Cut zucchini into lengthwise boards.
2. Scoop the zucchini meat.
3. Then mix up together ground chicken, goat cheese, salt, chili flakes, dried oregano, and fill the zucchini boats.
4. Then top them with sour cream and butter.
5. Wrap zucchini boats in the foil and transfer in the preheated to the 360F oven.
6. Bake zucchini for 30 minutes.
7. Then discard the foil and transfer cooked

zucchini boats in the serving plates.

Nutrition: calories 220, fat 14.8, fiber 1.2, carbs 4.2, protein 18

67. GREEK STYLE QUESADILLAS

Preparation Time: 10 minutes
Cooking time: 10 minutes
Servings: 4

Ingredients:

- 4 whole wheat tortillas
- 1 cup Mozzarella cheese, shredded
- 1 cup fresh spinach, chopped
- 2 tablespoon Greek yogurt
- 1 egg, beaten
- ¼ cup green olives, sliced
- 1 tablespoon olive oil
- 1/3 cup fresh cilantro, chopped

Directions:

1. In the bowl, combine together Mozzarella cheese, spinach, yogurt, egg, olives, and cilantro.
2. Then pour olive oil in the skillet.
3. Place one tortilla in the skillet and spread it with Mozzarella mixture. Top it with the second tortilla and spread it with cheese mixture again.
4. Then place the third tortilla and spread it with all remaining cheese mixture.
5. Cover it with the last tortilla and fry it for 5 minutes from each side over the medium heat.

Nutrition: calories 193, fat 7.7, fiber 3.2, carbs 23.6, protein 8.3

68. CREAMY PENNE

Preparation Time: 10 minutes
Cooking time: 25 minutes
Servings: 4

Ingredients:

- ½ cup penne, dried
- 9 oz chicken fillet
- 1 teaspoon Italian seasoning
- 1 tablespoon olive oil
- 1 tomato, chopped
- 1 cup heavy cream
- 1 tablespoon fresh basil, chopped
- ½ teaspoon salt
- 2 oz Parmesan, grated
- 1 cup water, for cooking

Directions:

1. Pour water in the pan, add penne, and boil it for 15 minutes. Then drain water.
2. Pour olive oil in the skillet and heat it up.
3. Slice the chicken fillet and put it in the hot oil.
4. Sprinkle chicken with Italian seasoning and roast for 2 minutes from each side.
5. Then add fresh basil, salt, tomato, and grated cheese.
6. Stir well.
7. Add heavy cream and cooked penne.
8. Cook the meal for 5 minutes more over the medium heat. Stir it from time to time.

Nutrition: calories 388, fat 23.4, fiber 0.2, carbs 17.6, protein 17.6

69. LIGHT PAPRIKA MOUSSAKA

Preparation Time: 15 minutes
Cooking time: 45 minutes
Servings: 3

Ingredients:

- 1 eggplant, trimmed
- 1 cup ground chicken
- 1/3 cup white onion, diced
- 3 oz Cheddar cheese, shredded
- 1 potato, sliced
- 1 teaspoon olive oil
- 1 teaspoon salt
- ½ cup milk
- 1 tablespoon butter
- 1 tablespoon ground paprika
- 1 tablespoon Italian seasoning
- 1 teaspoon tomato paste

Directions:

1. Slice the eggplant lengthwise and sprinkle with salt.
2. Pour olive oil in the skillet and add sliced potato.
3. Roast potato for 2 minutes from each side.

4. Then transfer it in the plate.
5. Put eggplant in the skillet and roast it for 2 minutes from each side too.
6. Pour milk in the pan and bring it to boil.
7. Add tomato paste, Italian seasoning, paprika, butter, and Cheddar cheese.
8. Then mix up together onion with ground chicken.
9. Arrange the sliced potato in the casserole in one layer.
10. Then add ½ part of all sliced eggplants.
11. Spread the eggplants with ½ part of chicken mixture.
12. Then add remaining eggplants.
13. Pour the milk mixture over the eggplants.
14. Bake moussaka for 30 minutes at 355F.

Nutrition: calories 387, fat 21.2, fiber 8.9, carbs 26.3, protein 25.4

70. CUCUMBER BOWL WITH SPICES AND GREEK YOGURT

Preparation Time: 10 minutes
Cooking time: 20 minutes
Servings: 3

Ingredients:

- 4 cucumbers
- ½ teaspoon chili pepper
- ¼ cup fresh parsley, chopped
- ¾ cup fresh dill, chopped
- 2 tablespoons lemon juice
- ½ teaspoon salt
- ½ teaspoon ground black pepper
- ¼ teaspoon sage
- ½ teaspoon dried oregano
- 1/3 cup Greek yogurt

Directions:

1. Make the cucumber dressing: blend the dill and parsley until you get green mash.
2. Then combine together green mash with lemon juice, salt, ground black pepper, sage, dried oregano, Greek yogurt, and chili pepper.
3. Churn the mixture well.
4. Chop the cucumbers roughly and combine them with cucumber dressing. Mix up well.
5. Refrigerate the cucumber for 20 minutes.

Nutrition: calories 114, fat 1.6, fiber 4.1, carbs 23.2, protein 7.6

71. TUFFED BELL PEPPERS WITH QUINOA

Preparation Time: 10 minutes
Cooking time: 35 minutes
Servings: 2

Ingredients:

- 2 bell peppers
- 1/3 cup quinoa
- 3 oz chicken stock
- ¼ cup onion, diced
- ½ teaspoon salt
- ¼ teaspoon tomato paste
- ½ teaspoon dried oregano
- 1/3 cup sour cream
- 1 teaspoon paprika

Directions:

1. Trim the bell peppers and remove the seeds.
2. Then combine together chicken stock and quinoa in the pan.
3. Add salt and boil the ingredients for 10 minutes or until quinoa will soak all liquid.
4. Then combine together cooked quinoa with dried oregano, tomato paste, and onion.
5. Fill the bell peppers with the quinoa mixture and arrange in the casserole mold.
6. Add sour cream and bake the peppers for 25 minutes at 365F.
7. Serve the cooked peppers with sour cream sauce from the casserole mold.

Nutrition: calories 237, fat 10.3, fiber 4.5, carbs 31.3, protein 6.9

72. MEDITERRANEAN BURRITO

Preparation Time: 10 minutes
Servings: 2

Ingredients:

- 2 wheat tortillas
- 2 oz red kidney beans, canned, drained
- 2 tablespoons hummus

- 2 teaspoons tahini sauce
- 1 cucumber
- 2 lettuce leaves
- 1 tablespoon lime juice
- 1 teaspoon olive oil
- ½ teaspoon dried oregano

Directions:

1. Mash the red kidney beans until you get a puree.
2. Then spread the wheat tortillas with beans mash from one side.
3. Add hummus and tahini sauce.
4. Cut the cucumber into the wedges and place them over tahini sauce.
5. Then add lettuce leaves.
6. Make the dressing: mix up together olive oil, dried oregano, and lime juice.
7. Drizzle the lettuce leaves with the dressing and wrap the wheat tortillas in the shape of burritos.

Nutrition: calories 288, fat 10.2, fiber 14.6, carbs 38.2, protein 12.5

73. SWEET POTATO BACON MASH

Preparation Time: 10 minutes
Cooking time: 20 minutes
Servings: 4

Ingredients:

- 3 sweet potato, peeled
- 4 oz bacon, chopped
- 1 cup chicken stock
- 1 tablespoon butter
- 1 teaspoon salt
- 2 oz Parmesan, grated

Directions:

1. Chop sweet potato and put it in the pan.
2. Add chicken stock and close the lid.
3. Boil the vegetables for 15 minutes or until they are soft.
4. After this, drain the chicken stock.
5. Mash the sweet potato with the help of the potato masher. Add grated cheese and butter.
6. Mix up together salt and chopped bacon. Fry the mixture until it is crunchy (10-15 minutes).
7. Add cooked bacon in the mashed sweet potato and mix up with the help of the spoon.
8. It is recommended to serve the meal warm or hot.

Nutrition: calories 304, fat 18.1, fiber 2.9, carbs 18.8, protein 17

74. PROSCIUTTO WRAPPED MOZZARELLA BALLS

Preparation Time: 10 minutes
Cooking time: 10 minutes
Servings: 4

Ingredients:

- 8 Mozzarella balls, cherry size
- 4 oz bacon, sliced
- ¼ teaspoon ground black pepper
- ¾ teaspoon dried rosemary
- 1 teaspoon butter

Directions:

1. Sprinkle the sliced bacon with ground black pepper and dried rosemary.
2. Wrap every Mozzarella ball in the sliced bacon and secure them with toothpicks.
3. Melt butter.
4. Brush wrapped Mozzarella balls with butter.
5. Line the tray with the baking paper and arrange Mozzarella balls in it.
6. Bake the meal for 10 minutes at 365F.

Nutrition: calories 323, fat 26.8, fiber 0.1, carbs 0.6, protein 20.6

75. GARLIC CHICKEN BALLS

Preparation Time: 15 minutes
Cooking time: 10 minutes
Servings: 4

Ingredients:

- 2 cups ground chicken
- 1 teaspoon minced garlic
- 1 teaspoon dried dill
- 1/3 carrot, grated
- 1 egg, beaten

- 1 tablespoon olive oil
- ¼ cup coconut flakes
- ½ teaspoon salt

Directions:

1. In the mixing bowl mix up together ground chicken, minced garlic, dried dill, carrot, egg, and salt.
2. Stir the chicken mixture with the help of the fingertips until homogenous.
3. Then make medium balls from the mixture.
4. Coat every chicken ball in coconut flakes.
5. Heat up olive oil in the skillet.
6. Add chicken balls and cook them for 3 minutes from each side. The cooked chicken balls will have a golden brown color.

Nutrition: calories 200, fat 11.5, fiber 0.6, carbs 1.7, protein 21.9

76. STUFFED TOMATOES WITH CHEESE AND MEAT

Preparation Time: 15 minutes
Cooking time: 40 minutes
Servings: 4

Ingredients:

- ½ cup ground beef
- ¼ onion, diced
- 1 teaspoon olive oil
- ½ teaspoon salt
- 3 oz Cheddar cheese, shredded
- 4 large tomatoes
- 1/3 cup water

1. Pour olive oil in the skillet.
2. Heat it up and add the onion. Cook it for 3 minutes.
3. Then add ground beef and salt. Stir well.
4. Cook the meat mixture for 15 minutes over the medium-high heat.
5. Then scoop the meat from the tomatoes.
6. Fill the tomatoes with ground beef mixture and top with shredded cheese.
7. Arrange the stuffed tomatoes in the baking tray and add water.
8. Bake the tomatoes for 20 minutes at 350F.

Nutrition: calories 164, fat 10.6, fiber 2.3, carbs 8, protein 10.2

77. STUFFED MEATBALLS WITH EGGS

Preparation Time: 15 minutes
Cooking time: 3.5 minutes
Servings: 4

Ingredients:

- 1 cup ground beef
- ½ cup ground pork
- 4 eggs, boiled, peeled
- 1 tablespoon semolina
- ½ teaspoon salt
- 1 teaspoon chili flakes
- 1 teaspoon turmeric
- ½ teaspoon white pepper
- ½ teaspoon garlic powder
- 1 tablespoon tomato paste
- 1/3 cup water
- 1 teaspoon butter

Directions:

1. In the mixing bowl, mix up together ground beef and ground pork.
2. Add semolina, salt, chili flakes, salt, chili flakes, turmeric, white pepper, and garlic powder.
3. Stir the mass until smooth.
4. Then make 4 balls from the meat mixture.
5. Fill every meatball with a boiled egg.
6. Mix up together water and tomato paste.
7. Place the meatballs in the casserole mold.
8. Add butter and tomato paste mixture.
9. Bake the meatballs for 35 minutes.

Nutrition: calories 269, fat 17.7, fiber 0.5, carbs 3.8, protein 22.8

78. DILL ORZO

Preparation Time: 10 minutes
Cooking time: 9 minutes
Servings: 2

Ingredients:

- ½ cup orzo
- 1 ½ cup chicken stock
- ¼ cup fresh dill, chopped
- 1 teaspoon butter, softened

Directions:

1. Place orzo in the pan. Add chicken stock.
2. Boil orzo for 9 minutes.
3. Meanwhile, churn together butter with fresh dill.
4. Combine together cooked orzo with dill butter.

Nutrition: calories 198, fat 3.4, fiber 2.3, carbs 35.7, protein 7

79. QUINOA TABBOULEH

Preparation Time: 15 minutes
Cooking time: 10 minutes
Servings: 8

Ingredients:

- 1 cup quinoa
- 1 ¼ cup water
- 4 teaspoons lemon juice
- ¼ teaspoon garlic clove, diced
- 5 tablespoons sesame oil
- 2 cucumbers, chopped
- 1/3 teaspoon ground black pepper
- 1/3 cup tomatoes, chopped
- ½ oz scallions, chopped
- ¼ teaspoon fresh mint, chopped

Directions:

1. Pour water in the pan. Add quinoa and boil it for 10 minutes.
2. Then close the lid and let it rest for 5 minutes more.
3. Meanwhile, in the mixing bowl mix up together lemon juice, diced garlic, sesame oil, cucumbers, ground black pepper, tomatoes, scallions, and fresh mint.
4. Then add cooked quinoa and carefully mix the side dish with the help of the spoon.
5. Store tabbouleh up to 2 days in the fridge.

Nutrition: calories 168, fat 9.9, fiber 2, carbs 16.9, protein 3.6

BAKED GRAPES WITH FETA

Preparation Time: 7 minutes
Cooking time: 10 minutes
Servings: 4

Ingredients:

- 1 ½ cup green grapes
- 2 oz Feta cheese, crumbled
- 1 teaspoon avocado oil

Directions:

1. Line the baking tray with baking paper.
2. Arrange the green grapes on it in one layer.
3. Sprinkle the grates with avocado oil and crumbled Feta.
4. Bake the grapes for 10 minutes at 355F.

Nutrition: calories 62, fat 3.3, fiber 0.4, carbs 6.6, protein 2.2

81. 4-INGREDIENTS SPINACH SALAD

Preparation Time: 7 minutes
Servings: 4

Ingredients:

- 2 cups fresh spinach
- 2 tomatoes
- 1 tablespoon Italian seasoning
- 1 teaspoon lemon juice

Directions:

1. Tear the fresh spinach and chop the tomatoes.
2. Place the ingredients in the salad bowl.
3. Add Italian seasoning and lemon juice.

Mix up the salad well.

Nutrition: calories 26, fat 1.2, fiber 1.1, carbs 3.3, protein 1

82. CELERIAC TORTILLA

Preparation Time: 10 minutes
Cooking time: 25 minutes
Servings: 4

Ingredients:

- 2 oz celery root, peeled
- 1 potato, peeled
- 1 tablespoon almond flour
- ½ teaspoon salt
- 1 egg, beaten
- 1 teaspoon olive oil

Directions:

1. Place potato and celery root in the tray and bake for 15 minutes at 355F. The baked vegetables should be tender.
2. Then transfer them in the food processor. Blend until smooth.
3. Add salt, almond flour, and egg. Knead the soft dough.
4. Cut the dough into 4 pieces and make the balls.
5. Using the rolling pin roll up the dough balls in the shape of tortillas
6. Heat up olive oil in the skillet.
7. Add first celeriac tortilla and roast it for 1.5 minutes from each side.
8. Repeat the steps with remaining tortilla balls.
9. Store the cooked tortillas in the towel before serving.

Nutrition: calories 104, fat 5.8, fiber 2, carbs 10.3, protein 4

83. CARAWAY MUSHROOM CAPS

Preparation Time: 8 minutes
Cooking time: 10 minutes
Servings: 4

Ingredients:

- 1 teaspoon caraway seeds
- 3 oz Portobella mushroom caps
- 2 teaspoons butter, softened
- ¼ teaspoon salt

Directions:

1. Trim and wash mushrooms caps if needed.
2. Preheat the oven to 360F.
3. Churn together butter with salt, and caraway seeds.
4. Fill the mushroom caps with butter mixture and transfer in the tray.
5. Bake Portobella caps for 10 minutes at 355F.

Nutrition: calories 24, fat 2, fiber 0.5, carbs 1.3, protein 0.7

84. STUFFED SWEET POTATO

Preparation Time: 10 minutes
Cooking time: 20 minutes
Servings:4

Ingredients:

- 4 sweet potatoes
- ¼ cup Cheddar cheese, shredded
- 2 teaspoons butter
- 1 tablespoon fresh parsley, chopped
- ½ teaspoon salt

Directions:

1. Make the lengthwise cut in every sweet potato and bake them for 10 minutes at 360F.
2. After this, scoop ½ part of every sweet potato flesh.
3. Fill the vegetables with salt, parsley, butter, and shredded cheese.
4. Return the sweet potatoes in the oven back and bake them for 10 minutes more at 355F.

Nutrition: calories 47, fat 4.3, fiber 0.1, carbs 0.4, protein 1.8

85. GARLIC GRATED BEETS

Preparation Time: 15 minutes
Cooking time: 25 minutes
Servings: 2

Ingredients:

- 1 beet, trimmed
- 1/3 teaspoon minced garlic

- 2 tablespoons walnuts
- 2 tablespoons Greek yogurt

Directions:

1. Preheat the oven to 360F.
2. Place the beet in the tray and bake it for 25 minutes. The baked beet should be tender.
3. Let the beet chill little. Peel it.
4. After this, grate it with the help of the grated and transfer in the bowl.
5. Add walnuts, Greek yogurt, and minced garlic. Mix up the mixture well.
6. Place it in the fridge for at least 10 minutes before serving.

Nutrition: calories 79, fat 4.8, fiber 1.5, carbs 6.4, protein 3.9

86. MUJADARA N

Preparation Time: 8 minutes
Cooking time: 15 minutes
Servings: 6
Ingredients:

- 1 cup of brown rice
- 2 yellow onions, sliced
- 1 tablespoon coconut oil
- 1 teaspoon canola oil
- ½ teaspoon honey
- 2 ½ cup chicken stock
- 1 teaspoon salt

Directions:

1. Pour chicken stock in the pan.
2. Add brown rice and close the lid.
3. Cook the rice for 15 minutes over the medium heat or until it will soak all the liquid (the time of cooking depends on the type and quality of brown rice).
4. Meanwhile, combine together canola oil and coconut oil in the skillet.
5. Heat up the mixture and add sliced onions and salt.
6. Cook them for 5-7 minutes or until they are light brown.
7. Then add honey and mix up well.
8. Cook the onions for 3 minutes more.
9. When the rice is cooked, combine it together with cooked rice and mix up well.

Nutrition: calories 162, fat 4.2, fiber 1.9, carbs 28.3, protein 3.1

87. OLIVES QUINOA WITH JALAPENO

Preparation Time: 7 minutes
Cooking time: 10 minutes
Servings: 4

Ingredients:

- 10 green olives, pitted
- ½ cup quinoa
- 1 cup of water
- ½ teaspoon salt
- 1 jalapeno pepper, chopped
- 1 teaspoon butter
- ½ teaspoon paprika

Directions:

1. Slice green olives and put them in the salad bowl.
2. Cook quinoa: boil it together with water for 10 minutes.
3. Then add salt and cool it to the room temperature.
4. Transfer the quinoa in salad bowls (to olives).
5. Add paprika.
6. Roast together jalapeno pepper and butter for 2 minutes.
7. Then add jalapeno pepper in the quinoa mixture. Mix it up well with the help of the spoon.

Nutrition: calories 91, fat 2.5, fiber 1.9, carbs 14.2, protein 3.1

88. CAULIFLOWER PUREE WITH BACON

Preparation Time: 10 minutes
Cooking time: 25 minutes
Servings:

Ingredients:

- ½ oz bacon, chopped
- 1 cup cauliflower, chopped
- 3 tablespoons water, hot
- 1 tablespoon cream cheese
- ¼ teaspoon salt

Directions:

1. Sprinkle bacon with salt and roast it for 5 minutes over the high heat. When the bacon is light crunchy, it is cooked.
2. After this, place chopped cauliflower in the tray.
3. Bake it for 25 minutes in the preheated to the 360F oven.
4. When the cauliflower is soft, transfer it in the food processor.
5. Add cream cheese and hot water.
6. Blend the vegetables until you get a fluffy puree.
7. The place the cooked puree in the serving plates and top with crunchy bacon.

Nutrition: calories 68, fat 4.8, fiber 13, carbs 2.9, protein 4

89. CITRUS SALAD

Preparation Time: 8 minutes
Servings: 3

Ingredients:

- 3 kalamata olives
- 1 orange, peeled
- 1 cup lettuce, chopped
- 1 teaspoon lemon juice
- 1 teaspoon dried oregano
- ½ teaspoon olive oil

Directions:

1. Chop kalamata olive roughly and put them in the big bowl.
2. Chop orange into the medium cubes and add it in the olives.
3. Then add lettuce.
4. Lemon juice dressing: in the shallow bowl combine together olive oil, dried oregano, and lemon juice.
5. Shake the salad well and drizzle with lemon juice dressing.

Nutrition: calories 45, fat 1.4, fiber 2, carbs 8.4, protein 0.8

90. SPANAKORIZO SPINACH RICE

Preparation Time: 10 minutes
Cooking time: 30 minutes
Servings: 4

Ingredients:

- 1 cup long grain rice
- 2 cups chicken stock
- 1 yellow onion, diced
- 1 tablespoon sunflower oil
- 1 cup fresh spinach, chopped
- 1 teaspoon salt
- 1 teaspoon ground black pepper
- ¼ teaspoon garlic, diced
- 1 teaspoon lemon juice

Directions:

1. Pour sunflower oil in the saucepan and heat it up.
2. Add diced onion and spinach.
3. Saute the ingredients for 5 minutes. Stir them from time to time.
4. Then add garlic, salt, ground black pepper, and lemon juice. Mix up well.
5. Add chicken stock and long grain rice.
6. Mix up ingredients carefully with the help of the spatula.
7. Close the lid and saute the rice for 20 minutes over the low heat.
8. When the rice is cooked, mix it up carefully and transfer in the serving plates.

Nutrition: calories 219, fat 4.2, fiber 1.5, carbs 40.6, protein 4.2

91. WALNUT SALAD

Preparation Time: 7 minutes
Servings: 6

Ingredients:

- 1 oz Feta cheese, crumbled
- 2 oz walnuts, chopped
- 1 cup fresh parsley, chopped
- 1 cup cucumbers, chopped
- ½ cup tomatoes, chopped
- ½ red onion, sliced
- 2 tablespoons sesame oil
- 1 tablespoon lemon juice
- 1 teaspoon Italian seasoning

Directions:

1. Make the dressing: mix up together Italian

seasoning, lemon juice, and sesame oil.
2. Then in the salad bowl combine together crumbled Feta cheese, walnuts, parsley, cucumbers, tomatoes, and onion.
3. Drizzle the dressing over the salad and mix it up with the help of two spatulas.

Nutrition: calories 126, fat 11.5, fiber 1.5, carbs 4, protein 3.6

92. BAKED OLIVES

Preparation Time: 5 minutes
Cooking time: 11 minutes
Servings: 3

Ingredients:

- 1 ½ cup olives
- 1 tablespoon olive oil
- 1 teaspoon dried oregano
- ¼ teaspoon dried thyme
- 1/3 teaspoon minced garlic
- ½ teaspoon salt

Directions:

1. Line the baking tray with baking paper.
2. Arrange the olives in the tray in one layer.
3. Then sprinkle them with olive oil, dried oregano, dried thyme, minced garlic, and salt.
4. Bake olives for 11 minutes at 420F.

Nutrition: calories 119, fat 11.9, fiber 2.4, carbs 4.7, protein 0.7

93. SLICED FIGS SALAD

Preparation Time: 10 minutes
Servings: 4

Ingredients:

- 1 tablespoon balsamic vinegar
- 1 teaspoon canola oil
- 2 tablespoons almonds, sliced
- 3 figs, sliced
- 2 cups fresh parsley
- 1 cup fresh arugula
- 2 oz Feta cheese, crumbled
- ½ teaspoon salt
- ½ teaspoon honey

Directions:

1. Make the salad dressing: mix up together balsamic vinegar, canola oil, salt, and honey.
2. Then put sliced almonds and figs in the big bowl.
3. Chop the parsley and add in the fig mixture too.
4. After this, tear arugula.
5. Combine together arugula with fig mixture.
6. Add salad dressing and shake the salad well.

Nutrition: calories 116, fat 6.1, fiber 2.8, carbs 13.2, protein 4.1

94. LEMON CUCUMBERS WITH DILL

Preparation Time: 5 minutes
Cooking time: 30 minutes
Servings: 3

Ingredients:

- 3 cucumbers
- 3 tablespoons lemon juice
- ¾ teaspoon lemon zest
- 3 teaspoons dill, chopped
- 1 tablespoon olive oil
- ¾ teaspoon chili flakes

Directions:

1. Peel the cucumbers and chop them roughly.
2. Place the cucumbers in the big glass jar.
3. Add lemon zest, lemon juice, dill, olive oil, and chili flakes.
4. Close the lid and shake well.
5. Marinate the cucumbers for 30 minutes.

Nutrition: calories 92, fat 5.2, fiber 1.8, carbs 11.9, protein 2.3

95. HONEY APPLE BITES

Preparation Time: 10 minutes
Cooking time: 15 minutes
Servings: 2

Ingredients:

- 1 tablespoon honey
- ½ teaspoon ground cardamom

- 2 apples

Directions:

1. Cut the apples into halves and remove the seeds.
2. Then cut the apples into 4 bites more.
3. Place the apple bites in the tray and sprinkle with ground cardamom and honey.
4. Bake apples for 15 minutes at 355F.

Nutrition: calories 149, fat 0.4, fiber 5.6, carbs 39.8, protein 0.7

96. CUCUMBER SALAD

Preparation Time: 10 minutes
Servings: 6

Ingredients:

- 2 cups tomatoes, chopped
- 1 cup cucumbers, chopped
- 1 red onion, chopped
- 1 cup fresh cilantro, chopped
- 1 red bell pepper, chopped
- 2 tablespoons sunflower oil
- 1 teaspoon salt

Directions:

1. In the bowl combine together tomatoes, cucumbers, onion, fresh cilantro, bell pepper, and salt.
2. Shake the salad mixture well.
3. Then add the sunflower oil.
4. Stir the salad directly before serving.

Nutrition: calories 69, fat 4.9, fiber 1.5, carbs 6.3, protein 1.1

97. SESAME SEEDS ESCAROLE

Preparation Time: 7 minutes
Cooking time: 7 minutes
Servings: 2

Ingredients:

- 1 head escarole
- 1 tablespoon sesame oil
- 1 teaspoon sesame seeds
- 1 teaspoon balsamic vinegar
- ¾ teaspoon ground black pepper
- ¼ cup of water

Directions:

1. Chop the escarole roughly.
2. Pour water in the skillet and bring it to boil.
3. Add chopped escarole. Saute it for 2 minutes over the high heat.
4. Then add sesame seeds, sesame oil, balsamic vinegar, and ground black pepper.
5. Mix up well and saute escarole for 1 minute more or until it starts to boil again.

Nutrition: calories 118, fat 8.1, fiber 8.3, carbs 9.5, protein 3.6

98. YOGURT EGGPLANTS

Preparation Time: 10 minutes
Cooking time: 18 minutes
Servings: 4

Ingredients:

- 1 cup Plain yogurt
- 1 tablespoon butter
- 1 teaspoon ground black pepper
- 1 teaspoon salt
- 2 eggplants, chopped
- 1 tablespoon fresh dill, chopped

Directions:

1. Heat up butter in the skillet.
2. Toss eggplants in the hot butter. Sprinkle them with salt and ground black pepper.
3. Roast the vegetables for 5 minutes over the medium-high heat. Stir them from time to time.
4. After this, add fresh dill and Plain Yogurt. Mix up well.
5. Close the lid and simmer eggplants for 10 minutes more over the medium-high heat.

Nutrition: calories 141, fat 4.2, fiber 9.9, carbs 21.2, protein 6.4

SEAFOOD

99. FISH PACKETS

Preparation Time: 15 minutes
Cooking time: 20 minutes
Servings:3

Ingredients:

- 3 tilapia fillets (4 oz each fish fillet)
- ½ teaspoon cayenne pepper
- ½ teaspoon salt
- 3 teaspoons olive oil
- 1 red onion, sliced
- 3 lemon slices
- 1 zucchini, chopped

Directions:

1. Make the medium packets from the foil and brush them with olive oil from inside.
2. Then sprinkle tilapia fillets with salt and cayenne pepper from each side and arrange in the foil packets.
3. Add sliced lemon on the top of the fish.
4. Then add sliced onion and zucchini.
5. Bake the fish packets for 20 minutes at 360F or until vegetables are tender.

Nutrition: calories 161, fat 5.9, fiber 1.8, carbs 6.4, protein 22.3

100. SALMON BAKED IN FOIL WITH FRESH THYME

Preparation Time: 10 minutes
Cooking time: 30 minutes
Servings:4

Ingredients:

- 4 fresh thyme sprig
- 4 garlic cloves, peeled, roughly chopped
- 16 oz salmon fillets (4 oz each fillet)
- ½ teaspoon salt
- ½ teaspoon ground black pepper
- 4 tablespoons cream
- 4 teaspoons butter
- ¼ teaspoon cumin seeds

Directions:

1. Line the baking tray with foil.
2. Sprinkle the fish fillets with salt, ground black pepper, cumin seeds, and arrange them in the tray with oil.
3. Add thyme sprig on the top of every fillet.
4. Then add cream, butter, and garlic.
5. Bake the fish for 30 minutes at 345F.

Nutrition: calories 198, fat 11.6, fiber 0.2, carbs 1.8, protein 22.4

101. POACHED HALIBUT IN ORANGE SAUCE

Preparation Time: 10 minutes
Cooking time: 10 minutes
Servings: 4

Ingredients:

- 1-pound halibut
- 1/3 cup butter
- 1 rosemary sprig
- ½ teaspoon ground black pepper
- 1 teaspoon salt
- 1 teaspoon honey
- ¼ cup of orange juice
- 1 teaspoon cornstarch

Directions:

1. Put butter in the saucepan and melt it.
2. Add rosemary sprig.
3. Sprinkle the halibut with salt and ground black pepper.
4. Put the fish in the boiling butter and poach it for 4 minutes.
5. Meanwhile, pour orange juice in the skillet. Add honey and bring the liquid to boil.
6. Add cornstarch and whisk until the liquid will start to be thick.
7. Then remove it from the heat.
8. Transfer the poached halibut in the plate and cut it on 4.
9. Place every fish serving in the serving plate and top with orange sauce.

Nutrition: calories 349, fat 29.3, fiber 0.1, carbs 3.2, protein 17.8

102. FISH EN PAPILLOTE

Preparation Time: 15 minutes
Cooking time: 20 minutes
Servings:3

Ingredients:

- 10 oz snapper fillet
- 1 tablespoon fresh dill, chopped
- 1 white onion, peeled, sliced
- ½ teaspoon tarragon
- 1 tablespoon olive oil
- 1 teaspoon salt
- ½ teaspoon hot pepper
- 2 tablespoons sour cream

Directions:

1. Make the medium size packets from parchment and arrange them in the baking tray.
2. Cut the snapper fillet on 3 and sprinkle them with salt, tarragon, and hot pepper.
3. Put the fish fillets in the parchment packets.
4. Then top the fish with olive oil, sour cream sliced onion, and fresh dill.
5. Bake the fish for 20 minutes at 355F.

Nutrition: calories 204, fat 8.2, fiber 1, carbs 4.6, protein 27.2

103. TUNA CASSEROLE

Preparation Time: 15 minutes
Cooking time: 35 minutes
Servings:4

Ingredients:

- ½ cup Cheddar cheese, shredded
- 2 tomatoes, chopped
- 7 oz tuna filet, chopped
- 1 teaspoon ground coriander
- ½ teaspoon salt
- 1 teaspoon olive oil
- ½ teaspoon dried oregano

Directions:

1. Brush the casserole mold with olive oil.
2. Mix up together chopped tuna fillet with dried oregano and ground coriander.
3. Place the fish in the mold and flatten well to get the layer.
4. Then add chopped tomatoes and shredded cheese.
5. Cover the casserole with foil and secure the edges.
6. Bake the meal for 35 minutes at 355F.

Nutrition: calories 260, fat 21.5, fiber 0.8, carbs 2.7, protein 14.6

104. OREGANO SALMON WITH CRUNCHY CRUST

Preparation Time: 10 minutes
Cooking time: 2 hours
Servings:2

Ingredients:

- 8 oz salmon fillet
- 2 tablespoons panko bread crumbs
- 1 oz Parmesan, grated
- 1 teaspoon dried oregano
- 1 teaspoon sunflower oil

Directions:

1. In the mixing bowl combine together panko bread crumbs, Parmesan, and dried oregano.
2. Sprinkle the salmon with olive oil and coat in the breadcrumbs mixture.
3. After this, line the baking tray with baking paper.
4. Place the salmon in the tray and transfer in the preheated to the 385F oven.
5. Bake the salmon for 25 minutes.

Nutrition: calories 245, fat 12.8, fiber 0.6, carbs 5.9, protein 27.5

105. SARDINE FISH CAKES

Preparation Time: 10 minutes
Cooking time: 10 minutes
Servings:4

Ingredients:

- 11 oz sardines, canned, drained
- 1/3 cup shallot, chopped
- 1 teaspoon chili flakes
- ½ teaspoon salt
- 2 tablespoon wheat flour, whole grain

- 1 egg, beaten
- 1 tablespoon chives, chopped
- 1 teaspoon olive oil
- 1 teaspoon butter

Directions:

1. Put the butter in the skillet and melt it.
2. Add shallot and cook it until translucent.
3. After this, transfer the shallot in the mixing bowl.
4. Add sardines, chili flakes, salt, flour, egg, chives, and mix up until smooth with the help of the fork.
5. Make the medium size cakes and place them in the skillet.
6. Add olive oil.
7. Roast the fish cakes for 3 minutes from each side over the medium heat.
8. Dry the cooked fish cakes with the paper towel if needed and transfer in the serving plates.

Nutrition: calories 221, fat 12.2, fiber 0.1, carbs 5.4, protein 21.3

106. CAJUN CATFISH

Preparation Time: 10 minutes
Cooking time: 10 minutes
Servings:4

Ingredients:

- 16 oz catfish steaks (4 oz each fish steak)
- 1 tablespoon cajun spices
- 1 egg, beaten
- 1 tablespoon sunflower oil

Directions:

1. Pour sunflower oil in the skillet and preheat it until shimmering.
2. Meanwhile, dip every catfish steak in the beaten egg and coat in Cajun spices.
3. Place the fish steaks in the hot oil and roast them for 4 minutes from each side.
4. The cooked catfish steaks should have a light brown crust.

Nutrition: calories 263, fat 16.7, fiber 0, carbs 0.1, protein 26.3

107. POACHED GENNARO/SEABASS WITH RED PEPPERS

Preparation Time: 10 minutes
Cooking time: 40 minutes
Servings:4

Ingredients:

- 2 red peppers, trimmed
- 11 oz Gennaro/seabass, trimmed
- 1 teaspoon salt
- ½ teaspoon ground black pepper
- 2 tablespoons butter
- 1 lemon

Directions:

1. Remove the seeds from red peppers and cut them on the wedges.
2. Then line the baking tray with parchment and arrange red peppers in a layer.
3. Rub Gennaro/seabass with ground black pepper and salt and place it on the peppers.
4. Then add butter.
5. Cut the lemon on the halves and squeeze the juice over the fish.
6. Bake the fish for 40 minutes at 350F.

Nutrition: calories 148, fat 10.3, fiber 1.2, carbs 7.3, protein 8.5

108. 4-INGREDIENTS SALMON FILLET

Preparation Time: 5 minutes
Cooking time: 25 minutes
Servings:1

Ingredients:

- 4 oz salmon fillet
- ½ teaspoon salt
- 1 teaspoon sesame oil
- ½ teaspoon sage

Directions:

1. Rub the fillet with salt and sage.
2. Place the fish in the tray and sprinkle it with sesame oil.
3. Cook the fish for 25 minutes at 365F.
4. Flip the fish carefully onto another side after 12 minutes of cooking.

Nutrition: calories 191, fat 11.6, fiber 0.1, carbs

0.2, protein 22

109. SPANISH COD IN SAUCE

Preparation Time: 10 minutes
Cooking time: 5.5 hours
Servings:2

Ingredients:

- 1 teaspoon tomato paste
- 1 teaspoon garlic, diced
- 1 white onion, sliced
- 1 jalapeno pepper, chopped
- 1/3 cup chicken stock
- 7 oz Spanish cod fillet
- 1 teaspoon paprika
- 1 teaspoon salt

Directions:

1. Pour chicken stock in the saucepan.
2. Add tomato paste and mix up the liquid until homogenous.
3. Add garlic, onion, jalapeno pepper, paprika, and salt.
4. Bring the liquid to boil and then simmer it.
5. Chop the cod fillet and add it in the tomato liquid.
6. Close the lid and simmer the fish for 10 minutes over the low heat.
7. Serve the fish in the bowls with tomato sauce.

Nutrition: calories 113, fat 1.2, fiber 1.9, carbs 7.2, protein 18.9

110. FISH SHAKSHUKA

Preparation Time: 5 minutes
Cooking time: 15 minutes
Servings:5

Ingredients:

- 5 eggs
- 1 cup tomatoes, chopped
- 3 bell peppers, chopped
- 1 tablespoon butter
- 1 teaspoon tomato paste
- 1 teaspoon chili pepper
- 1 teaspoon salt
- 1 tablespoon fresh dill
- 5 oz cod fillet, chopped
- 1 tablespoon scallions, chopped

Directions:

1. Melt butter in the skillet and add chili pepper, bell peppers, and tomatoes.
2. Sprinkle the vegetables with scallions, dill, salt, and chili pepper. Simmer them for 5 minutes.
3. After this, add chopped cod fillet and mix up well.
4. Close the lid and simmer the ingredients for 5 minutes over the medium heat.
5. Then crack the eggs over fish and close the lid.
6. Cook shakshuka with the closed lid for 5 minutes.

Nutrition: calories 143, fat 7.3, fiber 1.6, carbs 7.9, protein 12.8

111. MACKEREL SKILLET WITH GREENS

Preparation Time: 10 minutes
Cooking time: 15 minutes
Servings:4

Ingredients:

- 1 cup fresh spinach, chopped
- ½ cup endive, chopped
- 11 oz mackerel
- 1 tablespoon olive oil
- 1 teaspoon ground nutmeg
- ½ teaspoon salt
- ½ teaspoon turmeric
- ½ teaspoon chili flakes
- 3 tablespoons sour cream

Directions:

1. Pour olive oil in the skillet.
2. Add mackerel and sprinkle it with chili flakes, turmeric, and salt.
3. Roast fish for 2 minutes from each side.
4. Then add chopped endive, fresh spinach, and sour cream.
5. Mix up well and close the lid.
6. Simmer the meal for 10 minutes over the medium-low heat.

Nutrition: calories 260, fat 19.5, fiber 0.5, carbs

1.3, protein 19.2

112. SALMON BALLS WITH CREAM CHEESE

Preparation Time: 15 minutes
Cooking time: 15 minutes
Servings:5

Ingredients:

- 1-pound salmon fillet
- 2 teaspoons cream cheese
- 3 tablespoons panko breadcrumbs
- ½ teaspoon salt
- 1 oz Parmesan, grated
- ½ teaspoon ground black pepper
- 1 teaspoon dried oregano
- 1 tablespoon sunflower oil

Directions:

1. Grind the salmon fillet and combine it together with cream cheese, panko breadcrumbs, salt, Parmesan, ground black pepper, and dried oregano.
2. Then make the small balls from the mixture and place them in the non-sticky tray.
3. Sprinkle the balls with sunflower oil and bake in the preheated to the 365F oven for 15 minutes. Flip the balls on another side after 10 minutes of cooking.

Nutrition: calories 180, fat 10.2, fiber 0.5, carbs 2.8, protein 19.9

113. FISH CHILI WITH LENTILS

Preparation Time: 10 minutes
Cooking time: 30 minutes
Servings:4

Ingredients:

- 1 red pepper, chopped
- 1 yellow onion, diced
- 1 teaspoon ground black pepper
- 1 teaspoon butter
- 1 jalapeno pepper, chopped
- ½ cup lentils
- 3 cups chicken stock
- 1 teaspoon salt
- 1 tablespoon tomato paste
- 1 teaspoon chili pepper
- 3 tablespoons fresh cilantro, chopped
- 8 oz cod, chopped

Directions:

1. Place butter, red pepper, onion, and ground black pepper in the saucepan.
2. Roast the vegetables for 5 minutes over the medium heat.
3. Then add chopped jalapeno pepper, lentils, and chili pepper.
4. Mix up the mixture well and add chicken stock and tomato paste.
5. Stir until homogenous. Add cod.
6. Close the lid and cook chili for 20 minutes over the medium heat.

Nutrition: calories 187, fat 2.3, fiber 8.8, carbs 21.3, protein 20.6

114. CHILI MUSSELS

Preparation Time: 7 minutes
Cooking time: 10 minutes
Servings:4

Ingredients:

- 1-pound mussels
- 1 chili pepper, chopped
- 1 cup chicken stock
- ½ cup milk
- 1 teaspoon olive oil
- 1 teaspoon minced garlic
- 1 teaspoon ground coriander
- ½ teaspoon salt
- 1 cup fresh parsley, chopped
- 4 tablespoons lemon juice

Directions:

1. Pour milk in the saucepan.
2. Add chili pepper, chicken stock, olive oil, minced garlic, ground coriander, salt, and lemon juice.
3. Bring the liquid to boil and add mussels.
4. Boil the mussel for 4 minutes or until they will open shells.
5. Then add chopped parsley and mix up the meal well.
6. Remove it from the heat.

Nutrition: calories 136, fat 4.7, fiber 0.6, carbs

7.5, protein 15.3

115. FRIED SCALLOPS IN HEAVY CREAM

Preparation Time: 10 minutes
Cooking time: 7 minutes
Servings:4

Ingredients:

- ½ cup heavy cream
- 1 teaspoon fresh rosemary
- ½ teaspoon dried cumin
- ½ teaspoon garlic, diced
- 8 oz bay scallops
- 1 teaspoon olive oil
- ½ teaspoon salt
- ¼ teaspoon chili flakes

Directions:

1. Preheat olive oil in the skillet until hot.
2. Then sprinkle scallops with salt, chili flakes, and dried cumin and place in the hot oil.
3. Add fresh rosemary and diced garlic.
4. Roast the scallops for 2 minutes from each side.
5. After this, add heavy cream and bring the mixture to boil. Boil it for 1 minute.

Nutrition: calories 114, fat 7.3, fiber 0.2, carbs 2.2, protein 9.9

116. LETTUCE SEAFOOD WRAPS

Preparation Time: 10 minutes
Cooking time: 0 minutes
Servings:6

Ingredients:

- 6 lettuce leaves
- 8 oz salmon, canned
- 4 oz crab meat, canned
- 1 cucumber
- 2 tablespoons Plain yogurt
- ½ teaspoon minced garlic
- 1 tablespoon fresh dill, chopped
- ¼ teaspoon tarragon

Directions:

1. Mash the salmon and crab meat with the help of the fork.
2. Then add Plain yogurt, minced garlic, fresh dill, and tarragon.
3. Grate the cucumber and add it in the seafood mixture. Mix up well.
4. Fill the lettuce leaves with cooked mixture.

Nutrition: calories 80, fat 2.8, fiber 0.4, carbs 3.1, protein 10.5

117. MANGO TILAPIA FILLETS

Preparation Time: 10 minutes
Cooking time: 15 minutes
Servings:4

Ingredients:

- ¼ cup coconut flakes
- 5 oz mango, peeled
- 1/3 cup shallot, chopped
- 1 teaspoon ground turmeric
- 1 cup of water
- 1 bay leaf
- 12 oz tilapia fillets
- 1 chili pepper, chopped
- 1 tablespoon coconut oil
- ½ teaspoon salt
- 1 teaspoon paprika

Directions:

1. Blend together coconut flakes, mango, shallot, ground turmeric, and water.
2. After this, melt coconut oil in the saucepan.
3. Sprinkle the tilapia fillets with salt and paprika.
4. Then place them in the hot coconut oil and roast for 1 minute from each side.
5. Add chili pepper, bay leaf, and blended mango mixture.
6. Close the lid and cook fish for 10 minutes over the medium heat.

Nutrition: calories 153, fat 6.1, fiber 1.5, carbs 9.3, protein 16.8

118. SEAFOOD GRATIN

Preparation Time: 15 minutes
Cooking time: 40 minutes
Servings:5

Ingredients:

- 3 Russet potatoes, sliced
- ½ cup onion, chopped
- ½ cup milk
- 1 egg, beaten
- 3 tablespoon wheat flour, whole grain
- 1 cup shrimps, peeled
- ½ cup Mozzarella cheese, shredded
- ¼ cup Cheddar cheese, shredded
- 1 teaspoon olive oil
- 1 cup water, for cooking

Directions:

1. Pour water in the pan and bring it to boil.
2. Add sliced potatoes in the hot water and boil it for 3 minutes.
3. Then remove potatoes from water.
4. Mix up together beaten egg, milk, chopped onion, flour, and Cheddar cheese.
5. Preheat the mixture until cheese is melted.
6. Then place the potatoes in the gratin mold in one layer.
7. Add the layer of shrimps.
8. Pour Cheddar cheese mixture over shrimps and top the gratin with Mozzarella cheese.
9. Cover the gratin with foil and secure the edges.
10. Bake gratin for 35 minutes at 355F.

Nutrition: calories 205, fat 5.3, fiber 3.5, carbs 26.2, protein 14.1

119. GINGER SEABASS STIR-FRY

Preparation Time: 10 minutes
Cooking time: 10 minutes
Servings:4

Ingredients:

- 1 teaspoon fresh ginger, minced
- 10 oz seabass fillet (4 fillets)
- 1 tablespoon butter
- 1 teaspoon minced garlic
- ¼ teaspoon ground nutmeg
- ½ teaspoon salt

Directions:

1. Toss butter in the skillet and melt it.
2. Add minced garlic, ground nutmeg, salt, and fresh ginger.
3. Roast the mixture for 1 minute.
4. Then add seabass fillet.
5. Fryt the fish for 3 minutes from each side.

Nutrition: calories 205, fat 13.5, fiber 0.8, carbs 0.6, protein 19.7

120. TERIYAKI TUNA

Preparation Time: 10 minutes
Cooking time: 6 minutes
Servings:3

Ingredients:

- 3 tuna fillets
- 3 teaspoons teriyaki sauce
- ½ teaspoon minced garlic
- 1 teaspoon olive oil

Directions:

1. Whisk together teriyaki sauce, minced garlic, and olive oil.
2. Bruhs every tuna fillet with teriyaki mixture.
3. Preheat grill to 390F.
4. Grill the fish for 3 minutes from each side.

Nutrition: calories 382, fat 32.6, fiber 0, carbs 1.1, protein 21.4

121. SHRIMP KORMA

Preparation Time: 10 minutes
Cooking time: 15 minutes
Servings:2

Ingredients:

- 1 cinnamon stick
- 1/3 cup Plain yogurt
- 1 teaspoon minced ginger
- ½ teaspoon ground coriander
- ½ teaspoon salt
- 1 teaspoon olive oil
- 1 tablespoon tomato paste
- 1 teaspoon jalapeno pepper
- 1 cup shrimps, peeled
- ¼ cup of water
- 1 teaspoon turmeric
- ½ teaspoon paprika
- ½ teaspoon sage

Directions:

1. In the saucepan mix up together Plain yogurt, minced ginger, ground coriander, salt, tomato paste, and water.
2. Then pour olive oil in the skillet and preheat it.
3. Add jalapeno pepper and roast it for 2 minutes.
4. After this, transfer the roasted jalapeno in the saucepan.
5. Add turmeric, paprika, and sage.
6. Bring the liquid to boil and add shrimps.
7. Close the lid and cook korma for 10 minutes over the medium heat.

Nutrition: calories 148, fat 4.1, fiber 1.6, carbs 7.1, protein 21

122. TANDOORI SALMON SKEWERS

Preparation Time: 30 minutes
Cooking time: 15 minutes
Servings:5

Ingredients:

- 1.5-pound salmon fillet
- ½ cup Plain yogurt
- 1 teaspoon paprika
- 1 teaspoon turmeric
- 1 teaspoon red pepper
- 1 teaspoon salt
- 1 teaspoon dried cilantro
- 1 teaspoon sunflower oil
- ½ teaspoon ground nutmeg

Directions:

1. For the marinade: mix up together Plain yogurt, paprika, turmeric red pepper, salt, and ground nutmeg.
2. Chop the salmon fillet roughly and put it in the yogurt mixture.
3. Mix up well and marinate for 25 minutes.
4. Then skew the fish on the skewers.
5. Sprinkle the skewers with sunflower oil and place in the tray.
6. Bake the salmon skewers for 15 minutes at 375F.

Nutrition: calories 217, fat 9.9, fiber 0.6, carbs 4.2, protein 28.1

123. PRAWNS KEBABS

Preparation Time: 10 minutes
Cooking time: 5 minutes
Servings:2

Ingredients:

- 4 King prawns, peeled
- 1 tablespoon lemon juice
- ¾ teaspoon ground coriander
- ½ teaspoon salt
- 1 tablespoon tomato sauce
- 1 tablespoon olive oil

Directions:

1. Skew the shrimps on the skewers and sprinkle them with lemon juice, ground coriander, salt, and tomato sauce.
2. Then drizzle the shrimps with olive oil.
3. Preheat grill to 385F.
4. Grill the shrimp kebabs for 2 minutes from each side.

Nutrition: calories 106, fat 7.5, fiber 0.4, carbs 0.6, protein 9.1

124. LIME LOBSTERS

Preparation Time: 15 minutes
Cooking time: 15 minutes
Servings:3

Ingredients:

- 1-pound lobster, trimmed, peeled
- 2 tablespoons lime juice
- 1 teaspoon lime zest
- ½ teaspoon garlic powder
- ½ teaspoon chili flakes
- 3 tablespoons butter, melted
- 1 teaspoon dried dill
- ½ teaspoon salt

Directions:

1. Line the baking tray with baking paper and arrange lobsters in it.
2. Whisk together lime juice, lime zest, garlic powder, chili flakes, butter, dried dill, and salt.
3. Then brush the lobsters with butter mixture well.
4. Preheat the oven to 365F.

5. Place the tray with lobsters in the preheated oven and cook them for 15 minutes or until they are tender.

Nutrition: calories 241, fat 12.8, fiber 0.2, carbs 1, protein 29

125. ASIAN SESAME AND MISO SALMON

Preparation Time: 5 minutes
Cooking Time: 10 minutes
Serving: 6

Ingredients:

- 2 ½ pounds salmon fillets, skin removed
- 1 cup miso paste
- 2 tablespoons sesame seeds
- 1 teaspoon sesame oil
- ¼ cup water
- 1 thumb-size ginger, grated
- 3 tablespoons rice wine vinegar

Directions:

1. Place a heavy bottomed pot on medium high fire and heat pot for 2 minutes.
2. Add all ingredients and mix well.
3. Cover and bring to a boil. Boil for 2 minutes and then lower fire to a simmer. Simmer for 10 minutes.
4. Serve and enjoy.

Nutrition Facts Per Serving

Calories 343, Total Fat 12g, Saturated Fat 2g, Total Carbs 12g, Net Carbs 9g, Protein 44g, Sugar: 3g, Fiber 3g, Sodium 1805mg, Potassium 921mg

126. ORANGE HERBED SAUCED WHITE BASS

Preparation Time: 15 minutes
Cooking Time: 35 minutes
Serving: 6

Ingredients:

- 1 ½ tbsp fresh lemon juice
- ¼ cup thinly sliced green onions
- ½ cup orange juice
- 3 tbsp chopped fresh dill
- 6 3-oz skinless white bass fillets
- 1 ½ tbsp olive oil
- 1 large onion, halved, thinly sliced
- 1 large orange, unpeeled, sliced
- Additional unpeeled orange slices

Directions:

1. Grease a 13 x 9-inch glass baking dish and preheat oven to 400oF.
2. Arrange orange slices in single layer on baking dish, top with onion slices, seasoned with pepper and salt plus drizzled with oil.
3. Pop in the oven and roast for 25 minutes or until onions are tender and browned.
4. Remove from oven and increased oven temperature to 450oF.
5. Push onion and orange slices on sides of dish and place bass fillets in middle of dish. Season with 1 ½ tbsp dill, pepper and salt. Arrange onions and orange slices on top of fish and pop into the oven.
6. Roast for 8 minutes or until salmon is opaque and flaky.
7. In a small bowl, mix 1 ½ tbsp dill, lemon juice, green onions and orange juice.
8. Transfer salmon to a serving plate, discard roasted onions, drizzle with the newly made orange sauce and garnish with fresh orange slices.
9. Serve and enjoy.

Nutrition Facts Per Serving

Calories 159, Total Fat 6g, Saturated Fat 1g, Total Carbs 10g, Net Carbs 8g, Protein 17g, Sugar: 5g, Fiber 2g, Sodium 62mg, Potassium 388mg

127. GRILLED SALMON TERIYAKI

Preparation Time: 5 minutes
Cooking Time: 6 minutes
Serving: 2

Ingredients:

- ½ tsp coarsely ground black pepper
- 2 tbsp teriyaki sauce
- 2 8-oz Salmon fillets

Directions:

1. In a shallow dish, place salmon.
2. Add teriyaki sauce and marinate in room temperature for 10 minutes.

3. Preheat grill to medium high fire and grease grate.
4. Rub pepper on fleshy part of salmon and place on grate skin part touching grate.
5. Grill for 4 minutes. Turnover and grill for another 2 minutes or until salmon is cooked to desired doneness.
6. Serve and enjoy.

Nutrition Facts Per Serving

Calories 365, Total Fat 16g, Saturated Fat 3.3g, Total Carbs 3g, Net Carbs 2.8g, Protein 48g, Sugar: 2.5g, Fiber 0.2g, Sodium 1302mg, Potassium 797mg

128. PECAN CRUSTED TROUT

Preparation Time: 15 minutes
Cooking Time: 12 minutes
Serving: 4

Ingredients:

- 1 egg, beaten
- 4 4-oz trout fillets
- Whole wheat flour, as needed
- Black pepper to taste
- 1 tsp salt
- 1 tsp crush dried rosemary
- ½ tsp grated fresh ginger
- ½ cup crushed pecans
- cooking spray

Directions:

1. Grease baking sheet lightly with cooking spray and preheat oven to 400oF.
2. In a shallow bowl, combine black pepper, salt, rosemary and pecans. In another shallow bowl, add whole wheat flour. In a third bowl, add beaten egg.
3. To prepare fish, dip in flour until covered well. Shake off excess flour. Then dip into beaten egg until coated well. Let excess egg drip off before dipping trout fillet into pecan crumbs. Press the trout lightly onto pecan crumbs to make it stick to the fish.
4. Place breaded fish onto prepared pan. Repeat process for remaining fillets.
5. Pop into the oven and bake for 10 to 12 minutes or until fish is flaky.

Nutrition Facts Per Serving

Calories 247, Total Fat 14g, Saturated Fat 2g, Total Carbs 4g, Net Carbs 2g, Protein 26g, Sugar: 1g, Fiber 2g, Sodium 633mg, Potassium 659mg

129. OYSTERS ON THE SHELL

Preparation Time: 20 minutes
Cooking Time: 5 minutes
Serving: 4

Ingredients:

- 24 medium oysters
- 2 lemons
- tabasco sauce

Directions:

1. If you are a newbie when it comes to eating oysters, then I suggest that you blanch the oysters before eating.
2. For some, eating oysters raw is a great way to enjoy this dish because of the consistency and juiciness of raw oysters. Plus, adding lemon juice prior to eating the raw oysters cooks it a bit.
3. So, to blanch oysters, bring a big pot of water to a rolling boil. Add oysters in batches of 6-10 pieces. Leave on boiling pot of water between 3-5 minutes and remove oysters right away.
4. To eat oysters, squeeze lemon juice on oyster on shell, add tabasco as desired and enjoy.

Nutrition Facts Per Serving

Calories 250, Total Fat 7g, Saturated Fat 1.6g, Total Carbs 17g, Net Carbs 16g, Protein 29g, Sugar: 0.2g, Fiber 0.6g, Sodium 409mg, Potassium 547mg

130. BREADED AND SPICED HALIBUT

Preparation Time: 10 minutes
Cooking Time: 15 minutes
Serving: 4

Ingredients:

- 4 pieces of 6-oz halibut fillets
- ¼ tsp ground black pepper
- 1 tsp sea salt
- 1 tsp finely grated lemon zest

- 1 tbsp extra-virgin olive oil
- ¼ cup chopped fresh chives
- ¼ cup chopped fresh dill
- 1/3 cup chopped fresh parsley
- ¾ cup panko breadcrumbs

Directions:

1. Line a baking sheet with foil, grease with cooking spray and preheat oven to 400oF.
2. In a small bowl, mix black pepper, sea salt, lemon zest, olive oil, chives, dill, parsley and breadcrumbs. If needed add more salt to taste. Set aside.
3. Meanwhile, wash halibut fillets on cold tap water. Dry with paper towels and place on prepared baking sheet.
4. Generously spoon crumb mixture onto halibut fillets. Ensure that fillets are covered with crumb mixture. Press down on crumb mixture onto each fillet.
5. Pop into the oven and bake for 10-15 minutes or until fish is flaky and crumb topping are already lightly browned.

Nutrition Facts Per Serving

Calories 334, Total Fat 25g, Saturated Fat 4g, Total Carbs 1g, Net Carbs 0.7g, Protein 25g, Sugar: 0.2g, Fiber 0.3g, Sodium 751mg, Potassium 505mg

131. BAKED SALMON WITH GREENS

Preparation Time: 10 minutes
Cooking Time: 12 minutes
Serving: 2

Ingredients:

- 1 tbsp red-wine vinegar
- 1 tbsp extra-virgin olive oil
- Pepper and salt to taste
- ¼ cup red onion, sliced thinly
- 2/3 cup cherry tomatoes, halved
- 3 cups baby arugula leaves
- 1 ½ tbsp olive oil
- 1 ½ tbsp fresh lemon juice
- 2 center cut salmon fillets (6-oz each)

Directions:

1. In a shallow bowl, mix pepper, salt, 1 ½ tbsp olive oil and lemon juice. Toss in salmon fillets and rub with the marinade. Allow to marinate for at least 15 minutes.
2. Grease a baking sheet and preheat oven to 350oF.
3. Bake marinated salmon fillet for 10 to 12 minutes or until flaky with skin side touching the baking sheet.
4. Meanwhile, in a salad bowl mix onion, tomatoes and arugula.
5. Season with pepper and salt. Drizzle with vinegar and oil. Toss to combine and serve right away with baked salmon on the side.

Nutrition Facts Per Serving

Calories 565, Total Fat 36g, Saturated Fat 3g, Total Carbs 13g, Net Carbs 11g, Protein 46g, Sugar: 9g, Fiber 2g, Sodium 179mg, Potassium 1164mg

132. OYSTERS ROCKEFELLER

Preparation Time: 30 minutes
Cooking Time: 10 minutes
Serving: 8

Ingredients:

- 36 oysters on the half shell
- Pepper and salt to taste
- 1 pinch cayenne pepper
- 2 tbsp anise-flavored liqueur, like Pernod
- 2 tbsp chopped fresh parsley
- 2 tbsp chopped fresh tarragon
- 2 tbsp chopped celery
- 2 tbsp minced green onion
- ¼ cup breadcrumbs
- ½ cup olive oil, room temperature
- 1 cup chopped watercress
- 2 tsp salt

Directions:

1. In a large casserole dish, pour salt rock. Preheat oven to 500oF.
2. In food processor mix anise-flavored liqueur, Italian parsley, tarragon, celery, green onions, breadcrumbs, olive oil, cayenne pepper and watercress. Blend well until smooth and creamy. Season with pepper and salt to taste.

3. On top of casserole dish with rock salt, place 8 to 12 oysters on a half shell. Evenly place a teaspoonful of the processed mixture on top of each oyster. Pop in the oven and bake for 5 minutes or until oysters are firm.
4. Repeat process to the next batch of oysters until all are cooked. Serve oysters right away while still hot.

Nutrition Facts Per Serving

Calories 312, Total Fat 19g, Saturated Fat 3g, Total Carbs 13g, Net Carbs 12.6g, Protein 22g, Sugar: 0.4g, Fiber 0.5g, Sodium 825mg, Potassium 462mg

133. SMOKED HERRING SANDWICH

Preparation Time: 15 minutes
Cooking Time: 0 minutes
Serving: 4

Ingredients:

- 1 6-oz can kipper, drained
- 1/8 tsp pepper
- 1/8 tsp salt
- 1 clove garlic, minced
- 1 tsp lemon juice
- 1 tbsp chopped fresh parsley
- 1 celery stalk, finely chopped
- 1 small onion, finely chopped
- ½ cup reduced fat mayonnaise
- 8 lettuce leaves
- 4 slices of multi-grain bread

Directions:

1. Mix pepper, salt, garlic, lemon juice, parsley, celery, onion and mayonnaise in a medium bowl. Combine well.
2. Add drained kippers and mix well.
3. To assemble sandwich, cut each slice of bread diagonally to form a triangle. On one slice, add 1 lettuce leaf, slather with 2 tbsp of kipper mixture, top with another lettuce and cover with another triangular slice of bread.
4. Repeat process to remaining bread slices.
5. Serve and enjoy.

Nutrition Facts Per Serving

Calories 278, Total Fat 18g, Saturated Fat 3g, Total Carbs 14g, Net Carbs 11.5g, Protein 15g, Sugar: 2.7g, Fiber 2.5g, Sodium 346mg, Potassium 805mg

134. ROASTED SALMON GARDEN SALAD

Preparation Time: 10 minutes
Cooking Time: 10 minutes
Serving: 3

Ingredients:

- 2 tablespoon + 1 teaspoon olive oil, divided
- 3 tablespoon apple cider vinegar
- 1 cup diced fennel bulb
- 1 cup diced red onions
- 1 cup cucumber, peeled and diced
- ½ pound salmon
- Pepper and salt to taste

Directions:

1. Preheat oven to 400oF. Grease a small baking dish with 1 teaspoon olive oil. Place salmon with skin side down and season with pepper and salt. Pop in preheated oven and bake for 8 minutes or until salmon is flaky.
2. Remove salmon from oven. Coarsely flake salmon with two forks and discard skin of salmon. Let it cool.
3. Meanwhile, in a large salad bowl whisk well remaining olive oil and vinegar. Toss in fennel, onions, cooled salmon and cucumber. Toss to coat well and serve.

Nutrition Facts Per Serving

Calories 196, Total Fat 9g, Saturated Fat 2g, Total Carbs 12g, Net Carbs 8g, Protein 18g, Sugar: 6g, Fiber 4g, Sodium 372mg, Potassium 473mg

135. TUNA CAPRESE OPEN-FACED FLATBREAD

Preparation Time: 15 minutes
Cooking Time: 0 minutes
Serving: 1

Ingredients:

- 1 whole flatbread, whole wheat or gluten-free
- 1/2 cup spinach leaves
- 4 medium basil leaves
- 1 packet StarKist Selects Wild-Caught Yellowfin Tuna in E.V.O.O
- 1/2 whole avocado, sliced
- 4 small cherry tomatoes, diced
- 1-ounce mozzarella cheese, diced
- 1 tablespoon balsamic glaze
- salt and pepper, to taste

Directions:

1. Lay flatbread on a plate.
2. Evenly spread basil and spinach leaves on top of bread.
3. Spread avocado and tomato slices on top of the greens.
4. Add the packet of tuna on top and spread evenly.
5. Drizzle balsamic. Sprinkle cheese. Season with pepper and salt.
6. Serve and enjoy.

Nutrition Facts Per Serving

Calories 442, Total Fat 18g, Saturated Fat 3g, Total Carbs 48g, Net Carbs 33g, Protein 29g, Sugar: 10g, Fiber 15g, Sodium 709mg, Potassium 1414mg

136. TUNA-HUMMUS ON FLATBREAD

Preparation Time: 15 minutes
Cooking Time: 0 minutes
Serving: 1

Ingredients:

- 1 whole flat bread, whole wheat or gluten-free
- 1/2 cup spring mix
- 1/2 cup hummus
- 1 packet StarKist Selects Wild-Caught Yellowfin Tuna in E.V.O.O
- 2 mini bell peppers, diced
- 1 tablespoon pumpkin seeds, salted
- 1/2 whole lemon, juiced

Directions:

1. Lay flatbread on a plate.
2. Evenly spread hummus on top of bread.
3. Spread spring mix greens on top of hummus.
4. Add the packet of tuna on top and spread evenly.
5. Sprinkle bell pepper and pumpkin seeds.
6. Drizzle lemon juice.
7. Serve and enjoy.

Nutrition Facts Per Serving

Calories 432, Total Fat 18g, Saturated Fat 3g, Total Carbs 45g, Net Carbs 30g, Protein 29g, Sugar: 10g, Fiber 15g, Sodium 509mg, Potassium 914mg

137. TUNA & SUN-DRIED TOMATO-WICH

Preparation Time: 15 minutes
Cooking Time: 0 minutes
Serving: 1

Ingredients:

- 1 whole flat bread
- 1/2 whole avocado
- 1 packet StarKist Selects Wild Caught Yellowfin Tuna Sun Dried Tomato in E.V.O.O
- 1/4 cup sprouts or microgreens
- 1 tablespoon hemp seeds
- 1/2 whole lemon, juiced
- Salt and pepper to taste

Directions:

1. In a small bowl, mash avocado, hemp seeds and lemon juice. Lightly season with pepper and salt.
2. Lay flatbread on a plate.
3. Evenly spread avocado mixture on top of bread.
4. Add the packet of tuna on top and spread evenly.
5. Spread sprouts on top.
6. Serve and enjoy.

Nutrition Facts Per Serving

Calories 490, Total Fat 31g, Saturated Fat 4g, Total Carbs 23g, Net Carbs 20g, Protein 34g, Sugar: 3g, Fiber 7g, Sodium 201mg, Potassium

345mg

138. TUNA-AVO BOAT SALAD

Preparation Time: 10 minutes
Cooking Time: 0 minutes
Serving: 2

Ingredients:

- 2 tablespoons 0% plain Greek yogurt
- 4 teaspoons apple cider vinegar
- 1 teaspoon curry powder
- 1/4 teaspoon salt
- 1 medium pinch ground cinnamon
- 5-ounce can solid white albacore, drained and flaked
- 1/4 cup finely diced carrot
- 4 teaspoons chopped toasted cashews
- 2 tablespoons roughly chopped raisins
- 1 tablespoon chopped red onion
- 1 medium avocado, sliced in half and seed removed
- 2 teaspoons chopped parsley

Directions:

1. Mix well cinnamon, salt, curry, vinegar, and yogurt in a medium bowl. Whisk in tuna and mix well.
2. Add remaining ingredients in bowl except for parsley and avocado. Mix thoroughly and adjust seasoning to taste.
3. Evenly divide the tuna mixture inside the avocado hole left by the seed.
4. To enjoy, scoop out avocado flesh along with the tuna mixture with each bite.

Nutrition Facts Per Serving

Calories 241, Total Fat 13g, Saturated Fat 2g, Total Carbs 18g, Net Carbs 12g, Protein 18g, Sugar: 8g, Fiber 6g, Sodium 491mg, Potassium 653g

139. GRILLED SALMON-LETTUCE WRAPS

Preparation Time: 20 minutes
Cooking Time: 10 minutes
Serving: 6

Ingredients:

1/4 cup Avocado Sauce recipe link here

- 2 6-oz fresh salmon fish fillets
- 1 head of butter lettuce
- 2 cup coleslaw mix or shredded cabbage
- 1/4 cup fresh cilantro leaves, chopped
- 1 lime, juiced
- Salt and pepper to taste

Avocado Sauce Ingredients:

- 1/2 Avocado, pitted
- 1/2 cup Cilantro, fresh
- 1/2 Jalapeño, seeded (adjust to taste)
- 1/2 cup low fat mayo
- 1/4 cup Water
- 2 tbsp Lime juice, fresh (adjust to taste)
- 1 Garlic clove
- 1/2 tsp Salt

Directions:

1. In a blender, puree all avocado sauce ingredients. Adjust seasoning to taste and puree again. Transfer to a bowl and refrigerate until ready to use.
2. Preheat grill to medium high and lightly grease grate.
3. Season fish with pepper and salt to taste. Grill fish for 3 to 4 minutes per side. Transfer to a bowl and shred.
4. In bowl of fish, add shredded cabbage, juice of lime and mix well. If needed, adjust seasoning to taste.
5. To serve, slowly separate butter lettuce into one huge leaf. In one leaf, place a good amount of the salmon filling and a dollop of the avocado sauce. Roll leaf and enjoy.

Nutrition Facts Per Serving

Calories 247, Total Fat 10g, Saturated Fat 2.1g, Total Carbs 9g, Net Carbs 6g, Protein 31g, Sugar: 5g, Fiber 3g, Sodium 488mg, Potassium 907mg

140. BLACK BEAN 'N SALMON SALAD

Preparation Time: 15 minutes
Cooking Time: 0 minutes
Serving: 4

Ingredients:

- 2 cans (5oz each) wild salmon

(skinless/boneless), drained and flaked
- 1-15oz can black beans or lentils, drained and rinsed
- 1 clove garlic, minced
- ¼ cup scallions, minced
- ¼ cup celery, finely minced
- 1 tomato or 1cup cherry tomatoes, diced
- ½ lime, juiced
- ¼ tsp. sea salt
- 1 jalapeño, finely minced, ribs and seeds removed
- ¼ cup fresh cilantro, roughly chopped
- 1 ½ tbsp ground flaxseed

Salad Ingredients:
- 4 cup Spinach leaves
- 4 tsp EVO
- 1 avocado, diced

Directions:
1. In a large bowl, add all ingredients and mix well. Let it rest for 10 minutes to let the flavors meld. Mix once again.
2. Evenly divide spinach leaves on to 4 salad bowls.
3. Evenly divide salmon mixture on to each bowl.
4. Top with diced avocado and drizzle with olive oil.
5. Serve and enjoy.

Nutrition Facts Per Serving

Calories 433, Total Fat 21g, Saturated Fat 3g, Total Carbs 23g, Net Carbs 12g, Protein 41g, Sugar: 2g, Fiber 11g, Sodium 727mg, Potassium 1192mg

141. EASY 'N HEALTHY TUNA SALAD

Preparation Time: 5 minutes
Cooking Time: 5 minutes
Serving: 2

Ingredients:
- 5 oz olive oil packed tuna, drained
- 1 tbsp fresh chopped basil
- 1/2 stalk celery, minced
- 1 finely chopped scallion - green part only
- 2 tbsp lemon juice, or more to taste
- Extra virgin olive oil to taste
- Salt and pepper to taste
- 6 large leaves of Boston Bibb Lettuce

Directions:
1. Mix all ingredients in a bowl except for the lettuce.
2. Adjust seasoning if needed and mix well once more.
3. Evenly divide lettuce leaves on two plates.
4. Evenly divide tuna salad on top of the leaves.
5. Serve and enjoy.

Nutrition Facts Per Serving

Calories 209, Total Fat 11g, Saturated Fat 2g, Total Carbs 3g, Net Carbs 1g, Protein 20g, Sugar: -g, Fiber 2g, Sodium 260mg, Potassium 291g

142. FRESH TOMATO 'N TUNA SALAD SANDWICH

Preparation Time: 10 minutes
Cooking Time: 0 minutes
Serving: 3

Ingredients:
- 1/2 cup celery (finely chopped)
- 2 5 ounces can tuna in water (drained)
- 2 teaspoons whole grain mustard
- 1/4 cup light mayonnaise
- 1/2 teaspoon turmeric
- Salt and pepper to taste
- 3 Whole pita bread
- 1 avocado, peeled, pitted and sliced
- 2 roma tomatoes sliced

Directions:
1. Mix all ingredients in a bowl except for the pita bread, avocado and tomatoes.
2. Adjust seasoning if needed and mix well once more.
3. Evenly divide tuna salad on top of each pita bread.
4. Top evenly by avocado and tomato slices. Fold pita bread in half to form half-moons.
5. Serve and enjoy.

Nutrition Facts Per Serving

Calories 323, Total Fat 10.1g, Saturated Fat 2g, Total Carbs 26.8g, Net Carbs 21.9g, Protein 30.1g, Sugar: 4.9g, Fiber 4.9g, Sodium 433mg, Potassium 234g

143. BAKED SALMON BURGER PATTY

Preparation Time: 15 minutes
Cooking Time: 15 minutes
Serving: 3

Ingredients:

- 1-pound salmon skin removed and chopped into cubes
- 1 Tbsp stone ground mustard
- 1 Tbsp avocado oil
- 1 tsp ground paprika
- 1/2 tsp sea salt
- 3 whole wheat flat bread
- 3 lettuce leaves
- 1 roma tomato sliced into 3 circles
- 3 onion rings

Directions:

1. Preheat oven to 450oF.
2. Lightly grease a cookie sheet with cooking spray.
3. In a food processor, add salmon, mustard, oil, paprika, and salt. Process until you form a thick paste. Scraping sides and bottom.
4. Evenly divide mixture into three and form into equal patties.
5. Place on prepared sheet and bake for 20 minutes. Flip burger halfway through cooking time.
6. Assemble burger, serve and enjoy.

Nutrition Facts Per Serving

Calories 372, Total Fat 15g, Saturated Fat 3g, Total Carbs 17g, Net Carbs 14g, Protein 43g, Sugar: 1g, Fiber 3g, Sodium 1097mg, Potassium 591mg

144. BAKED HALIBUT WITH AVOCADO-BLUEBERRY SALSA

Preparation Time: 20 minutes
Cooking Time: 25 minutes
Serving: 4

Ingredients:

- 1-pound halibut cut into 4 fillets
- 1 Tbsp fresh ginger peeled and grated
- 1/4 cup orange juice
- 1/4 tsp sea salt
- 2 tsp orange zest
- 3 Tbsp avocado oil
- 3 Tbsp coconut aminos

Avocado-Blueberry Salsa Ingredients:

- 1 cup fresh blueberries
- 1 avocado peeled and diced
- 1/3 cup red bell pepper chopped
- 2 Tbsp chives chopped
- 2 Tbsp lime juice
- 1 pinch sea salt to taste

Directions:

1. In a blender, puree ginger, orange juice, salt, orange zest, oil, and aminos until smooth and creamy. Pour into Ziplock bag along with halibut and marinade for at least an hour.
2. Preheat oven to 400oF. Lightly grease a casserole dish with cooking spray. Transfer halibut and marinade into dish. Bake for 20 minutes. And then broil for 5 minutes. Place dish in middle rack of oven.
3. Meanwhile, in a bowl, mix well all salsa ingredients. Serve on top of cooked halibut.
4. Enjoy.

Nutrition Facts Per Serving

Calories 457, Total Fat 34g, Saturated Fat 5g, Total Carbs 22g, Net Carbs 17g, Protein 18g, Sugar: 16g, Fiber 5g, Sodium 254mg, Potassium 669mg

145. RICE 'N TUNA CASSEROLE

Preparation Time: 20 minutes
Cooking Time: 20 minutes
Serving: 6

Ingredients:

- 2 cups white rice, cooked according to

manufacturer's Directions:

- 1 1/3 cup unsweetened almond milk
- 2 large eggs
- 3 Tbsp avocado oil mayonnaise
- 2 Tbsp stone ground mustard
- 3 cans tuna drained
- 1 cup low-fat mozzarella cheese divided

Directions:

1. In a bowl, whisk well milk, eggs, mayonnaise, 2 cups cheese and mustard.
2. Stir in tuna and mix well.
3. Stir in cooked rice and mix well.
4. Evenly spread in a lightly greased casserole dish. Sprinkle remaining cheese on top and bake in a preheated 400oF oven for 20 minutes.
5. Remove from oven and let it rest for 5 minutes.
6. Serve and enjoy.

Nutrition Facts Per Serving

Calories 318, Total Fat 15g, Saturated Fat 5g, Total Carbs 18g, Net Carbs 17g, Protein 27g, Sugar: 3g, Fiber 1g, Sodium 408mg, Potassium 296mg

146. SARDINE SALAD PICKLED PEPPER BOATS

Servings: 4
Preparation Time: 10 minutes

Ingredients

- 1 tablespoon fresh parsley, chopped
- 2 (3.75-ounce) cans sardines, drained
- 2 tablespoons fresh lemon
- 4 pickled peppers, slice into halves
- 1 cup scallions, chopped
- 1 teaspoon deli mustard
- Salt and freshly ground black pepper, to taste

Directions

1. In a mixing container, thoroughly combine mustard, sardines, lemon juice, scallions, salt and black pepper.
2. Merge until everything is well incorporated.
3. Now, fill pickle boats with sardine salad. Enjoy well-chilled garnished with fresh parsley.
4. Nutrition: Calories120 ,Protein 12.3g ,Fat 5.4g ,Carbs 5.8g ,Sugar 2.4g

147. ASIAN-INSPIRED TILAPIA CHOWDER

Servings: 6
Preparation Time: 30 minutes

Ingredients

- 1 teaspoon five-spice powder
- 1 celery stalk, diced
- 1 garlic clove, smashed
- 1/2 teaspoon paprika
- 1/4 cup fresh mint, chopped
- 3/4 cup full-fat milk
- 2 ½ cups hot water
- 1/2 cup scallions, sliced
- 1 bell pepper, deveined and sliced
- 3 teaspoons olive oil
- 1 ¼ pounds tilapia fish fillets, cut into small chunks
- 1 tablespoon fish sauce

Directions

1. First of, heat olive oil in a stockpot that is preheated over a normal high heat. Heat the scallions and garlic until they are softened.
2. Add celery, water, fish sauce, peppers, and Five-spice powder. Close with the lid, turn the heat to medium-low and simmer for about 13 minutes longer.
3. Stir in fish chunks and heat an additional 12 minutes or until the fish is heated through. Include milk, stir well, and dispose of from heat.
4. Now, ladle into individual serving plates. Spray with paprika and serve garnished with fresh mint. Bon appétit!

Nutrition: Calories165 ,Protein 25.4g ,Fat 5.5g ,Carbs 4g ,Sugar 2.7g

148. SMOKED SALMON AND CHEESE STUFFED TOMATOES

Servings: 6

Preparation Time: 30 minutes

Ingredients

- 2 tablespoons cilantro, chopped
- 1/2 cup aioli
- 10 ounces smoked salmon, flaked
- 2 garlic cloves, minced
- 6 medium-sized tomatoes
- Sea salt and ground black pepper, to taste
- 1 teaspoon yellow mustard
- 1 red onion, finely chopped
- 1 tablespoon white vinegar
- 1 ½ cups Monterey Jack cheese, shredded

Directions

1. Preheat an oven to 4000F.
2. In a mixing container, thoroughly merge the garlic, salmon, onion, cilantro, aioli, mustard, vinegar, salt, and pepper.
3. Cut your tomatoes in half horizontally; now, scoop out pulp and seeds.
4. Now, Stuff tomatoes with the filling, and bake until they are thoroughly heated or cooked and tops are golden, for about 20 minutes.
5. Include the shredded cheese and put it in the oven for a further 5 minutes. Bon appétit!

Nutrition: Calories303 ,Protein 17g ,Fat 22.9g ,Carbs 6.8g ,Sugar 2.2g

149. CHILEAN SEA BASS WITH CAULIFLOWER AND CHUTNEY

Servings: 4
Preparation Time: 30 minutes

Ingredients

- 1 ½ pounds wild Chilean sea bass
- 1 onion, thinly sliced
- Sea salt and freshly ground black pepper, to taste
- 2 bell peppers, thinly sliced
- 1 pound cauliflower, cut into florets
- 1 teaspoon cayenne pepper
- 2 tablespoons olive oil, for drizzling

For Tomato Chutney:

- 2 garlic cloves, sliced
- 1 teaspoon olive oil
- 1 cup ripe on-the-vine plum tomatoes
- 1/4 teaspoon black pepper
- 1/2 teaspoon kosher salt

Directions

1. Heat 1 tablespoon of olive oil in a pan that is preheated over a normal flame.
2. Now, heat the bell peppers, cauliflower florets, and onion until they are slightly tender; After that, season with black pepper, salt, and cayenne pepper; set aside.
3. Now, preheat another tablespoon of olive oil. Sear sea bass on each side for about 5 minutes.
4. To make chutney, heat 1 teaspoon of olive oil in a pan over a normal high heat. Sauté the garlic until just browned and also aromatic.
5. Include the plum tomatoes and cook, occasionally stirring, until heated through, or for about 10 minutes. Season with salt and pepper.
6. Share seared fish among 4 serving plates. Serve garnished with sautéed cauliflower mixture and tomato chutney. Enjoy!

Nutrition: Calories 291 ,Protein 42.5g ,Fat 9.5g ,Carbs 3.5g ,Sugar 1.4g

150. GRILLED HALLOUMI AND TUNA SALAD

Servings: 4
Preparation Time: 15 minutes

Ingredients

- 1/2 cup radishes, thinly sliced
- 1 cup halloumi cheese
- 2 cucumbers, thinly sliced
- 2 tablespoons sunflower seeds
- 1 red onion, thinly sliced
- 1/2 head Romaine lettuce
- 1 ½ tablespoons extra-virgin olive oil
- Sea salt and black pepper, to taste
- Dried rosemary, to taste
- 1 can light tuna fish in water, rinsed
- 2 medium-sized Roma tomatoes, sliced
- 1 tablespoon lime juice

Directions

1. Grill halloumi cheese over normal high heat and cut into cubes.
2. Now, toss grilled halloumi cheese with the remaining ingredients. Bon appétit!

Nutrition: Calories199 ,Protein 14.2g ,Fat 10.6g ,Carbs 6.1g ,Sugar 4.2g

151. COLORFUL TUNA SALAD WITH BOCCONCINI

Servings: 4
Preparation Time: 10 minutes

Ingredients

- 1 green bell pepper, sliced
- 2 cans tuna in brine, drained
- 1/4 teaspoon black peppercorns, preferably freshly ground
- 1 tablespoon oyster sauce
- 1 head iceberg lettuce
- 1 teaspoon Pasilla chili pepper, finely chopped
- 2 garlic cloves, minced
- 2 teaspoons peanut butter
- 1/2 cup radishes, sliced
- 1 yellow bell pepper, sliced
- 1/2 cup Kalamata olives, pitted and sliced
- 1/2 cup yellow onion, thinly sliced
- 1 teaspoon olive oil
- 8 ounces bocconcini
- 1 cucumber, sliced
- 1 tomato, diced
- 1 teaspoon champagne vinegar

Directions

1. Merge cucumbers, iceberg lettuce, peppers, onion, tuna, radishes, tomatoes and Kalamata olives in a salad container.
2. In a small mixing dish, thoroughly merge champagne vinegar, olive oil, peanut butter, oyster sauce black peppercorns, and garlic.
3. Include this vinaigrette to the salad bowl; ensure to toss until everything is well coated.
4. Now, top with bocconcini and serve well-chilled. Bon appétit!

Nutrition: Calories 273 ,Protein 34.2g ,Fat 11.7g ,Carbs 6.7g ,Sugar 2.5g

152. TUNA FILLETS WITH GREENS

Servings: 6
Preparation Time: 20 minutes

Ingredients

- 3 tablespoons olive oil, plus more for drizzling
- 1 fresh lime, sliced
- 6 tuna fillets
- Salt and ground black pepper, to your liking
- 2 teaspoons yellow mustard
- 2 cups baby spinach
- 1 yellow onion, thinly sliced
- 1 tablespoons apple cider vinegar
- Salt and red pepper flakes, to taste
- 1 cup rocket lettuce
- 1/2 cup radishes, thinly sliced

Directions

1. Begin by preheating your oven to 4500F. Now, coat a baking dish with parchment paper or a Silpat mat.
2. Drizzle each tuna fillet with olive oil; season with pepper and salt.
3. Transfer tuna fillets to the baking dish. Top with lime slices and bake 8 to 12 minutes.
4. In a mixing container, whisk the vinegar, salt, mustard and red pepper flakes.
5. Position baby spinach, onion rocket lettuce, and radishes on 6 serving plates. Now, drizzle with vinegar/mustard mixture. Finally, top with tuna fillets. Bon appétit!

Nutrition: Calories 444 ,Protein 21.9g ,Fat 38.2g ,Carbs 4.7g ,Sugar 1.5g

153. ONE-POT SEAFOOD STEW

Servings: 4
Preparation Time: 20 minutes

Ingredients

- 2 garlic cloves, pressed
- 1/2 pound shrimp

- 1 teaspoon Italian seasonings
- 1 celery stalk, chopped
- 1 cup hot water
- 2 tomatoes, pureed
- 2 tablespoons dry white wine
- 1/2 teaspoon lemon zest
- 1/2 pound mussels
- 1 teaspoon saffron threads
- Salt and ground black pepper, to taste
- 1/2 stick butter, at room temperature
- 2 cups shellfish stock
- 2 onions, chopped

Directions

1. Dissolve the butter in a stockpot over a normal heat. Heat the onion and garlic until aromatic.
2. After that, stir in pureed tomatoes; cook for about 8 minutes or until heated through.
3. Include the remaining ingredients and bring to a rapid boil. Decrease the heat to a simmer and heat an additional 4 minutes.
4. Ladle into individual bowls and enjoy warm.

Nutrition: Calories209 ,Protein 15.2g ,Fat 12.6g ,Carbs 6.6g ,Sugar 3.1g

154. SEAFOOD AND ANDOUILLE MEDLEY

Servings: 4
Preparation Time: 25 minutes

Ingredients

- 2 andouille sausages, cut crosswise into 1/2-inch-thick slices
- 1/2 stick butter, melted
- 2 tomatoes, pureed
- 2 tablespoons fresh cilantro, chopped
- 1/2 pound skinned sole, cut into chunks
- 1/3 cup dry white wine
- 1 shallot, chopped
- 2 garlic cloves, finely minced
- 1 tablespoon oyster sauce
- 3/4 cup clam juice
- 20 sea scallops

Directions

1. Dissolve the butter in a heavy-bottomed pot over medium-high heat. Heat the sausages until no longer pink; reserve.
2. Suceeding the above, sauté the garlic and shallots in pan drippings until they are softened; reserve.
3. Include the oyster sauce, pureed tomatoes, clam juice and wine; simmer for another duration of 12 minutes.
4. Include the scallops, skinned sole, and reserved sausages. Let it simmer, partially covered, for duration of 6 minutes.
5. Enjoy garnished with fresh cilantro. Bon appétit!

Nutrition: Calories481 ,Protein 46.6g ,Fat 26.9g ,Carbs 5g ,Sugar 1.1g

155. QUATRE ÉPICES SALMON FILLETS WITH CHEESE

Servings: 6
Preparation Time: 20 minutes

Ingredients

- 1 teaspoon whole grain mustard
- 1 teaspoon seasoned salt
- 2 tablespoons avocado oil
- 3 tablespoons mayonnaise
- 6 salmon fillets
- 1 cup cauliflower
- 1 garlic clove, finely minced
- 1 teaspoon Quatre épices
- 1 cup Colby cheese, grated
- 1/2 red onion, thinly sliced
- 1 tablespoon fresh lemon juice

Directions

1. Preheat your oven to 4000F. Now, line a baking dish with aluminum foil.
2. Spray salmon fillets with salt and Quatre épices on all sides and put on a piece of foil. Position cauliflower and onions around them.
3. Suceeding the above, wrap the fish and vegetables with foil. Bake for the duration of 10 minutes until salmon fillets flake easily with a fork.
4. In a mixing container, thoroughly merge

mayo, garlic, cheese, mustard, lemon juice, and avocado oil.
5. Transfer this mixture over the fish and veggies. Bake for a further duration of 5 to 6 minutes or until the top is golden. Enjoy warm garnished with fresh chives.

Nutrition: Calories 354 ,Protein 39.6g ,Fat 20.2g ,Carbs 4.5g ,Sugar 1.4g

156. EASY PARMESAN CRUSTED TILAPIA

Servings: 4
Preparation Time: 15 minutes

Ingredients

- 3/4 cup grated Parmesan cheese
- 1/3 teaspoon salt
- 1/4 teaspoon red pepper flakes, crushed
- 1 pound tilapia fillets, cut into 4
- 1/3 teaspoon ground black pepper
- 2 tablespoons olive oil

Directions

1. Start with seasoning the fish fillets with salt, black pepper and red pepper flakes.
2. Now, brush tilapia fillets with olive oil; press them into the Parmesan cheese.
3. Put fish fillets on a foil-lined baking sheet. Bake for approximately 10 minutes or until fish fillets is opaque.

Nutrition: Calories222 ,Protein 27.9g ,Fat 12.6g ,Carbs 0.9g ,Sugar 0g

157. CREAMY ANCHOVY SALAD

Servings: 4
Preparation Time: 10 minutes

Ingredients

- 3/4 cup mayonnaise
- 2 cans anchovies, chopped
- 1 teaspoon yellow mustard
- 1 head of Romaine lettuce
- 1 cup red onions, chopped
- 1 cucumber, thinly sliced
- 1/4 cup fresh chives, roughly chopped
- Sea salt and ground black pepper, to taste
- 1/2 teaspoon smoked cayenne pepper

Directions

1. Position lettuce leaves in a salad bowl. Include anchovies, onions and cucumber. Season using salt and pepper.
2. After, stir in mayonnaise and mustard. Spray with cayenne pepper and toss until everything is well merged.
3. Enjoy well-chilled and garnished with fresh chives. Bon appétit!

Nutrition: Calories195 ,Protein 7.8g ,Fat 14.7g ,Carbs 6g ,Sugar 2.5g

158. MOMS' AROMATIC FISH CURRY

Servings: 6
Preparation Time: 25 minutes

Ingredients

- 2 pounds blue grenadier, cut into large pieces
- 2 tablespoons fresh lime juice
- 2 tablespoons olive oil
- 1 cup shallots, chopped
- 1 cup coconut milk
- 4 Roma tomatoes, pureed
- 2 green chilies, minced
- 1/2 tablespoon fresh ginger, grated
- 8 fresh curry leaves
- 2 green cardamom pods
- Salt and black pepper, to taste
- 2 garlic cloves, finely chopped
- 1 teaspoon dried basil
- 1 tablespoon ground coriander

Directions

1. Begin with drizzling blue grenadier with lime juice.
2. Now, heat the oil in a nonstick skillet over a moderate flame. Heat curry leaves and shallots until the shallot is softened, for about 4 minutes.
3. Succeeding that, include the chilies, ginger and garlic and heat an additional minute or until fragrant. Include the remaining ingredients, except for coconut milk, and simmer for a duration of 10 minutes or until heated through.
4. After that, stir in the fish; pour in 1 cup of

coconut milk and heat, covered, for about 6 minutes longer. Serve warm and enjoy!

Nutrition: Calories 270 ,Protein 22.3g ,Fat 16.9g ,Carbs 5.6g ,Sugar 2.2g

159. PAN-SEARED TROUT FILLETS WITH CHIMICHURRI

Servings: 6
Preparation Time: 15 minutes

Ingredients

- 2 tablespoons ghee
- 1/2 tablespoon yellow mustard
- 6 trout fillets
- 1/2 teaspoon turmeric powder
- Celery salt and ground black pepper, to taste
- For Chimichurri Sauce:
- 1/2 teaspoon salt
- 3 garlic cloves, minced
- 1/3 cup wine vinegar
- 1/3 cup extra-virgin olive oil
- 1/2 cup fresh flat-leaf parsley, minced
- 1/2 shallot, finely chopped
- 1 Fresno chili pepper, finely chopped
- 1 tablespoon fresh oregano leaves, finely chopped

Directions

1. Heat ghee in a large stainless skillet that is preheated over a normal high heat. Season trout fillets with pepper, salt, and turmeric powder; now, brush with yellow mustard.
2. Sear the trout fillet for duration of 4 to 5 minutes on each side.
3. In the meantime, salt, pulse wine vinegar, garlic, Fresno chili pepper, shallot, parsley, and oregano in your food processor.
4. With the food processor running slowly, gradually include olive oil and blend until it becomes uniform and smooth. You can keep Chimichurri in the refrigerator for a maximum of 2 days.
5. Enjoy warm fish fillets with Chimichurri sauce on the side. Bon appétit!

Nutrition: Calories265 ,Protein 17.1g ,Fat 20.9g ,Carbs 4g ,Sugar 0.2g

160. SUNDAY AMBER JACK FILLETS WITH PARMESAN SAUCE

Servings: 6
Preparation Time: 20 minutes

Ingredients

- 1/4 cup fresh tarragon chopped
- 2 tablespoons ghee, at room temperature
- 1 teaspoon sea salt
- 1/4 teaspoon cayenne pepper, or more to taste
- 1 lemon, cut into wedges
- 6 amber jack fillets
- 1/2 teaspoon ground black pepper
- For the Sauce:
- Salt and ground black pepper, to taste
- 3 teaspoons ghee,at room temperature
- 1/3 cup beef bone broth
- 1/3 cup Parmesan cheese,grated
- 1 teaspoon garlic, finely minced
- 3/4 cup heavy cream

Directions

1. Dissolve the ghee in a large bottomed non-stick frying pan.
2. Coat both sides of your fish with the black pepper, salt, cayenne pepper and chopped tarragon.
3. Now, fry the fish fillets for about 10 minutes or until the edges are turning opaque and the segments flake apart.
4. In order to make the sauce, dissolve 3 teaspoons of ghee in a pan over moderate heat. Now, sauté the garlic until aromatic, for about 3 minutes.
5. Include the broth and cream; commence on cooking and constantly stirring, about 6 minutes.
6. Stir in Parmesan cheese and continue stirring until everything is thoroughly heated. Now, season with salt and pepper to taste.
7. Serve fish fillets with the sauce garnished with fresh lemon wedges.

Nutrition: Calories 285 ,Protein 23.8g ,Fat 20.4g ,Carbs 1.2g ,Sugar 0.1g

161. CRAB MEAT, PROSCIUTTO AND VEGETABLE DELIGHT

Servings: 4
Preparation Time: 10 minutes

Ingredients

- 1 tablespoon tahini
- 1/2 lemon, zested and juiced
- 3 tablespoons olive oil
- 2 (6-ounce) cans lump crabmeat, drained
- 1/2 cup fresh Italian parsley, chopped
- 2 ounces thinly sliced prosciutto, chopped
- 10 cherry tomato, halved
- Coarse salt and ground black pepper, to your liking
- 4 cups baby spinach
- 10 ripe olives, pitted and halved

Directions

1. In a small-sized mixing bowl, whisk the lemon zest, oil, tahini, lemon juice, salt, and pepper.
2. In a salad container, gently toss crab meat with spinach, prosciutto, cherry tomatoes, and olives. Drizzle with the prepared dressing and toss to merge.
3. Finally, serve garnished with fresh parsley in individual salad bowls.

Nutrition: Calories232 ,Protein 18.9g ,Fat 15.6g ,Carbs 6g ,Sugar 1g

162. FISH WITH CREMINI MUSHROOMS AND SOUR CREAM SAUCE

Servings: 4
Preparation Time: 20 minutes

Ingredients

- 2 tablespoons olive oil
- 4 skinless halibut fillets
- 2 garlic cloves, chopped
- 1/2 cup fresh parsley, chopped
- Coarse salt and freshly ground black pepper, to taste
- 1 ½ cups clam juice
- 1 onion, chopped
- 1/2 pound cremini mushrooms, thinly sliced
- 1 tablespoon ghee
- 1 cup sour cream

Directions

1. Heat 1 tablespoon of olive oil in a pan over a normal high heat. Also, Sauté the onion until it's softened.
2. Succeeding the above, stir in the mushrooms, salt, and black pepper; cook for the duration of 5 minutes.
3. Now, wipe out your pan and heat the remaining tablespoon of oil. Sear fish fillets over average-high heat for approximately 4 minutes per side. Pour into a plate with mushroom mixture.
4. Dissolve ghee over a moderately high flame. Heat the garlic until slightly browned.
5. Transfer in clam juice and work it back and forth, constantly stirring over high heat until reduced by half.
6. Dispose of sauce from heat; let it cool slightly before quickly whisking in the sour cream. Finally, serve with cremini mushrooms and fish, garnished with fresh parsley. Bon appétit!

Nutrition: Calories585 ,Protein 66.8g ,Fat 30.5g ,Carbs 5.5g ,Sugar 2.1g

163. SPRING SALAD WITH HARISSA CRAB MAYO

Servings: 4
Preparation Time: 15 minutes

Ingredients

For the Crab Mayo:

- 3/4 cup olive oil
- 2 egg yolks
- 1/2 teaspoon dried dill weed
- 2 tablespoons fresh lemon juice
- 1/2 teaspoon harissa
- 1/2 tablespoon whole grain mustard
- 1 clove garlic, crushed
- A pinch of salt
- A pinch of freshly ground black pepper
- 1 pound white crab meat

For the Salad:

- 1/2 cup chervil
- 1 head Iceberg lettuce
- 1 bell pepper, julienned
- A bunch of scallions, chopped
- 1 cup radishes, sliced

Directions

1. Firstly, whisk the egg yolks and mustard; gradually pour in the oil, in a tiny stream, until you have a thick combination.
2. Now, include the lemon juice, salt, garlic, dill black pepper, and crabmeat. Place in your refrigerator until ready to serve.
3. In a salad container, place all salad ingredients. Toss with prepared crab mayo and enjoy well-chilled. Bon appétit!

Nutrition: Calories 293 ,Protein 9.3g ,Fat 27.1g ,Carbs 6.3g ,Sugar 3.1g

164. GRILLED CLAMS WITH TOMATO SAUCE

Servings: 4
Preparation Time: 25 minutes

Ingredients

- 40 littleneck clams
- For the Sauce:
- 1 onion, chopped
- 2 tablespoons olive oil
- 2 tomatoes, pureed
- 1/2 teaspoon cayenne pepper
- 1/3 cup dry sherry
- 1 teaspoon crushed garlic
- Sea salt and freshly ground black pepper, to taste
- 1 lemon, cut into wedges

Directions

1. Heat grill to average-high.Heat until clams open, about 6 minutes.
2. Heat the oil in sauté pan over average heat. Heat the onion and garlic until aromatic.
3. Include pureed tomatoes, black pepper, salt and cayenne pepper and heat an additional 10 minutes or until everything is thoroughly cooked.
4. Dispose of from heat and include dry sherry; stir to combine. Enjoy with grilled clams, garnished with fresh lemon wedges.

Nutrition: Calories 134 ,Protein 8.3g ,Fat 7.8g ,Carbs 5.9g ,Sugar 3.2g

165. PRAWN AND AVOCADO COCKTAIL SALAD

Servings: 6
Preparation Time: 10 minutes

Ingredients

- 1/2 cup Lebanese cucumber, chopped
- 1/2 cup mayonnaise
- 1 avocado, pitted and sliced
- 1 pound large king prawns, peeled leaving tails intact
- A few drops red Tabasco pepper sauce
- 1 small-sized red onion, thinly sliced
- 2 teaspoons fresh lime juice
- 1 tablespoon Worcestershire sauce
- 1/2 head iceberg lettuce leaves

Directions

1. Boil a pot of salted water; heat the prawns for 3 minutes. Drain and pour into a mixing bowl.
2. In the mixing container, merge the prawns with chopped cucumber and red onion. In another container, thoroughly merge mayonnaise with lime juice, Worcestershire sauce and Tabasco pepper sauce.
3. Include the mayo mixture to the prawn mixture. Put in your refrigerator until serving time.
4. To serve, position lettuce leaves and avocado slices on a serving platter. Mound the salad onto lettuce leaves and enjoy well chilled.

Nutrition: Calories 236 ,Protein 16.3g ,Fat 14.3g ,Carbs 5.3g ,Sugar 2.2g

166. CHINESE-STYLE MILK FISH WITH MUSHROOM-PEPPER COULIS

Servings: 4

Preparation Time: 35 minutes

Ingredients

For the Fish:

- 1/3 cup Rosé wine
- 1/2 teaspoon salt
- 1⁄2 teaspoon red pepper flakes, crushed
- 2 milk fishes, scaled
- 2 tablespoons olive oil
- 1/4 teaspoon ground black pepper
- 2 tablespoons Chinese dark soy sauce
- For the Mushroom/Pepper Coulis:
- 1 bell pepper, deveined and chopped
- 3 tablespoons consommé
- 1/2 onion, peeled and chopped
- 1/8 teaspoon freshly grated nutmeg
- 1/2 tablespoon champagne vinegar
- 1/4 teaspoon ground black pepper
- 2 ounces Cremini mushrooms, chopped
- 1/2 teaspoon kosher
- 1 ½ ounces olive oil

Directions

1. Heat olive oil in a pan over averagely-high heat. Season milk fish with black pepper, salt, and red pepper flakes.
2. Now, fry milk fish in batches for about 5 minutes per side or until golden brown; reserve, keeping warm.
3. Include Rosé wine and Chinese dark soy sauce to the same pan. Succeeding the previous, bring to a rolling boil, reduce heat to average-low and let it simmer an additional duration of 5 minutes.
4. Include milk fish back to the pan and continue to heat, basting with wine sauce, for about 3 minutes.
5. To make your coulis, heat olive oil in a skillet that is preheated over a normal heat. After that, cook the onions until translucent.
6. Turn the heat to medium-low and include the peppers and mushrooms along with a splash of consommé; heat, constantly stirring, another 13 minutes or until they are softened.
7. Process the sautéed mixture in your blender until creamy and uniform.
8. Include the remaining ingredients, stir to combine well and serve with prepared fish.

Nutrition: Calories 415 ,Protein 34.5g ,Fat 28g ,Carbs 4.4g ,Sugar 2.3g

167. TUNA AND VEGETABLE KEBABS

Servings: 4
Preparation Time: 15 minutes

Ingredients

- 1/2 teaspoon rosemary
- 1 pound 1 1/4 -inch-thick tuna, cut into bite-sized cubes
- 1 onion, cut into wedges
- 1 cup grape tomatoes
- 2 tablespoons soy sauce
- 1/2 teaspoon thyme
- Salt and crushed black peppercorns
- 1 zucchini, diced
- 2 tablespoons olive oil

Directions

1. Firstly, preheat your grill on high. Season tuna cubes and vegetables with peppercorns, salt, rosemary, and thyme. After that, drizzle with the oil and soy sauce.
2. Succeeding the above, alternate seasoned tuna cubes, zucchini, onion, and tomatoes on each of 8 metal skewers.
3. Now, grill 5 minutes for medium-rare, turning frequently. Bon appetite!

Nutrition: Calories257 ,Protein 27.5g ,Fat 12.5g ,Carbs 7g ,Sugar 5.1g

168. MACKEREL STEAK CASSEROLE WITH CHEESE AND VEGGIES

Servings: 4
Preparation Time: 30 minutes

Ingredients

- 2 cloves garlic, thinly sliced
- Salt and black pepper, to your liking
- 1 tablespoon Old Bay seasoning
- 1 cup mozzarella, shredded

- 1/2 stick butter
- 1 pound mackerel steaks
- 1/2 cup fresh chives, chopped
- 1/4 cup clam juice
- 2 onions, thinly sliced
- 3 tomatoes, thinly sliced

Directions

1. Firstly, preheat your oven to 4500F.
2. Dissolve the butter in a pan that is previously preheated over a normal flame. Heat the garlic and onions until they are tender.
3. Include clam juice and tomatoes and cook for 4 minutes more. Put this vegetable mixture into a casserole dish.
4. Then, Lay the fish steaks on top of the vegetable layer. Spray with seasonings. Close with foil and roast for about 10 minutes until the fish is opaque in the center.
5. Now, top with shredded cheese and bake another 5 minutes. Enjoy warm garnished with fresh chopped chives. Bon appétit!

Nutrition: Calories 301 ,Protein 33.3g ,Fat 14g ,Carbs 6g ,Sugar 2.3g

169. CLASSIC SEAFOOD CHOWDER

Servings: 5
Preparation Time: 15 minutes

Ingredients

- 2 tablespoons green onion, chopped
- 1 teaspoon minced garlic
- 1/2 stick butter
- 2 cups heavy cream
- 3 bouillon cubes
- 1 teaspoon dried rosemary
- 1 egg, lightly beaten
- 1/2 pound crab meat
- 3/4 pound shrimp, peeled and deveined
- 1 quart water
- 1/3 cup dry white wine
- 1 tablespoon tomato paste
- Salt and ground black pepper, to taste

Directions

1. Dissolve the butter in a large pot that is preheated over medium-high heat.
2. Heat or cook the onion and garlic until they are tender and aromatic.
3. Include the shrimp, crab meat, bouillon cubes, wine and water. Heat until the seafood is thoroughly warmed, for about 5 minutes.
4. Decrease the heat to low and include the remaining ingredients. Simmer, frequently stirring, for an additional 2 to 3 minutes. Bon appétit!

Nutrition: Calories 404 ,Protein 23.9g ,Fat 30g ,Carbs 5.3g ,Sugar 1.1g

170. SMOKY CHOLULA SEAFOOD DIP

Servings: 8
Preparation Time: 10 minutes

Ingredients

- Sea salt and ground black pepper, to taste
- 1/2 cup mayonnaise
- 1 tablespoon Cholula
- 12 ounces seafood, canned and drained
- 1/2 teaspoon dried dill weed
- 2 cloves garlic, finely minced
- 1/4 teaspoon white pepper
- A few drops of liquid smoke
- 1 teaspoon smoked paprika

Directions

1. In a mixing container, gently stir garlic, mayo, and canned seafood.
2. Include the remaining ingredients and stir with a wide spatula until everything is well merged.
3. Close the lid and place it in your refrigerator until it is thoroughly chilled. Enjoy well-chilled with fresh or pickled veggies. Bon appétit!

Nutrition: Calories 108 ,Protein 8.2g ,Fat 5.4g ,Carbs 5g ,Sugar 1g

171. SMOKED CREAMY FISH FAT BOMBS

Servings: 6

Preparation Time: 15 minutes

Ingredients

- 1/4 cup of mayonnaise
- 1 cup cream cheese
- 1 Tbsp of mustard
- 1 filet smoked fish, boneless, crumbled
- 2 Tbsp grated cheese
- 1 tsp fresh parsley, chopped

Directions:

1. Combine all Ingredients and beat in a food processor.
2. Make 6 balls and place them on a lined pan with parchment paper.
3. Refrigerate for 3 hours.
4. Serve cold.

Nutrition:

Calories: 221 Carbohydrates: 2g Proteins: 20g Fat: 15g Fiber: 0.1g

172. STEAMED BREAM WITH FENNEL

Servings: 4
Preparation Time: 10 minutes
Cooking Time: 20 minutes

Ingredients

- 2 Tbsp of olive oil
- 4 Tbsp of water
- 2 large spring onion, sliced
- 1 sprig of fresh rosemary, only the leaves, chopped
- 1 clove of garlic, crushed
- 4 fillets of sea bream (about 1 1/2 lbs.)
- Juice of 1 lemon
- 4 Tbsp of fresh fennel
- Salt and ground pepper

Directions:

1. Heat the olive oil in a large skillet.
2. Add the spring onions, cover and cook for 7 - 8 minutes on medium heat.
3. Next, add the garlic, water rosemary, salt, pepper, stir and cook for 2 - 3 minutes.
4. In a large pot heat water and set a steamer with the fish.
5. Cover the pot and steam the fish for 8 minutes.
6. Remove fish on a plate, and cover with the spring onion sauce.
7. Sprinkle with chopped fennel, and drizzle with fresh lemon juice.

Nutrition:

Calories: 281 Carbohydrates: 5g Proteins: 38g Fat: 12g Fiber: 3g

173. EGG AND FISH FRY

Servings: 3
Preparation Time: 15 minutes
Cooking Time: 15 minutes

Ingredients

- 1 lbs. Fish fillet- skinless and boneless (Tilapia, Catfish or any white fish)
- 1/2 Lime juice
- Sea salt
- 1 green onion
- 1/2-inch ginger
- 3 cloves garlic
- 1/2 cup cilantro
- 2 green chilies
- 1 egg
- 1 cup ground almonds
- Oil for frying

Directions:

1. Cut the fish fillet into pieces, rinse and pat dry.
2. Put the fish fillets in a plastic bag and marinate with lime juice and the salt.
3. Make a fine paste with onion, ginger, garlic, green chilies and cilantro, using a food processor, Vitamix or blender.
4. Add the paste to the marinade and shake to combine well.
5. Remove the fish pieces only, and discard the excess marinate.
6. Whisk the egg with 2-3 tbsp of water to have a smooth consistency.
7. Spread the ground almonds on a flat surface.
8. Dip the fish piece in the egg mixture, and then roll into ground almonds.
9. Heat the oil in deep frying skillet.
10. 1Fry the fish fillets until get a nice golden-

brown color.

11. 1Remove from the skillet and place on a paper towel to absorb the excess oil.
12. 1Serve hot.

Nutrition:

Calories: 381 Carbohydrates: 9g Proteins: 44g Fat: 19g Fiber: 2g

174. TUNA SALAD WITH AVOCADO, SESAME AND MINT

Servings: 6
Preparation Time: 15 minutes
Cooking Time: 15 minutes

Ingredients

- 1 cucumber, sliced
- 1 pepper green, hot
- 1 avocado
- 1 zucchini, sliced
- Juice and zest of 2 limes
- 1/4 cup of olive oil
- Salt and ground pepper
- 1 lbs. of tuna, fresh
- 2 Tbsp of sesame seeds
- 2 - 3 Tbsp of fresh mint, finely chopped

Directions:

1. Cut the cucumber in the middle and then at 4 slices.
2. Clean and slice the pepper, avocado, zucchini and place in a large bowl.
3. Pour with fresh lime juice and drizzle with olive oil.
4. Cut the tuna fish into large pieces, and season with the salt and pepper.
5. Heat some oil in a skillet at high heat, and fry tuna slices for 2-3 minutes.
6. Remove the tuna from the pan and transfer in a salad bowl; gently stir.
7. Sprinkle with sesame seeds and fresh mint and serve immediately.

Nutrition:

Calories: 331 Carbohydrates: 9g Proteins: 24g Fat: 23g Fiber: 4.5g

175. ALMOND BREADED CRAYFISH WITH HERBS

Servings: 6
Preparation Time: 15 minutes
Cooking Time: 5 minutes

Ingredients

- 1 cup of grated almonds
- The zest of one orange
- 1 bunch of parsley
- 3/4 cup of olive oil
- Salt and ground pepper
- 30 crayfish, cleaned
- 2 lemons For serving

Directions:

1. Place grated almonds, orange zest, parsley, 3 tablespoons of oil, and the salt and ground pepper in a blender.
2. Pour the almond mixture to the deep plate and roll on each crayfish.
3. Heat the oil in a large skillet over high heat.
4. Cook crayfish for 5 minutes turning 2 - 3 times.
5. Serve hot with lemon wedges.

Nutrition:

Calories: 489 Carbohydrates: 9g Proteins: 12g Fat: 40g Fiber: 2g

176. AROMATIC CUTTLEFISH WITH SPINACH

Servings: 6
Preparation Time: 10 minutes
Cooking Time: 1 hour

Ingredients

- 2 lbs. of cuttlefish
- 3/4 cup of olive oil
- 3 cups of water
- 3/4 cup of fresh anis
- 1 lbs. of fresh spinach
- 2 spring onions cut into thin slices
- 1 small tomato, grated
- Juice of 1 large lemon
- Salt and pepper to taste

Directions:

1. Clean and rinse thoroughly the cuttlefish.
2. Heat the oil in a large skillet and sauté the

onion for 1-2 minutes over medium heat.
3. Add the cuttlefish and cook until get the color.
4. Pour 3 cups of water, close the pot lid and simmer for at least 40-45 minutes.
5. Add the spinach, anis, grated tomato, salt and ground pepper.
6. Close the lid again and continue cooking at low temperature until the herbs soften.
7. Pour in the lemon juice and mix well. Serve warm.

Nutrition:

Calories: 378 Carbohydrates: 5.5g Proteins: 27g Fat: 28g Fiber: 2g

177. BAKED SHRIMP SAGANAKI WITH FETA

Servings: 6
Preparation Time: 10 minutes
Cooking Time: 15 minutes

Ingredients

- 1 cup of olive oil
- 1 large grated tomato
- 1 green onion, sliced
- 2 lbs. of large shrimp
- 2 cups of feta cheese, crumbled
- Salt and ground pepper to taste
- 1 cup of fresh parsley, chopped For serving

Directions:

1. Preheat the oven to 350° F/175° C.
2. In a large skillet heat the olive oil and cook the green onion and tomato.
3. Season with the salt and pepper and cook for 2 minutes.
4. Add shrimp and stir for 2 minutes.
5. Finally, sprinkle feta cheese evenly over the shrimp.
6. Place in oven and bake for 6 -8 minutes.
7. Serve hot with chopped parsley.

Nutrition:

Calories: 516 Carbohydrates: 5g Proteins: 28g Fat: 48g Fiber: 1g

178. BREADED CATFISH FILLETS

Servings: 4
Preparation Time: 15 minutes
Cooking Time: Time: 10 minutes

Ingredients

- 1/2 cup ground almonds
- 1/2 tsp sea salt
- 1/8 tsp freshly-ground black pepper
- 1/2 tsp of garlic powder
- 1 1/2 lbs. catfish fillets
- 2 eggs, beaten
- Olive oil for frying

Directions:

1. In a bowl, combine ground almonds, salt, garlic powder and pepper. Dip catfish fillets in beaten egg, then coat well with the almond mixture.
2. Heat the oil in a large skillet and cook breaded fish for 4 minutes from each side over medium heat.
3. Turn only once during cooking.
4. Serve hot.

Nutrition:

Calories: 410 Carbohydrates: 5.5g Proteins: 32g Fat: 29g Fiber: 2g

179. CALAMARI AND SHRIMP STEW

Servings: 4
Preparation Time: 10 minutes
Cooking Time: Time: 15 minutes

Ingredients

- 3 Tbsp olive oil
- 1 green onion, finely chopped
- 3 cloves garlic, minced
- 3 lbs. shrimp cleaned and deveined
- 1 lbs. of calamari rings, frozen
- 1/4 can of white wine
- 1/2 can fresh parsley, finely chopped
- 1 grated tomato
- Salt and freshly ground black pepper

Directions:

1. In a large skillet, heat the olive oil and sauté chopped green onion and garlic for 2-3 minutes or until softened.
2. Add the shrimps and calamari rings.

3. Stir and cook for about 3 - 4 minutes over medium heat.
4. Add the wine, parsley and grated tomato.
5. Season the salt and pepper to taste.
6. Cover and cook for 4 -5 minutes.
7. Serve hot with chopped parsley.

Nutrition:

Calories: 184 Carbohydrates: 4.5g Proteins: 24g Fat: 7g Fiber: 0.7g

180. CATALONIAN SHRIMP STEW

Servings: 4
Preparation Time: 5 minutes
Cooking Time: Time: 15 minutes

Ingredients

- 1/2 cup olive oil
- 1 1/2 lbs. shrimp, peeled and deveined
- 36 garlic cloves, minced
- 1/4 cup fresh lemon juice
- 1 tsp red pepper flakes (to taste)
- 4 Tbsp of fresh parsley, chopped
- Salt and fresh ground pepper

Directions:

1. In a large skillet heat the on high heat. Add shrimp and garlic and sauté for about 2-3 minutes.
2. Add the lemon juice, pepper flakes, and salt and pepper to taste. Adjust seasonings to your liking.
3. Serve hot with chopped parsley.

Nutrition:

Calories: 403 Carbohydrates: 8.5g Proteins: 25g Fat: 29g Fiber: 0.6g

181. CUTTLEFISH WITH GREEN OLIVES AND FENNEL

Servings: 6
Preparation Time: 10 minutes
Cooking Time: Time: 20 minutes

Ingredients

- 2/3 glass of olive oil
- 2 green onions, finely chopped
- 2 cloves of garlic, minced
- 2 lbs. of cuttlefish cleaned (or squid, calamari if cuttlefish is unavailable or difficult to find. Adjust cooking times accordingly)
- 2/3 glass of red wine
- 1/2 cup of water
- 11 oz of green olives, pitted
- 1 bunch of fresh fennel, chopped
- Salt and ground black pepper

Directions:

1. Wash the cuttlefish very well and cut into thick pieces.
2. Heat the oil in a large skillet over medium-high heat.
3. Add green onion, garlic and cuttlefish; sauté for 2 - 3 minutes.
4. Pour the wine and water and stir for 5 -6 minutes over low heat.
5. In a meantime, in a separate pot, boil the fennel for 3 minutes.
6. Strain the fennel and add along with olives in a skillet with cuttlefish; stir.
7. Season with the salt and pepper, cover and cook for 2 - 3 minutes. Serve hot.

Nutrition:

Calories: 433 Carbohydrates: 9g Proteins: 26g Fat: 30g Fiber: 3.5g

182. DELICIOUS SHRIMP WITH BROCCOLI

Servings: 4
Preparation Time: 10 minutes
Cooking Time: Time: 20 minutes

Ingredients

- 2 Tbsp sesame oil
- 2 large cloves garlic, minced
- 1 cup water
- 2 Tbsp coconut aminos (from coconut sap)
- 2 tsp fresh ginger root, grated
- 2 cups fresh broccoli florets
- 1 1/2 lbs. shrimp, peeled and deveined
- Lemon wedges For serving

Directions:

1. Heat the oil in a large skillet or wok over medium-high heat.

2. Cook the garlic for about 3 - 4 minutes.
3. Reduce the heat to low; add water, coconut aminos, and ginger.
4. Bring the mixture to a boil, and shrimp; cook and stir until the shrimp turn pink, about 3 to 4 minutes.
5. Add broccoli and cook for 10 minutes.
6. Serve hot with lemon wedges.

Nutrition:

Calories: 220 Carbohydrates: 9g Proteins: 27g Fat: 10g Fiber: 2.7g

183. FRIED MUSSELS WITH MUSTARD AND LEMON

Servings: 6
Preparation Time: 10 minutes
Cooking Time: 10 minutes

Ingredients

- 1/4 cup garlic-infused olive oil
- 2 spring onions, finely chopped
- 1 small green pepper, chopped
- 2 cherry tomatoes
- 1 tsp oregano
- 1 1/2 lbs. mussels with shells, freshly cleaned
- 1 cup water
- 2 Tbsp mustard (Dijon, English, ground stone)
- Freshly ground pepper to taste
- Pinch of cayenne pepper (optional)
- 2 lemons, juice, zest and slices

Directions:

1. Heat the oil in a large frying skillet over high heat.
2. Sauté fresh onion, pepper, oregano and chopped tomatoes for 2-3 minutes.
3. Add the mussels and water and cover.
4. Cook for 2-3 minutes on high heat; shake the pan to open the mussels.
5. Combine the mustard with the lemon and pour over mussels. Cook for 1 minute and sprinkle some black pepper and cayenne pepper if used.
6. Serve with lemon juice and lemon juice.

Nutrition:

Calories: 301 Carbohydrates: 9.5g Proteins: 22g Fat: 19g Fiber: 4g

184. FRIED WINE OCTOPUS PATTIES

Servings: 6
Preparation Time: 10 minutes
Cooking Time: 10 minutes

Ingredients

- 2 lbs. octopus fresh or frozen, cleaned and cut in small cubes
- 1 cup of ground almond
- 1 cup of red wine
- 2 spring onions finely chopped
- 1 Tbsp of oregano
- Salt and ground black pepper
- 1 cup of olive oil

Directions:

1. In a deep bowl, combine the octopus cubes, ground almond, red wine, spring onions, oregano, and the salt and the pepper.
2. Knead until combined well.
3. Form the mixture into balls or patties.
4. Heat the oil in a large and deep fry pan.
5. Fry octopus patties until get a golden color.
6. Transfer the octopus patties on a platter lined with kitchen paper towel.
7. Serve warm.

Nutrition:

Calories: 526 Carbohydrates: 8g Proteins: 28g Fat: 49.5g Fiber: 3g

185. GRILLED KING PRAWNS WITH PARSLEY SAUCE

Servings: 4
Preparation Time: 10 minutes
Cooking Time: 15 minutes

Ingredients

- 40 king prawns, heads off and unpeeled
- 1/4 cup olive oil
- 2 green onions (scallions), finely chopped
- 2 Tbsp of fresh parsley, finely chopped
- 3 Tbsp water

- Salt and pepper to taste

Directions:

1. Cut prawns in half so that the meat is exposed in the shell.
2. In a large skillet heat the olive oil and sauté the green onion for 2 - 3 minutes or until softened.
3. Add chopped parsley, water, salt and pepper: stir for 2 minutes and remove from the heat.
4. Preheat your grill (pellet, gas, charcoal) to HIGH according to manufacturer Instructions.
5. Brush prawns with onion - parsley mixture, and grill for 3 - 4 each side.
6. Serve hot.

Nutrition:

Calories: 209 Carbohydrates: 3g Proteins: 38g Fat: 4g Fiber: 0.3g

186. CAJUN LIME GRILLED SHRIMP

Servings: 6
Preparation Time: 10 minutes
Cooking Time: 15 minutes

Ingredients

- 3 Tbsp Cajun seasoning
- 2 lime, juiced
- 2 Tbsp olive oil
- 1 lbs. peeled and deveined medium shrimp (30-40 per pound)

Directions:

1. Mix together the Cajun seasoning, lime juice, and olive oil in a resalable plastic bag.
2. Add the shrimp, coat with the marinade, squeeze out excess air, and seal the bag.
3. Marinate in the refrigerator for 20 minutes.
4. Preheat your grill (pellet, gas, charcoal) to HIGH according to manufacturer Instructions.
5. Remove the shrimp from the marinade and shake off excess. Discard the remaining marinade.
6. Grill shrimp until they are bright pink on the outside and the meat is no longer transparent in the center, about 2 minutes per side.
7. Serve hot.

Nutrition:

Calories: 318 Carbohydrates: 8.7g Proteins: 32g Fat: 17g Fiber: 3g

187. IBERIAN SHRIMP FRITTERS

Servings: 4
Preparation Time: 10 minutes
Cooking Time: 5 minutes

Ingredients

- 1 green onion, finely diced
- 1 lbs. raw shrimp, peeled, deveined, and finely chopped
- 1 cup almond flour
- 2 Tbsp fresh parsley (chopped)
- 1 tsp baking powder
- 1 tsp hot paprika
- Salt and freshly ground black pepper, to taste
- 1/4 cup olive oil
- Lemon wedges, For serving

Directions:

1. In a large and deep bowl, combine green onions, shrimp, almond flour, parsley, baking powder, paprika, and pinch of the salt and pepper.
2. Form mixture in patties/balls/fritters.
3. Heat the oil in a large skillet over high heat.
4. Fry shrimp fritters for about 5 minutes in total turning once or twice.
5. Using a spatula, transfer fritters to plate lined with kitchen paper towels to drain.
6. Serve immediately with lemon wedges.

Nutrition:

Calories: 271 Carbohydrates: 3.5g Proteins: 16g Fat: 22g Fiber: 1g

188. MUSSELS WITH HERBED BUTTER ON GRILL

Servings: 4
Preparation Time: 15 minutes

Cooking Time: 10 minutes

Ingredients

- 1/2 cup of butter unsalted, softened
- 2 Tbsp fresh parsley, chopped
- 1 Tbsp of fresh dill
- 2 Tbsp of spring/green onions finely chopped
- 2 tsp lemon juice
- Salt and freshly ground pepper
- 2 lbs. of fresh mussels
- Lemon For serving

Directions:

1. In a bowl, combine butter, softened at room temperature, parsley, dill, spring onions and lemon juice.
2. Season with the salt and pepper to taste.
3. Preheat your grill (pellet, gas, charcoal) to HIGH according to manufacturer Instructions.
4. Grill mussels for 8 - 10 minutes or until shells open.
5. Remove mussels on serving plate, pour with herbed butter, and serve with lemon.

Nutrition:

Calories: 401 Carbohydrates: 8g Proteins: 28g Fat: 29g Fiber: 0.3g

189. MUSSELS WITH SAFFRON

Servings: 4
Preparation Time: 5 minutes
Cooking Time: 8 minutes

Ingredients

- 2 lbs. of mussels, cleaned
- 1 onion, finely chopped
- 4 Tbsp heavy cream
- 1/2 cup of dry white wine
- Pepper to taste
- 1 pinch of saffron
- 2 Tbsp of fresh parsley, finely chopped

Directions:

1. In a large pot, boil the mussels with white wine, chopped onion and ground black pepper.
2. In a separate saucepot, boil the cream with a pinch of saffron for 2 minutes.
3. Drain the mussels and combine with the cream and saffron.
4. Serve immediately with parsley.

Nutrition:

Calories: 259 Carbohydrates: 9g Proteins: 28g Fat: 8g Fiber: 0.6g

190. MUSSELS WITH SPINACH STIR-FRY

Servings: 6
Preparation Time: 10 minutes
Cooking Time: 30 minutes

Ingredients

- 1/2 cup of fresh butter
- 2 spring onions, finely sliced
- 2 cloves of garlic, minced
- 1 1/2 lbs. of fresh mussels
- 2 lbs. of fresh spinach, roughly chopped
- 1/2 cup of fresh parsley, chopped
- 3 Tbsp of fresh dill
- Salt and ground black pepper
- 1 cup of red wine
- 1 cup of water

Directions:

1. Heat the butter in a large pot or skillet; sauté the green onions and minced garlic for 2 - 3 minutes.
2. Add mussels, spinach, parsley, dill, and the salt and pepper; stir.
3. Pour wine and water, cover and cook for 25 - 30 minutes over medium-low heat.
4. Serve hot.

Nutrition:

Calories: 277 Carbohydrates: 9g Proteins: 18g Fat: 19g Fiber: 3g

191. SHRIMP AND OCTOPUS SOUP

Servings: 6
Preparation Time: 10 minutes
Cooking Time: 35 minutes

Ingredients

- 2 quarts water
- 2 lbs. octopus, cut into 1-inch pieces

- 1 Tbsp olive oil
- 1 small carrot, cut into slices
- 1 cup fresh celery finely chopped
- 1 cup cauliflower floret
- 1/2 cup green onion, or to taste
- 1 Tbsp of coconut aminos
- Salt to taste
- Lemon juice For serving (to taste)

Directions:

1. Place the water in a large soup pot and bring to a boil over medium-high heat.
2. Add octopus and continue boiling for about 20 minutes.
3. Add all remaining Ingredients and cook for 12 - 15 minutes over medium-low heat.
4. Serve hot with lemon juice.

Nutrition:

Calories: 98 Carbohydrates: 4g Proteins: 14g Fat: 3g Fiber: 0.7g

192. SHRIMP WITH CURRY AND COCONUT MILK

Servings: 6
Preparation Time: 5 minutes
Cooking Time: 30 minutes

Ingredients

- 1 Tbsp of olive oil
- 2 green onions, finely chopped
- 2 cloves garlic, minced
- 1 hot red pepper, cut into small pieces
- 1 tsp of fresh grated ginger
- 1 Tbsp of curry powder
- 1 grated tomato
- 1 1/2 cups of unsweetened coconut milk
- Salt and ground black pepper
- 1 1/2 lbs. of shrimp, cleaned and deveined
- Fresh coriander For serving

Directions:

1. Heat the oil in large skillet over high heat.
2. Sauté the onions, garlic, hot red pepper, and freshly ground ginger; stir.
3. Add curry powder and stir for 1 to 2 minutes.
4. Add grated tomato, coconut milk, the salt and ground pepper, lower the heat, cover and cook for 5 minutes.
5. Add shrimp, cover and cook for about 15 minutes stirring two to three times.
6. Serve hot with chopped coriander.

Nutrition:

Calories: 227 Carbohydrates: 8.5g Proteins: 21g Fat: 12g Fiber: 2.5g

193. SPICY RAZOR CLAMS

Servings: 6
Preparation Time: 5 minutes
Cooking Time: 10 minutes

Ingredients

- 1/2 cup olive oil
- 3 cloves garlic, minced
- 2 hot red chili pepper, finely sliced
- 3 lbs. razor clams, cleaned and rinsed thoroughly
- 1 cup white wine
- 1 1/2 cups of parsley leaves, finely chopped
- 1 pinch sea salt to taste

Directions:

1. Heat the oil in a large skillet, and sauté garlic and hot red peppers for 4 minutes.
2. Increase heat at high; add razor clams and wine, and cook, covered, until clams are just cooked through, about 3 minutes.
3. Add the parsley and season with the salt; toss razor clams to coat with sauce.
4. Transfer clams to a serving platter and drizzle with remaining sauce.
5. Serve hot.

Nutrition:

Calories: 198 Carbohydrates: 8g Proteins: 30g Fat: 4g Fiber: 0.3g

194. SQUID WITH HOMEMADE PESTO SAUCE

Servings: 4
Preparation Time: 10 minutes
Cooking Time: 10 minutes

Ingredients

- 2 lbs. squid fresh, cut in small pieces
- 1 cup of bone broth
- 3 bay leaves
- 2 Tbsp of fresh thyme, finely chopped
- 1 cup of fresh basil, finely chopped
- 4 cloves of garlic, sliced
- 1/3 cup of finely sliced or ground almonds
- 1/3 cup of olive oil
- 2 Tbsp of grated Parmesan cheese

Directions:

1. In a pot, boil the squid with bone broth, bay leaves and fresh thyme for about 10 minutes.
2. Remove the squid from the pot, drain and place on a serving platter.
3. Place the basil, garlic, sliced almonds and olive oil in your blender; blend until all Ingredients smooth.
4. Add the grated Parmesan, and blend for 30 further seconds.
5. Serve squid pieces with fresh pesto sauce and enjoy your lunch!

Nutrition:

Calories: 456 Carbohydrates: 9g Proteins: 42g Fat: 28g Fiber: 2g

195. TRADITIONAL HUNGARIAN HALÁSZLÉ

Preparation Time: 20 minutes
Servings: 2

Nutrition: 252 Calories; 12.6g Fat; 5g Carbs; 28.2g Protein; 1.9g Fiber

Ingredients

- 1 red onion, chopped
- 2 bell peppers, chopped
- 2 vine-ripe tomatoes, pureed
- 1/2 pound tilapia, cut into bite-sized pieces
- 2 tablespoons sour cream

Directions

1. Heat 1 tablespoon of canola oil in a soup pot over medium-high flame. Now, sauté the peppers and onion until tender and fragrant.
2. Stir in tomatoes and tilapia. Turn the heat to medium-low and let it simmer, partially covered, for about 10 minutes.
3. Serve in soup bowls, garnished with well-chilled sour cream.

196. SALMON FILLETS IN MARSALA SAUCE

Preparation Time: 20 minutes
Servings: 6

Nutrition: 347 Calories; 18.5g Fat; 4g Carbs; 39.9g Protein; 1g Fiber

Ingredients

- 2 ½ pounds salmon fillets
- 4 tablespoons Marsala wine
- 2 bell peppers, deseeded and sliced
- 1/2 cup scallions, chopped
- 2 cups marinara sauce

Directions

1. In a Dutch oven, heat 2 tablespoons of peanut oil over a moderate heat. Sauté the bell peppers and scallions for 3 to 4 minutes until they have softened.
2. Add a splash of wine to deglaze the pan. Stir in marinara sauce and salmon.
3. Reduce the heat to medium-low and let it simmer for 15 to 20 minutes or until the salmon easily flakes with a fork. Enjoy!

197. OLD BAY PRAWNS WITH SOUR CREAM

Preparation Time: 20 minutes
Servings: 2

Nutrition: 269 Calories; 9.6g Fat; 7.2g Carbs; 38.2g Protein; 2.5g Fiber

Ingredients

- 3/4 pound prawns, peeled and deveined
- 1 teaspoon Old Bay seasoning mix
- 1 bell pepper, deveined and minced
- 1 cup pound broccoli florets
- 2 dollops of sour cream, for garnish

Directions

1. Begin by preheating your oven to 380 dergees F. Toss the prawns with the Old

Bay seasoning mix.

2. Place them on a parchment-lined roasting pan. Scatter the bell peppers and broccoli florets around them.
3. Drizzle 2 teaspoon of olive oil over everything.
4. Roast in the preheated oven for about 10 minutes or until the prawns are pink, rotating the pan periodically to ensure even cooking.
5. Serve with sour cream and enjoy!

198. DAD'S FISH JAMBALAYA

Preparation Time: 15 minutes
Servings: 2
Nutrition: 232 Calories; 3.6g Fat; 6.7g Carbs; 38.1g Protein; 2.1g Fiber

Ingredients

- 1 teaspoon canola oil
- 1 small-sized leek, chopped
- 1 pound sole fish fillets, cut into bite-sized strips
- 1 cup marinara sauce
- 1 cup spinach, torn into pieces

Directions

1. Heat canola oil in a heavy-bottomed pot over a moderate heat. Sauté the leeks until they have softened.
2. Stir in the fish fillets, marinara sauce, and 1 cup of water (clam juice). Reduce the temperature to medium-low.
3. Let it simmer, covered, for about 5 minutes or until the cooking liquid has reduced and thickened slightly.
4. Stir in the spinach and continue to simmer for 2 to 3 minutes more. Serve in individual bowls. Bon appétit!

199. MEDITERRANEAN HADDOCK WITH CHEESE SAUCE

Preparation Time: 30 minutes
Servings: 4

Nutrition: 260 Calories; 19.1g Fat; 1.3g Carbs; 19.6g Protein; 0.3g Fiber

Ingredients

- 1 pound haddock fillets
- 2 scallions, chopped
- 1/4 cup cream cheese, at room temperature
- 1/4 cup mayonnaise
- 1 tablespoon olive oil

Directions

1. Begin by preheating an oven to 365 degrees F. Toss the haddock with the olive oil, salt, and black pepper.
2. Wrap your fish with foil and bake for about 25 minutes.
3. Then, prepare the sauce by whisking the scallions, cream cheese and mayo. Serve and enjoy!

200. FISH CAKES WITH CLASSIC HORSERADISH SAUCE

Preparation Time: 20 minutes
Servings: 4

Nutrition: 206 Calories; 8.3g Fat; 1.9g Carbs; 27.3g Protein; 0.1g Fiber

Ingredients

- 1 pound cod fillets
- 8 tablespoons Ricotta cheese
- 4 tablespoons parmesan cheese, grated
- 1 teaspoon creamed horseradish
- 2 eggs, beaten

Directions

1. Steam the cod fillets for about 10 minutes or until easily flakes with a fork. Chop your fish and mix with eggs and parmesan cheese.
2. Form the mixture into 4 fish cakes. Heat 2 tablespoons of olive oil in a frying skillet. Once hot, cook the fish cakes over medium-high heat for 3 to 4 minutes on each side.
3. Make the sauce by whisking Ricotta cheese and creamed horseradish. Bon appétit!

201. CLASSIC FISH CURRY

Preparation Time: 20 minutes
Servings: 4

Nutrition: 226 Calories; 6.9g Fat; 3.1g Carbs;

34.8g Protein; 1.8g Fiber

Ingredients

- 1 ½ pounds tilapia
- 1 tablespoon peanut oil
- 1 shallot, chopped
- 1 tablespoon curry paste
- 1 cup tomato onion masala sauce

Directions

1. Heat the peanut oil in a wok over medium-high heat. Cook the shallot for 2 to 3 minutes until tender and fragrant.
2. Pour in tomato onion masala sauce along with 1 cup of chicken broth. Bring to a boil.
3. Reduce the heat to a simmer and stir in the curry paste and tilapia; season with the salt and pepper to your liking.
4. Continue to simmer, partially covered, for 10 to 12 minutes until heated through. Serve hot and enjoy!

202. 34SEA BASS WITH DILL SAUCE

Preparation Time: 25 minutes
Servings: 2

Nutrition: 374 Calories; 17g Fat; 6.2g Carbs; 43.2g Protein; 2.2g Fiber

Ingredients

- 1/4 cup Greek yogurt
- 1 tablespoon fresh dill, chopped
- 1 pound sea bass fillets
- 1 cup red onions, sliced
- 2 bell peppers, deveined and sliced

Directions

1. Start by preheating your oven to 390 degrees F.
2. Toss sea bass fillets, bell peppers, and the onions with 1 tablespoon of olive oil; season with the salt and pepper.
3. Place the fish and vegetables in a lightly greased baking dish. Bake for 20 to 22 minutes, rotating the pan once or twice
4. Make the sauce by whisking Greek yogurt and chopped dill. Serve warm fish and vegetables with the sauce on the side and enjoy!

203. SALMON LETTUCE TACOS

Preparation Time: 20 minutes
Servings: 5

Nutrition: 304 Calories; 14.1g Fat; 5.3g Carbs; 38.6g Protein; 3.4g Fiber

Ingredients

- 10 lettuce leaves
- 2 pounds salmon
- 1 tomato, halved
- 1 avocado, pitted and peeled
- 4 tablespoons green onions

Directions

1. Toss the salmon with salt and black pepper to your liking.
2. Drizzle the salmon with 2 tablespoons of olive oil and grill over medium-high heat for about 15 minutes. Flake the fish with two forks.
3. Divide the fish among the lettuce leaves.
4. Puree avocado, tomato, and green onions in your blender until your desired consistency is reached; add 1 tablespoon of olive oil to your blender, if desired.
5. Top each taco with the avocado sauce, drizzle with fresh lemon juice and serve.

204. TRADITIONAL MAHI MAHI CEVICHE

Preparation Time: 15 minutes
Servings: 4

Nutrition: 424 Calories; 29.8g Fat; 5.8g Carbs; 32.5g Protein; 1.6g Fiber

Ingredients

- 1 ½ pounds mahi-mahi fish, cut into bite-sized cubes
- 2 Roma tomatoes, sliced
- 1 bell pepper, sliced
- 2 garlic cloves, minced
- 4 scallions, chopped

Directions

1. Season mahi-mahi fish with salt and black pepper to taste. Brush them with nonstick

cooking oil.

2. In a preheated grill pan, cook mahi-mahi fish for about 10 minutes until golden-brown on edges.
3. Toss mahi-mahi fish with the garlic, scallions, tomatoes, and bell pepper. Toss with 4 tablespoons of extra-virgin olive oil and 2 tablespoons of fresh lemon juice.
4. Divide between individual bowls and serve.

205. FRIED COD FILLETS

Preparation Time: 15 minutes
Servings: 3

Nutrition: 406 Calories; 29.5g Fat; 4.1g Carbs; 31.9g Protein; 2.2g Fiber

Ingredients

- 2 tablespoons butter
- 3 cod fillets
- 1 cup Romano cheese, preferably freshly grated
- 1 teaspoon dried rosemary, crushed
- 1/2 cup almond meal

Directions

1. Place the fish, almond meal, salt, black pepper, and rosemary in a resealable bag; shake to coat well. Press cod fillets into the grated Romano cheese.
2. Melt the butter in a nonstick skillet over medium-high heat.
3. Cook the fish until it is nearly opaque, about 5 minutes on each side. Bon appétit!

206. SHRIMP AND HAM JAMBALAYA

Preparation Time: 25 minutes
Servings: 4

Nutrition: 170 Calories; 4.8g Fat; 5.6g Carbs; 25.9g Protein; 1.4g Fiber

Ingredients

- 1 shallot, chopped
- 1 ½ cups vegetable broth
- 1 ½ cups tomatoes, crushed
- 1 cup ham, cut into 1/2-inch cubes
- 3/4 pound shrimp

Directions

1. Heat up a lightly oiled stockpot over medium-high heat. Sweat the shallot for about 4 minutes until tender and fragrant.
2. Add in vegetable broth, tomatoes, and ham, and bring to a boil. Reduce heat to medium-low, cover and continue to simmer for 12 minutes more.
3. Stir in the shrimp and continue to simmer until they are pink and thoroughly cooked about 5 minutes.
4. Serve warm and enjoy!

207. HERRING AND SPINACH SALAD

Preparation Time: 10 minutes
Servings: 3

Nutrition: 134 Calories; 7.9g Fat; 5.4g Carbs; 1g Fiber; 10.2g Protein;

Ingredients

- 1/2 cup baby spinach
- 6 ounces pickled herring pieces, drained and flaked
- 1 teaspoon garlic, minced
- 1 red onion, chopped
- 1 bell pepper, chopped

Directions

1. In a salad bowl, combine the spinach, herring, garlic, red onion, and bell pepper.
2. Toss your salad with 2 tablespoons of fresh lime juice. Season with the salt and pepper to your liking.
3. Serve immediately and enjoy!

208. HADDOCK AND PARMESAN FISH BURGERS

Preparation Time: 20 minutes
Servings: 4

Nutrition: 174 Calories; 11.4g Fat; 1.5g Carbs; 0.2g Fiber; 15.4g Protein;

Ingredients

- 8 ounces smoked haddock
- 4 lemon wedges
- 1 egg
- 1/4 cup scallions, chopped

- 1/4 cup Parmesan cheese, grated

Directions

1. Heat 1 tablespoon of olive oil in a frying pan over medium-high flame. Once hot, cook the haddock for 5 to 6 minutes; flake the fish with a fork, discarding the skin and bones
2. Add in cheese, eggs, and scallions; season with sea salt and pepper to taste.
3. Heat 1 tablespoon of olive oil until sizzling. Now, fry your burgers for 5 to 6 minutes until they are thoroughly cooked. Garnish with lemon wedges and enjoy!

209. GREEK-STYLE HALIBUT FILLETS

Preparation Time: 35 minutes
Servings: 4

Nutrition: 397 Calories; 32.1g Fat; 1.5g Carbs; 24.6g Protein; 0.6g Fiber

Ingredients

- 1 ½ pounds halibut fillets
- 1 tablespoon Greek seasoning blend
- 2 tablespoons fresh lemon juice
- 2 tablespoons olive oil
- 1/2 cup Kalamata olives, pitted and sliced

Directions

1. Begin by preheating your oven to 385 degrees F.
2. Toss the halibut fillets with Greek seasoning blend, lemon juice, and olive oil. Place the halibut fillets in a lightly-greased baking dish.
3. Bake for about 15 minutes, flip the fillets over and bake an additional 15 minutes.
4. Garnish with Kalamata olives and serve immediately!

210. COD FISH À LA NAGE

Preparation Time: 20 minutes
Servings: 5

Nutrition: 177 Calories; 6.4g Fat; 4g Carbs; 24.9g Protein; 1g Fiber

Ingredients

- 1 ½ pounds cod fish fillets
- 2 tablespoons olive oil
- 1 medium-sized zucchini, diced
- 2 vine-ripe tomatoes, pureed
- 1 Spanish onion, chopped

Directions

1. Heat the olive oil in a Dutch oven over medium-high heat. Cook the Spanish onion until softened.
2. Add in zucchini and pureed tomatoes; pour in 2 cups of water and bring to a boil. Turn the heat to medium-low. Allow it to simmer for about 12 minutes.
3. Stir in cod fish and continue to cook, covered, for about 6 minutes (an instant-read thermometer should register 140 degrees F).
4. Serve the fish with cooking juice. Bon appétit!

211. TILAPIA IN GARLIC BUTTER SAUCE

Preparation Time: 15 minutes
Servings: 6

Nutrition: 215 Calories; 13.5g Fat; 0.4g Carbs; 23.5g Protein; 0.1g Fiber

Ingredients

- 6 tilapia fillets, patted dry
- 1 teaspoon fresh lime juice
- 1 teaspoon garlic, minced
- 1 tablespoon parsley, chopped
- 6 tablespoons butter

Directions

1. Spritz a frying pan skillet with nonstick cooking oil. Preheat the frying pan over medium-high flame.
2. Once hot, fry the tilapia for 5 to 6 minutes; flip it over using a wide spatula and continue to cook for 5 minutes more.
3. Season with salt and black pepper to taste.
4. In a mixing bowl, whisk the butter, garlic, parsley, and lime juice. Serve warm fish with a dollop of chilled butter sauce. Bon appétit!

212. CHINESE FISH SALAD

Preparation Time: 15 minutes

Servings: 2

Nutrition: 277 Calories; 15.1g Fat; 4.9g Carbs; 24.4g Protein; 0.9g Fiber

Ingredients

- 1/2 pound salmon fillets
- 2 tablespoons low-carb salad dressing
- 1 tomato, sliced
- 1 medium-sized white onion, sliced
- 1 cup Chinese cabbage, sliced

Directions

1. Place 1/2 cup of water and in a saucepan over a moderate flame.
2. Now, cook the salmon fillets for about 7 minutes and reserve.
3. Place the Chinese cabbage, tomato, and onion in a serving bowl. Toss the salad with low-carb dressing. Top with reserved salmon fillets and serve!

213. 36INDIAN FISH FRY

Preparation Time: 15 minutes
Servings: 3

Nutrition: 443 Calories; 28.3g Fat; 2.6g Carbs; 42.5g Protein; 1g Fiber

Ingredients

- 3 carp fillets
- 1/2 teaspoon garam masala
- 3 tablespoons full-fat coconut milk
- 1 egg
- 2 tablespoons olive oil

Directions

1. Pat the fish fillets dry with pepper towels. Toss fish fillets with garam masala along with sea salt and black pepper.
2. In a mixing dish, beat the coconut milk and egg until pale and frothy. Dip the fillets into the milk/egg mixture.
3. Heat olive oil in a frying pan over medium-high heat. Fry the fish fillets until they begin to flake when tested with a fork.
4. Serve with curry leaves if desired and enjoy!

214. 36TILAPIA AND SHRIMP SOUP

Preparation Time: 25 minutes
Servings: 5

Nutrition: 215 Calories; 7g Fat; 5.6g Carbs; 26.4g Protein; 2.6g Fiber

Ingredients

- 1 cup celery, chopped
- 2 cups cauliflower, grated
- 2 cups tomato sauce with onion and garlic
- 1 pound tilapia, skinless and chopped into small chunks
- 1/2 pound medium shrimp, deveined

Directions

1. Melt 2 tablespoons of butter in a soup pot over medium-high flame. Once hot, cook celery and cauliflower for 4 to 5 minutes or until tender.
2. Add in tomato sauce along with 4 cups of chicken broth and bring to a boil. Now, turn the heat to medium-low.
3. Stir in the tilapia and continue to cook, partially covered, for about 10 minutes. Stir in the shrimp and continue to simmer for 3 to 4 minutes or until shrimp is pink.
4. Ladle into soup bowls and serve hot!

215. 36PROVENÇAL FISH AND PRAWN STEW

Preparation Time: 20 minutes
Servings: 5

Nutrition: 176 Calories; 6.5g Fat; 5.1g Carbs; 23.8g Protein; 0.8g Fiber

Ingredients

- 1/3 pound prawns
- 1 pound grouper fish
- 1/3 pound cockles, scrubbed
- 1 shallot, sliced
- 1 cup tomato sauce with onion and garlic

Directions

1. Heat 2 tablespoons of olive oil in a heavy-bottomed pot over medium-high heat. Sauté the shallot for 3 to 4 minutes or until it has softened.
2. Stir in tomato sauce along with 5 cups of

white fish stock. When the stew reaches boiling, add in salt and black pepper.

3. Reduce the heat to medium-low and stir in the grouper and cockles; continue to simmer for 2 to 3 minutes.
4. Fold in the prawns and continue to simmer approximately 3 minutes or until they are pink.
5. Garnish each serving with fresh lemon juice if desired and enjoy!

216.36MEXICAN-STYLE GRILLED SALMON

Preparation Time: 1 hour | 4

Nutrition: 331 Calories; 21.4g Fat; 2.2g Carbs; 30.4g Protein; 0.4g Fiber

Ingredients

- 2 cloves garlic, pressed
- 1 tablespoon Taco seasoning mix
- 2 tablespoons fresh lemon juice
- 4 (5-ounce) salmon steaks
- 4 tablespoons olive oil

Directions

1. Place all ingredients in a ceramic dish. Cover and allow it to marinate in your refrigerator for 35 to 40 minutes.
2. Grill the salmon steaks for about 6 minutes per side, basting with the reserved marinade.
3. Serve warm and enjoy!

217. 36PORTUGUESE CALDEIRADA DE PEIXE

Preparation Time: 25 minutes
Servings: 3

Nutrition: 191 Calories; 9.1g Fat; 2.8g Carbs; 23.9g Protein; 1.1g Fiber

Ingredients

- 3/4 pound sole fillets, cut into 1-inch pieces
- 1 shallot, chopped
- 1 cup tomatoes, pureed
- 1 teaspoon curry paste
- 1 tablespoon butter, at room temperature

Directions

1. In a heavy-bottomed pot, melt the butter a moderate flame. Sauté the shallot until tender and translucent.
2. Add in pureed tomatoes and curry paste and along with 2 cups of water. When your stew reaches boiling, immediately reduce the temperature to a simmer.
3. Continue to simmer, covered, for 10 to 15 minutes, stirring periodically.
4. Stir in sole fillets and continue to simmer for about 7 minutes or until the internal temperature of your fish reaches 145 degrees F. Enjoy!

218. 36SEA BASS WITH PEPPERS

Preparation Time: 20 minutes
Servings: 6

Nutrition: 218 Calories; 7.3g Fat; 7g Carbs; 29.3g Protein; 2g Fiber

Ingredients

- 2 pounds sea bass fillets, chopped into small chunks
- 2 cups marinara sauce, low-carb
- 1 leek, chopped
- 1 bell pepper, chopped
- 1 serrano pepper, chopped

Directions

1. Melt 2 tablespoons of butter in a soup pot over medium-high heat. Sauté the leek and peppers for about 4 to 5 minutes or until they have softened.
2. Add in marinara sauce and sea bass along with 4 cups fish stock. Turn the heat to a simmer.
3. Let it cook, partially covered, for 10 to 12 minutes. Bon appétit!

219. 36COD FISH SALAD (INSALATA DI BACCALÀ)

Preparation Time: 15 minutes
Servings: 5

Nutrition: 276 Calories; 6.9g Fat; 6.4g Carbs; 42.7g Protein; 1.7g Fiber

Ingredients

- 5 cod fillets
- 2 cups lettuce, cut into small pieces
- 1/4 cup balsamic vinegar
- 1 red onion, sliced
- 1/2 pound green cabbage, shredded

Directions

1. Heat 1 tablespoon of the olive oil in a large saucepan over a moderate flame.
2. Once hot, cook the fish for about 10 minutes or until it is golden brown on top. Flake the fish and reserve.
3. Then, whisk 3 tablespoons of olive oil and balsamic vinegar; season with salt and black pepper; stir in 1 tablespoon of stone-ground mustard, if desired.
4. Combine the lettuce, green cabbage, and onion in a serving bowl. Dress the salad and top with cod fish. Enjoy!

220. GROUND CHICKEN & PEAS CURRY

Servings: 3-4
Preparation Time: 15 minutes
Cooking Time: 6-10 minutes

Ingredients:

For Marinade:

- 3 tablespoons essential olive oil
- 2 bay leaves
- 2 onions, grinded to some paste
- ½ tablespoon garlic paste
- ½ tablespoon ginger paste
- 2 tomatoes, chopped finely
- 1 tablespoon ground cumin
- 1 tablespoon ground coriander
- 1 teaspoon ground turmeric
- 1 teaspoon red chili powder
- Salt, to taste
- 1-pound lean ground chicken
- 2 cups frozen peas
- 1½ cups water
- 1-2 teaspoons garam masala powder

Directions:

1. In a deep skillet, heat oil on medium heat.
2. Add bay leaves and sauté for approximately half a minute.
3. Add onion paste and sauté for approximately 3-4 minutes.
4. Add garlic and ginger paste and sauté for around 1-1½ minutes.
5. Add tomatoes and spices and cook, stirring occasionally for about 3-4 minutes.
6. Stir in chicken and cook for about 4-5 minutes.
7. Stir in peas and water and bring to a boil on high heat.
8. Reduce the heat to low and simmer approximately 5-8 minutes or till desired doneness.
9. Stir in garam masala and remove from heat.
10. Serve hot.

Nutrition:

Calories: 450, Fat: 10g, Carbohydrates: 19g, Fiber: 6g, Protein: 38g

221. CHICKEN MEATBALLS CURRY

Servings: 3-4
Preparation Time: 20 min
Cooking Time: 25 minutes

Ingredients:

For Meatballs:

- 1-pound lean ground chicken
- 1 tablespoon onion paste
- 1 teaspoon fresh ginger paste
- 1 teaspoons garlic paste
- 1 green chili, chopped finely
- 1 tablespoon fresh cilantro leaves, chopped
- 1 teaspoon ground coriander
- ½ teaspoon cumin seeds
- ½ teaspoon red chili powder
- ½ teaspoon ground turmeric
- Salt, to taste

For Curry:

- 3 tablespoons extra-virgin olive oil
- ½ teaspoon cumin seeds
- 1 (1-inch) cinnamon stick
- 3 whole cloves
- 3 whole green cardamoms
- 1 whole black cardamom
- 2 onions, chopped
- 1 teaspoon fresh ginger, minced
- 1 teaspoons garlic, minced
- 4 whole tomatoes, chopped finely
- 2 teaspoons ground coriander
- 1 teaspoon garam masala powder
- ½ teaspoon ground nutmeg
- ½ teaspoon red chili powder
- ½ teaspoon ground turmeric
- Salt, to taste
- 1 cup water

- Chopped fresh cilantro, for garnishing

Directions:

1. For meatballs in a substantial bowl, add all ingredients and mix till well combined.
2. Make small equal-sized meatballs from mixture.
3. In a big deep skillet, heat oil on medium heat.
4. Add meatballs and fry approximately 3-5 minutes or till browned from all sides.
5. Transfer the meatballs in a bowl.
6. In the same skillet, add cumin seeds, cinnamon stick, cloves, green cardamom and black cardamom and sauté approximately 1 minute.
7. Add onions and sauté for around 4-5 minutes.
8. Add ginger and garlic paste and sauté approximately 1 minute.
9. Add tomato and spices and cook, crushing with the back of spoon for approximately 2-3 minutes.
10. Add water and meatballs and provide to a boil.
11. Reduce heat to low.
12. Simmer for approximately 10 minutes.
13. Serve hot with all the garnishing of cilantro.

Nutrition:

Calories: 421, Fat: 8g, Carbohydrates: 18g, Fiber: 5g, Protein: 34g

222. GROUND CHICKEN WITH BASIL

Servings: 8
Preparation Time: fifteen minutes
Cooking Time: 16 minutes

Ingredients:

- 2 pounds lean ground chicken
- 3 tablespoons coconut oil, divided
- 1 zucchini, chopped
- 1 red bell pepper, seeded and chopped
- ½ of green bell pepper, seeded and chopped
- 4 garlic cloves, minced
- 1 (1-inch) piece fresh ginger, minced
- 1 (1-inch) piece fresh turmeric, minced
- 1 fresh red chile, sliced thinly
- 1 tablespoon organic honey
- 1 tablespoon coconut aminos
- 1½ tablespoons fish sauce
- ½ cup fresh basil, chopped
- Salt and freshly ground black pepper, to taste
- 1 tablespoon fresh lime juice

Directions:

1. Heat a large skillet on medium-high heat.
2. Add ground beef and cook for approximately 5 minutes or till browned completely.
3. Transfer the beef in a bowl.
4. In a similar pan, melt 1 tablespoon of coconut oil on medium-high heat.
5. Add zucchini and bell peppers and stir fry for around 3-4 minutes.
6. Transfer the vegetables inside bowl with chicken.
7. In exactly the same pan, melt remaining coconut oil on medium heat.
8. Add garlic, ginger, turmeric and red chile and sauté for approximately 1-2 minutes.
9. Add chicken mixture, honey and coconut aminos and increase the heat to high.
10. Cook, stirring occasionally for approximately 4-5 minutes or till sauce is nearly reduced.
11. Stir in remaining ingredients and take off from heat.

Nutrition:

Calories: 407, Fat: 7g, Carbohydrates: 20g, Fiber: 13g, Protein: 36g

223. CHICKEN &VEGGIE CASSEROLE

A winner recipe of your casserole to get a supper party. Honey sauce adds an abundant flavoring in chicken, mushroom and broccoli.
Servings: 4
Preparation Time: 15 minutes
Cooking Time: half an hour

Ingredients:

- 1/3 cup Dijon mustard

- 1/3 cup organic honey
- 1 teaspoon dried basil
- ¼ teaspoon ground turmeric
- 1 teaspoon dried basil, crushed
- Salt and freshly ground black pepper, to taste
- 1¾ pound chicken breasts
- 1 cup fresh white mushrooms, sliced
- ½ head broccoli, cut into small florets

Directions:

1. Preheat the oven to 350 degrees F. Lightly, grease a baking dish.
2. In a bowl, mix together all ingredients except chicken, mushrooms and broccoli.
3. Arrange chicken in prepared baking dish and top with mushroom slices.
4. Place broccoli florets around chicken evenly.
5. Pour 1 / 2 of honey mixture over chicken and broccoli evenly.
6. Bake for approximately twenty minutes.
7. Now, coat the chicken with remaining sauce and bake for approximately 10 minutes.

Nutrition:

Calories: 427, Fat: 9g, Carbohydrates: 16g, Fiber: 7g, Protein: 35g

224. CHICKEN & CAULIFLOWER RICE CASSEROLE

Amuse your loved ones with this particular easy but flavorful recipe of casserole at dinner time. Blend of spices, ginger and garlic gives a fragrant twist to the chicken casserole.
Servings: 8-10
Preparation Time: fifteen minutes
Cooking Time: an hour fifteen minutes

Ingredients:

- 2 tablespoons coconut oil, divided
- 3-pound bone-in chicken thighs and drumsticks
- Salt and freshly ground black pepper, to taste
- 3 carrots, peeled and sliced
- 1 onion, chopped finely
- 2 garlic cloves, chopped finely
- 2 tablespoons fresh cinnamon, chopped finely
- 2 teaspoons ground cumin
- 1 teaspoon ground coriander
- 12 teaspoon ground cinnamon
- ½ teaspoon ground turmeric
- 1 teaspoon paprika
- ¼ tsp red pepper cayenne
- 1 (28-ounce) can diced tomatoes with liquid
- 1 red bell pepper, seeded and cut into thin strips
- ½ cup fresh parsley leaves, minced
- Salt, to taste
- 1 head cauliflower, grated to some rice like consistency
- 1 lemon, sliced thinly

Directions:

1. Preheat the oven to 375 degrees F.
2. In a large pan, melt 1 tablespoon of coconut oil high heat.
3. Add chicken pieces and cook for about 3-5 minutes per side or till golden brown.
4. Transfer the chicken in a plate.
5. In a similar pan, sauté the carrot, onion, garlic and ginger for about 4-5 minutes on medium heat.
6. Stir in spices and remaining coconut oil.
7. Add chicken, tomatoes, bell pepper, parsley and salt and simmer for approximately 3-5 minutes.
8. In the bottom of a 13x9-inch rectangular baking dish, spread the cauliflower rice evenly.
9. Place chicken mixture over cauliflower rice evenly and top with lemon slices.
10. With a foil paper, cover the baking dish and bake for approximately 35 minutes.
11. Uncover the baking dish and bake approximately 25 minutes.

Nutrition:

Calories: 412, Fat: 12g, Carbohydrates: 23g, Fiber: 7g, Protein: 34g

225. CHICKEN MEATLOAF WITH VEGGIES

Servings: 4
Preparation Time: 20 minutes
Cooking Time: 1-1¼ hours

Ingredients:

For Meatloaf:

- ½ cup cooked chickpeas
- 2 egg whites
- 2½ teaspoons poultry seasoning
- Salt and freshly ground black pepper, to taste
- 10-ounce lean ground chicken
- 1 cup red bell pepper, seeded and minced
- 1 cup celery stalk, minced
- 1/3 cup steel-cut oats
- 1 cup tomato puree, divided
- 2 tablespoons dried onion flakes, crushed
- 1 tablespoon prepared mustard

For Veggies:

- 2-pounds summer squash, sliced
- 16-ounce frozen Brussels sprouts
- 2 tablespoons extra-virgin extra virgin olive oil
- Salt and freshly ground black pepper, to taste

Directions:

1. Preheat the oven to 350 degrees F. Grease a 9x5-inch loaf pan.
2. In a mixer, add chickpeas, egg whites, poultry seasoning, salt and black pepper and pulse till smooth.
3. Transfer a combination in a large bowl.
4. Add chicken, veggies oats, ½ cup of tomato puree and onion flakes and mix till well combined.
5. Transfer the amalgamation into prepared loaf pan evenly.
6. With both hands, press, down the amalgamation slightly.
7. In another bowl mix together mustard and remaining tomato puree.
8. Place the mustard mixture over loaf pan evenly.
9. Bake approximately 1-1¼ hours or till desired doneness.
10. Meanwhile in a big pan of water, arrange a steamer basket.
11. Bring to a boil and set summer time squash I steamer basket.
12. Cover and steam approximately 10-12 minutes.
13. Drain well and aside.
14. Now, prepare the Brussels sprouts according to package's directions.
15. In a big bowl, add veggies, oil, salt and black pepper and toss to coat well.
16. Serve the meatloaf with veggies.

Nutrition:

Calories: 420, Fat: 9g, Carbohydrates: 21g, Fiber: 14g, Protein: 36g

226. ROASTED SPATCHCOCK CHICKEN

Servings: 4-6
Preparation Time: twenty or so minutes
Cooking Time: 50 minutes

Ingredients:

- 1 (4-pound) whole chicken
- 1 (1-inch) piece fresh ginger, sliced
- 4 garlic cloves, chopped
- 1 small bunch fresh thyme
- Pinch of cayenne
- Salt and freshly ground black pepper, to taste
- ¼ cup fresh lemon juice
- 3 tablespoons extra virgin olive oil

Directions:

1. Arrange chicken, breast side down onto a large cutting board.
2. With a kitchen shear, begin with thigh and cut along 1 side of backbone and turn chicken around.
3. Now, cut along sleep issues and discard the backbone.
4. Change the inside and open it like a book.
5. Flatten the backbone firmly to flatten.
6. In a food processor, add all ingredients except chicken and pulse till smooth.
7. In a big baking dish, add the marinade mixture.
8. Add chicken and coat with marinade generously.
9. With a plastic wrap, cover the baking dish and refrigerate to marinate for overnight.

10. Preheat the oven to 450 degrees F. Arrange a rack in a very roasting pan.
11. Remove the chicken from refrigerator make onto rack over roasting pan, skin side down.
12. Roast for about 50 minutes, turning once in the middle way.

Nutrition:

Calories: 419, Fat: 14g, Carbohydrates: 28g, Fiber: 4g, Protein: 40g

227. ROASTED CHICKEN WITH VEGGIES & ORANGE

Servings: 4
Preparation Time: 20 min
Cooking Time: 1 hour
Ingredients:

- 1 teaspoon ground ginger
- ½ teaspoon ground cumin
- ½ teaspoon ground coriander
- 1 teaspoon paprika
- Salt and freshly ground black pepper, to taste
- 1 (3 ½-4-pound) whole chicken
- 1 unpeeled orange, cut into 8 wedges
- 2 medium carrots, peeled and cut 1nto 2-inch pieces
- 2 medium sweet potatoes, peeled and cut into ½-inch wedges
- ½ cup water

Directions:

1. Preheat the oven to 450 degrees F.
2. In a little bowl, mix together the spices.
3. Rub the chicken with spice mixture evenly.
4. Arrange the chicken in a substantial Dutch oven and put orange, carrot and sweet potato pieces around it.
5. Add water and cover the pan tightly.
6. Roast for around 30 minutes.
7. Uncover and roast for about half an hour.

Nutrition:

Calories: 432, Fat: 10g, Carbohydrates: 20g, Fiber: 15g, Protein: 34g

228. ROASTED CHICKEN BREAST

Servings: 4-6
Preparation Time: 15 minutes
Cooking Time: 40 minutes

Ingredients:

- ½ of small apple, peeled, cored and chopped
- 1 bunch scallion, trimmed and copped roughly
- 8 fresh ginger slices, chopped
- 2 garlic cloves, chopped
- 3 tablespoons essential olive oil
- 12 teaspoon sesame oil, toasted
- 3 tablespoons using apple cider vinegar
- 1 tablespoon fish sauce
- 1 tablespoon coconut aminos
- Salt and freshly ground black pepper, to taste
- 4-pounds chicken thighs

Directions:

1. In a blender, add all ingredients except chicken thighs and pulse till smooth.
2. Transfer a combination and chicken right into a large Ziploc bag and seal it.
3. Shake the bag to coat the chicken with marinade well.
4. Refrigerate to marinade for about 12 hours.
5. Preheat the oven to 400 degrees F. Arrange a rack in foil paper lined baking sheet.
6. Place the chicken thighs on rack, skin-side down.
7. Roast for about 40 minutes, flipping once within the middle way.

Nutrition:

Calories: 451, Fat: 17g, Carbohydrates: 277g, Fiber: 4g, Protein: 42g

229. ROASTED CHICKEN DRUMSTICKS

Servings: 4-6
Preparation Time: fifteen minutes
Cooking Time: 50 minutes

Ingredients:

- 1 medium onion, chopped

- 1-2 tablespoons fresh turmeric, chopped
- 1-2 tablespoons fresh ginger, chopped
- 2 lemongrass stalks (bottom third), peeled and chopped
- 1-2 jalapeños, seeded and chopped
- 1 teaspoon fresh lime zest, grated
- 1 tablespoon curry powder
- 1¼ cups unsweetened coconut milk
- 3 tablespoons fresh lime juice
- 1 tablespoon coconut aminos
- 1 tablespoon fish sauce
- 4-pound chicken kegs
- Chopped fresh cilantro, for garnishing

Directions:

1. In a blender, add all ingredients except chicken legs and pulse till smooth.
2. Transfer a combination in a large baking dish.
3. Add chicken and coat with marinade generously.
4. Cover and refrigerate to marinade approximately 12 hours.
5. Remove chicken from refrigerator and in room temperature approximately 25-half an hour before cooking.
6. Preheat the oven to 350 degrees F.
7. Uncover the baking dish and roast or about 50 minutes.

Nutrition:

Calories: 432, Fat: 13g, Carbohydrates: 19g, Fiber: 6g, Protein: 35g

230. GRILLED CHICKEN

Servings: 8
Preparation Time: 15 minutes
Cooking Time: 41 minutes

Ingredients:

- 1 (3-inch) piece fresh ginger, minced
- 6 small garlic cloves, minced
- 1½ tablespoons tamarind paste
- 1 tablespoon organic honey
- ¼ cup coconut aminos
- 2½ tablespoons extra virgin olive oil
- 1½ tablespoons sesame oil, toasted
- ½ teaspoon ground cardamom
- Salt and freshly ground white pepper, to taste
- 1 (4-5-pound) whole chicken, cut into 8 pieces

Directions:

1. In a large glass bowl, mix together all ingredients except chicken pieces.
2. With a fork, pierce the chicken pieces completely.
3. Add chicken pieces in bowl and coat with marinade generously.
4. Cover and refrigerate to marinate for approximately a couple of hours to overnight.
5. Preheat the grill to medium heat. Grease the grill grate.
6. Place the chicken pieces on grill, bone-side down.
7. Grill, covered approximately 20-25 minutes.
8. Change the side and grill, covered approximately 6-8 minutes.
9. Change alongside it and grill, covered for about 5-8 minutes.

Nutrition:

Calories: 423, Fat: 12g, Carbohydrates: 20g, Fiber: 3g, Protein: 42g

231. GRILLED CHICKEN BREAST

Servings: 4
Preparation Time: 15 minutes
Cooking Time: 20 minutes

Ingredients:

- 2 scallions, chopped
- 1 (1-inch) piece fresh ginger, minced
- 2 minced garlic cloves
- 1 cup fresh pineapple juice
- ¼ cup coconut aminos
- ¼ cup extra-virgin organic olive oil
- 1 teaspoon ground cinnamon
- 1 teaspoon ground cumin
- 1 teaspoon ground turmeric
- Salt, to taste
- 4 skinless, boneless chicken breasts

Directions:

1. In a big Ziploc bag add all ingredients and

seal it.

2. Shake the bag to coat the chicken with marinade well.
3. Refrigerate to marinade for about twenty or so minutes to an hour.
4. Preheat the grill to medium-high heat. Grease the grill grate.
5. Place the chicken pieces on grill and grill for about 10 min per side.

Nutrition:

Calories: 445, Fat: 9g, Carbohydrates: 21g, Fiber: 4g, Protein: 39g

232. GRILLED CHICKEN WITH PINEAPPLE & VEGGIES

Servings: 4
Preparation Time: twenty or so minutes
Cooking Time: 22 minutes

Ingredients:

For Sauce:

- 1 garlic oil, minced
- ¾ teaspoon fresh ginger, minced
- ½ cup coconut aminos
- ¼ cup fresh pineapple juice
- 2 tablespoons freshly squeezed lemon juice
- 2 tablespoons balsamic vinegar
- ¼ teaspoon red pepper flakes, crushed
- Salt and freshly ground black pepper, to taste

For Grilling:

- 4 skinless, boneless chicken breasts
- 1 pineapple, peeled and sliced
- 1 bell pepper, seeded and cubed
- 1 zucchini, sliced
- 1red onion, sliced

Directions:

1. For sauce in a pan, mix together all ingredients on medium-high heat.
2. Bring to a boil reducing the heat to medium-low.
3. Cook approximately 5-6 minutes.
4. Remove from heat and keep aside to cool down the slightly.
5. Coat the chicken breasts about ¼ from the sauce.
6. Keep aside for approximately half an hour.
7. Preheat the grill to medium-high heat. Grease the grill grate.
8. Place the chicken pieces on grill and grill for around 5-8 minutes per side.
9. Now, squeeze pineapple and vegetables on grill grate.
10. Grill the pineapple for around 3 minutes per side.
11. Grill the vegetables for approximately 4-5 minutes, stirring once inside middle way.
12. Cut the chicken breasts into desired size slices.
13. Divide chicken, pineapple and vegetables in serving plates.
14. Serve alongside remaining sauce.

Nutrition:

Calories: 435, Fat: 12g, Carbohydrates: 25g, Fiber: 13g, Protein: 38g

233. GROUND TURKEY WITH VEGGIES

Servings: 4
Preparation Time: 15 minutes
Cooking Time: 12 minutes

Ingredients:

- 1 tablespoon sesame oil
- 1 tablespoon coconut oil
- 1-pound lean ground turkey
- 2 tablespoons fresh ginger, minced
- 2 minced garlic cloves
- 1 (16-ounce) bag vegetable mix (broccoli, carrot, cabbage, kale and Brussels sprouts)
- ¼ cup coconut aminos
- 2 tablespoons balsamic vinegar

Directions:

1. In a big skillet heat both oils on medium-high heat.
2. Add turkey, ginger and garlic and cook approximately 5-6 minutes.
3. Add vegetable mix and cook approximately 4-5 minutes.
4. Stir in coconut aminos and vinegar and cook for about 1 minute.
5. Serve hot.

Nutrition:

Calories: 234, Fat: 9g, Carbohydrates: 9g, Fiber: 3g, Protein: 29g

234. GROUND TURKEY WITH ASPARAGUS

Servings: 8
Preparation Time: 15 minutes
Cooking Time: fifteen minutes

Ingredients:

- 1¾ pound lean ground turkey
- 2 tablespoons sesame oil
- 1 medium onion, chopped
- 1 cup celery, chopped
- 6 garlic cloves, minced
- 2 cups asparagus, trimmed and cut into 1-inch pieces
- 1/3 cup coconut aminos
- 2½ teaspoons ginger powder
- 2 tablespoons organic coconut crystals
- 1 tablespoon arrowroot starch
- 1 tablespoon cold water
- ¼ teaspoon red pepper flakes, crushed

Directions:

1. Heat a substantial nonstick skillet on medium-high heat.
2. Add turkey and cook for approximately 5-7 minutes or till browned.
3. With a slotted spoon transfer the turkey inside a bowl and discard the grease from skillet.
4. In exactly the same skillet, heat oil on medium heat.
5. Add onion, celery and garlic and sauté for about 5 minutes.
6. Add asparagus and cooked turkey minimizing the temperature to medium-low.
7. Meanwhile inside a pan mix together coconut aminos, ginger powder and coconut crystals n medium heat and convey to some boil.
8. In a smaller bowl, mix together arrowroot starch and water.
9. Slowly, add arrowroot mixture, stirring continuously.
10. Cook approximately 2-3 minutes.
11. Add the sauce in s killed with turkey mixture and stir to blend.
12. Stir in red pepper flakes and cook for approximately 2-3 minutes.
13. Serve hot.

Nutrition:

Calories: 309, Fat: 20g, Carbohydrates: 19g, Fiber: 2g, Protein: 28g

235. GROUND TURKEY WITH PEAS & POTATO

Servings: 4
Preparation Time: fifteen minutes
Cooking Time: 35 minutes

Ingredients:

- 3-4 tablespoons coconut oil
- 1-pound lean ground turkey
- 1-2 fresh red chiles, chopped
- 1 onion, chopped
- Salt, to taste
- 2 minced garlic cloves
- 1 (1-inch) piece fresh ginger, grated finely
- 1 tablespoon curry powder
- 1 teaspoon ground coriander
- 1 teaspoon ground cumin
- 1 teaspoon ground turmeric
- 2 large Yukon gold potatoes, peeled and cubed into 1-inch size
- ½ cup water
- 1 cup fresh peas, shelled
- 2-4 plum tomatoes, chopped
- ½ cup fresh cilantro, chopped

Directions:

1. In a substantial pan, heat oil on medium-high heat.
2. Add turkey and cook for about 4-5 minutes.
3. Add chiles and onion and cook for about 4-5 minutes.
4. Add garlic and ginger and cook approximately 1-2 minutes.
5. Stir in spices, potatoes and water and convey to your boil
6. Reduce the warmth to medium-low.

7. Simmer, covered approximately 15-twenty or so minutes.
8. Add peas and tomatoes and cook for about 2-3 minutes.
9. Serve using the garnishing of cilantro.

Nutrition:

Calories: 452, Fat: 14g, Carbohydrates: 24g, Fiber: 13g, Protein: 36g

236. TURKEY & PUMPKIN CHILI

Servings: 4-6
Preparation Time: 15 minutes
Cooking Time: 41 minutes

Ingredients:

- 2 tablespoons extra-virgin olive oil
- 1 green bell pepper, seeded and chopped
- 1 small yellow onion, chopped
- 2 garlic cloves, chopped finely
- 1-pound lean ground turkey
- 1 (15-ounce) pumpkin puree
- 1 (14 ½-ounce) can diced tomatoes with liquid
- 1 teaspoon ground cumin
- ½ teaspoon ground turmeric
- ½ teaspoon ground cinnamon
- 1 cup water
- 1 (15-ounce) can chickpeas, rinsed and drained

Directions:

1. In a big pan, heat oil on medium-low heat.
2. Add the bell pepper, onion and garlic and sauté approximately 5 minutes.
3. Add turkey and cook for about 5-6 minutes.
4. Add tomatoes, pumpkin, spices and water and convey to your boil on high heat.
5. Reduce the temperature to medium-low heat and stir in chickpeas.
6. Simmer, covered for approximately a half-hour, stirring occasionally.
7. Serve hot.

Nutrition:

Calories: 437, Fat: 17g, Carbohydrates: 29g, Fiber: 16g, Protein: 42g

237. TURKEY & VEGGIES CHILI

Servings: 8
Preparation Time: 15 minutes
Cooking Time: 35 minutes

Ingredients:

- 3 tablespoons essential olive oil, divided
- 1½ pound lean ground turkey
- 2 tablespoons tomato paste
- 1 teaspoon dried oregano, crushed
- 1 teaspoon ground coriander
- 1 teaspoon ground cumin
- ½ teaspoon ground cinnamon
- ½ teaspoon ground turmeric
- 1½ cups chicken broth
- 3 cups cooked sprouted beans trio
- ½ cup mild salsa
- 2 carrots, peeled and chopped
- 1 (14½-ounce) can crushed tomatoes
- 1 medium onion, chopped
- 2 garlic cloves, chopped finely
- 3 medium zucchinis, chopped
- 1 cup cheddar cheese
- 4 scallions, chopped

Directions:

1. In a sizable pan, heat 1 tablespoon of oil on medium-high heat.
2. Add turkey and with the spoon, plunge into pieces.
3. Add tomato paste, oregano and spices and cook for about 4-5 minutes.
4. Add broth and provide to a boil,
5. Reduce the temperature to medium and simmer for around 5 minutes.
6. Add beans trio, salsa, carrots and tomatoes and simmer for about 10 minutes.
7. Meanwhile in a substantial skillet, heat remaining oil on medium-high heat.
8. Add onion and garlic and sauté for about 5 minutes.
9. Add zucchini and cook for approximately 5 minutes, stirring occasionally.
10. Transfer the zucchini mixture within the chili mixture and transfer the warmth to low.
11. Simmer for around 15 minutes.

Nutrition:

Calories: 411, Fat: 10g, Carbohydrates: 19g, Fiber: 14g, Protein: 37g

238. GROUND TURKEY WITH LENTILS

Servings: 8
Preparation Time: 15 minutes
Cooking Time: 35 minutes

Ingredients:

- 3 tablespoons olive oil, divided
- 1 onion, chopped
- 1 tablespoon fresh ginger, minced
- 4 garlic cloves, minced
- 2 Roma tomatoes, seeded and chopped
- 3 celery stalks, chopped
- 1 large carrot, peeled and chopped
- 1 cup dried red lentils, rinsed, soaked for thirty minutes and drained
- 2 cups chicken broth
- 1 teaspoon black mustard seeds
- 1½ teaspoons cumin seeds
- 1 teaspoon ground turmeric
- ½ teaspoon paprika
- 1-pound lean ground turkey
- 1 Serrano chile, seeded and chopped
- 2 scallions, chopped
- Chopped fresh cilantro, for garnishing

Directions:

1. In a Dutch oven, heat 1 tablespoon of oil on medium heat.
2. Add onion, ginger and garlic and sauté for around 5 minutes.
3. Stir in tomatoes, celery, carrot, lentils and broth and convey to your boil
4. Reduce the warmth to medium-low.
5. Simmer, covered for around thirty minutes.
6. Meanwhile in a skillet, heat remaining oil on medium heat.
7. Add mustard seeds and cumin seeds and sauté approximately 30 seconds.
8. Add turmeric and paprika and sauté approximately 25 seconds.
9. Transfer a combination into a small bowl and aside.
10. In exactly the same skillet, add turkey and cook for around 4-5 minutes.
11. Add Serrano chile and scallion and cook for about 3-4 minutes.
12. Add spiced oil mixture and stir to mix well.
13. Transfer the turkey mixture in simmering lentils and simmer for around 5-10 minutes more.

Nutrition:

Calories: 422, Fat: 9g, Carbohydrates: 17g, Fiber: 14g, Protein: 37g

239. ROASTED WHOLE TURKEY

Servings: 8-10
Preparation Time: 15 minutes
Cooking Time: 3 hours 30 minutes

Ingredients:

For Turkey Marinade:

- 1 (2-inch) piece fresh ginger, grated finely
- 3 large garlic cloves, crushed
- 1 green chili, chopped finely
- 1 teaspoon fresh lemon zest, grated finely
- 5-ounce plain Greek yogurt
- 3 tablespoons tomato puree
- 2 tablespoons fresh lemon juice
- 1 tablespoon ground cumin
- 1½ tablespoons garam masala
- 2 teaspoons ground turmeric

For Turkey:

- 1 (9-pound) whole turkey, giblets and neck removed
- Salt and freshly ground black pepper, to taste
- 1 garlic clove, halved
- 1 lime, halved
- ½ of lemon

Directions:

1. In a bowl, mix together all marinade ingredients.
2. With a fork, pierce the turkey completely.
3. In a sizable baking dish, put the turkey.
4. Rub the turkey with marinade mixture evenly.
5. Refrigerate to marinate for overnight.
6. Remove from refrigerator and make aside approximately a half-hour before serving.

7. Preheat the oven to 390 degrees F.
8. Sprinkle turkey with salt and black pepper evenly and stuff the cavity with garlic, lime and lemon.
9. Arrange the turkey in a big roasting pan and roast for approximately a half-hour.
10. Now, reduce the temperature of oven to 350 degrees F.
11. Roast for around 3 hours. (if skin becomes brown during roasting, then cover with foil paper)

Nutrition:

Calories: 434, Fat: 12g, Carbohydrates: 20g, Fiber: 3g, Protein: 39g

240. GRILLED TURKEY BREAST

A moist and flavorful turkey breast with crispy touch. This barbequed turkey breast will likely be an excellent addition within your menu list.
Servings: 4
Preparation Time: 15 minutes
Cooking Time: 6-10 min

Ingredients:

- 1 large shallot, quartered
- (¾-inch) piece fresh ginger, chopped
- 2 small garlic cloves, chopped
- 1 tablespoon honey
- ¼ cup extra virgin olive oil
- ¼ cup coconut aminos
- 2 tablespoons fresh lime juice
- Freshly ground black pepper, to taste
- 4 turkey breast tenderloins

Directions:

1. In a food processor, add shallot, ginger and garlic and pulse till minced.
2. Add remaining ingredients except turkey tenderloins and pulse till well combined.
3. Transfer the mixture in a sizable bowl.
4. Add turkey tenderloins and coat with mixture generously.
5. Keep aside, covered for approximately 30 minutes.
6. Preheat the grill to medium heat. Grease the grill grate.
7. Grill for about 6-8 minutes per side.

Nutrition:

Calories: 412, Fat: 14g, Carbohydrates: 17g, Fiber: 3g, Protein: 38g

241. DUCK WITH BOK CHOY

Servings: 4-6
Preparation Time: 15 minutes
Cooking Time: 12 minutes

Ingredients:

- 2 tablespoons coconut oil
- 1 onion, sliced thinly
- 2 teaspoons fresh ginger, grated finely
- 2 minced garlic cloves
- 1 tablespoon fresh orange zest, grated finely
- ¼ cup chicken broth
- 2/3 cup fresh orange juice
- 1 roasted duck, meat picked
- 3-pound Bok choy leaves
- 1 orange, peeled, seeded and segmented

Directions:

1. In a sizable skillet, melt coconut oil on medium heat.
2. Add onion, ginger and garlic and sauté for around 3 minutes.
3. Add ginger and garlic and sauté for about 1-2 minutes.
4. Stir in orange zest, broth and orange juice.
5. Add duck meat and cook for around 3 minutes.
6. Transfer the meat pieces in a plate.
7. Add Bok choy and cook for about 3-4 minutes.
8. Divide Bok choy mixture in serving plates and top with duck meat.
9. Serve with the garnishing of orange segments.

Nutrition:

Calories: 433, Fat: 12g, Carbohydrates: 21g, Fiber: 9g, Protein: 34g

242. GRILLED DUCK BREAST & PEACH

Servings: 2
Preparation Time: 15 minutes
Cooking Time: 24 minutes

Ingredients:

- 2 shallots, sliced thinly
- 2 tablespoons fresh ginger, minced
- 2 tablespoons fresh thyme, chopped
- Salt and freshly ground black pepper, to taste
- 2 duck breasts
- 2 peaches, pitted and quartered
- ½ teaspoon ground fennel seeds
- ½ tablespoon extra-virgin olive oil

Directions:

1. In a substantial bowl, mix together shallots, ginger, thyme, salt and black pepper.
2. Add duck breasts and coat with marinade evenly.
3. Refrigerate to marinate for about 2-12 hours.
4. Preheat the grill to medium-high heat. Grease the grill grate.
5. In a sizable bowl, add peaches, fennel seeds, salt, black pepper and oil and toss to coat well.
6. Place the duck breast on grill, skin side down and grill for around 6-8 minutes per side.
7. Transfer the duck breast onto a plate.
8. Now, grill the peaches for around 3 minutes per side.
9. Serve the duck breasts with grilled peaches.

Nutrition:

Calories: 450, Fat: 14g, Carbohydrates: 25g, Fiber: 12g, Protein: 42g

243. SLOW COOKER TURKEY LEGS

Servings 6
Preparation Time: 6 hours

Ingredients

- 2 turkey legs
- 1 tablespoon mustard
- 1 tablespoon butter
- 1/2 teaspoon smoked paprika
- 1 teaspoon dried rosemary
- Salt and pepper, to taste
- 1 chopped leek
- 1/2 teaspoon minced garlic
- For the Gravy:
- 1/2 stick butter
- 1 cup heavy cream
- Salt and pepper, to taste

Directions

1. Rub turkey legs with the mustard and butter.
2. Preheat a skillet over a medium-high heat Fry the turkey legs on all sides, making sure that they are brown all over.
3. Put the turkey legs in the slow cooker, but keep the fat to one side. Add the paprika, rosemary, pepper, salt, leeks and garlic.
4. Put the slow cooker on low and cook for 6 hours.
5. Heat the reserved fat with 1/2 stick of butter on a medium flame. Add the cream to the fat and stir until the mixture is hot.
6. Add salt and pepper and stir until the sauce is thickened and hot. Serve the sauce on top of the chicken drumsticks. Enjoy.

Nutrition: Calories280 ,Protein 15.8g ,Fat 22.2g ,Carbs 4.3g ,Sugar 1.7g

244. TURKEY AND CAULIFLOWER SOUP LIKE GRANDMA USED TO MAKE

Servings 4
Preparation Time: 35 minutes

Ingredients

- 2 tablespoons coconut oil
- 2 chopped garlic cloves
- 2 chopped shallots
- 4 ½ cups chicken stock
- 1/2 head cauliflower florets
- 1 pound turkey thighs
- 2 bay leaves
- 1 rosemary sprig
- 1/2 teaspoon celery seeds
- Salt and ground black pepper, to taste
- 1/2 teaspoon cayenne pepper
- 4 dollops of sour cream

Directions

1. Preheat a heavy pot over a medium flame and heat the oil. Sauté the garlic and shallots until they are fragrant.
2. Pour in the chicken stock and bring to the boil.
3. Add the turkey, cauliflower, bay leaves, celery seeds, rosemary, salt, pepper and cayenne pepper.
4. Simmer on a moderate-low heat for 25 – 30 minutes.
5. Pour the soup into 4 bowls and put a dollop of sour cream on each Enjoy!

Nutrition: Calories274 ,Protein 26.7g ,Fat 14.4g ,Carbs 5.6g ,Sugar 3.1g

245. CHICKEN LEFTOVERS CHOWDER

Servings 4
Preparation Time: 35 minutes

Ingredients

- 2 tablespoons coconut oil
- 2 roughly chopped cloves of garlic
- A bunch of chopped scallions
- 1/2 pound shredded and skinned leftover roast chicken
- 2 rosemary sprigs
- 1 bay leaf
- 1 thyme sprig
- 1 tablespoon chicken bouillon granules
- 3 cups water
- 1/2 cup whipped cream
- 1 1/2 cups milk
- 1 lightly beaten whole egg
- 1 tablespoons dry sherry

Directions

1. Preheat a stockpot over a moderate flame and melt the coconut oil. Sauté the garlic and scallions until softened and fragrant.
2. Add the chicken, rosemary, bay leaf, thyme, chicken bouillon granules and water. Partially cover and bring to the boil. Then simmer for 20 minutes.
3. Turn the heat down to low and add the whipped cream and milk. Simmer until it has thickened. Put in the egg and stir for a couple of minutes.
4. Taste to make sure the seasoning is right. Ladle into individual bowls and drizzle each with the sherry. Enjoy!

Nutrition: Calories350 ,Protein 20g ,Fat 25.8g ,Carbs 5.5g ,Sugar 2.8g

246. AMAZING TURKEY KEBABS

Servings 6
Preparation Time: 30 minutes

Ingredients

- 1 1/2 pounds diced British turkey thigh
- 2 tablespoons butter, at room temperature
- 1 tablespoon dry ranch seasoning
- 1 red onion, cut into wedges
- 1 sliced zucchini
- 2 sliced orange bell peppers
- 1 sliced red bell pepper
- 1 sliced green bell pepper
- 1 cup sliced radishes
- 1 sliced cucumber
- 2 tablespoons red wine vinegar
- 1 tablespoon roughly chopped fresh parsley

Directions

1. Rub the butter on the turkey and then add the seasoning. Put the turkey pieces on skewers.
2. Alternate the onion, zucchini and bell peppers on the skewers and put in the fridge while you get the grill ready.
3. Put the kebabs on the grill and cook for 9 minutes, turning every now and then.
4. While they are cooking mix the radishes and cucumbers with the parsley and red wine vinegar.
5. Serve the kebabs with the salad straight away and enjoy!

Nutrition: Calories 293 ,Protein 34.5g ,Fat 13.8g ,Carbs 3.7g ,Sugar 1.9g

247. HEALTHY CHICKEN SALAD

Servings 4
Preparation Time: 20 minutes

Ingredients

- 2 chicken breasts
- 1/3 teaspoon crushed red pepper flakes
- 1/2 teaspoon sea salt
- 1/4 teaspoon dried thyme, or to taste
- 1 large pitted and sliced avocado
- 2 egg yolks
- 1 tablespoon Worcestershire sauce
- 1/3 cup olive oil
- 1 tablespoon lime juice
- 1/2 teaspoon mustard powder
- 1/3 teaspoon sea salt

Directions

1. Put your grill on high. Season the chicken breasts with pepper, salt and thyme. Cook each side of the chicken for 3 – 5 minutes until browned.
2. Cut the grilled chicken into strips.
3. Put the sliced avocado onto 4 plates.
4. Make the dressing. Combine the egg yolks, Worcestershire sauce, olive oil, lime juice, mustard powder and sea salt.
5. Put the chicken strips on top of the avocado and then pour the dressing over them. Enjoy!

Nutrition: Calories 400 ,Protein 22.7g ,Fat 34.2g ,Carbs 4.8g ,Sugar 0.4g

248. SPICY CHICKEN AND HEMP SEEDS

Servings 6
Preparation Time: 55 minutes

Ingredients

- 3 chicken breasts cut into strips
- Salt and pepper to taste
- 1/2 stick butter
- 2 cloves minced garlic
- 2 tablespoons tomato paste
- 1/2 teaspoon sugar-free hot chili sauce
- 3 teaspoons apple cider vinegar
- 2 tablespoons soy sauce
- 2 eggs
- 1/4 cup hemp seeds
- Fresh chives

Directions

1. Put your oven on to 4100F and grease a baking dish with cooking spray.
2. Rub the chicken wings with the salt, pepper and butter.
3. Mix together the garlic, tomato paste, chili sauce, vinegar and soy sauce. Pour this over the chicken wings and leave to marinate for 30 minutes in your fridge.
4. Whisk together the hemp seeds and eggs. Put the chicken strips into this mixture and then put them on the baking dish.
5. Cook for 20 – 25 minutes and turn over once. Broil the chicken strips if you want them to be crispier.
6. Serve the chicken strips with a chive garnish.

Nutrition: Calories 374.9 ,Protein 24g ,Fat 28.5g ,Carbs 5.6g ,Sugar 2g

249. CHICKEN WITH A MUSTARD AND CREAM SAUCE

Servings 4
Preparation Time: 25 minutes

Ingredients

- 1 pound chicken fillets
- Salt and pepper, to taste
- 1 tablespoon melted butter
- 1 teaspoon garlic paste
- 1/2 cup chopped scallions
- 1/4 cup dry white wine
- 1/2 cup double cream
- ¼ cup low-sodium chicken broth
- 2 tablespoons whole grain mustard
- 1/2 cup roughly chopped fresh cilantro

Directions

1. Rub the chicken fillets with as much salt and pepper you want.
2. Preheat a pan over a medium flame and melt the butter. Fry the chicken fillets until they are just done. Set the chicken to one side.
3. Cook the garlic and scallions in the pan and stir every now and again. Cook until they are fragrant; about 4 minutes.
4. Put the heat up to moderate-high and pour in the wine. Scrape any bits that

might be stuck to the saucepan.

5. Pour in the broth and reduce the liquid to half. Stir in the mustard and double cream.
6. Place the chicken on 4 serving plates and pour the sauce over them. Garnish with the fresh cilantro.

Nutrition: Calories 311 ,Protein 33.6g ,Fat 16.9g ,Carbs 2.1g ,Sugar 0.4g

250. DELICIOUS AND EASY CHICKEN DRUMETTES

Servings 4
Preparation Time: 30 minutes

Ingredients

- 2 tablespoons tallow
- 4 chicken drumettes
- Salt, to taste
- 2 minced cloves garlic
- 1/2 cups chopped leeks
- 1 rosemary sprig
- 1 thyme sprig
- 1 teaspoon mixed peppercorns
- 1 tablespoon Worcestershire sauce
- 2 crushed tomatoes
- 1 teaspoon cayenne pepper
- 1 teaspoon dried marjoram
- 1/2 teaspoon mustard seeds
- 1 cup turkey stock

Directions

1. Put a saucepan on a moderate-high heat and melt the tallow, Put the salt on the chicken drumettes.
2. Fry the chicken drumettes until they are brown on all sides. Put to one side.
3. In the pan drippings cook the garlic and leeks over a moderate heat for 4 – 6 minutes.
4. Add the remaining ingredients and the chicken and simmer for 15 – 20 minutes partially covered. Serve hot.

Nutrition: Calories 165 ,Protein 12.4g ,Fat 9.8g ,Carbs 4.7g ,Sugar 2.9g

251. SALSA CHICKEN SAUSAGE

Servings 4
Preparation Time: 15 minutes

Ingredients

- 2 teaspoons lard at room temperature
- 4 sliced chicken sausage
- 1/4 cup Sauvignon Blanc
- 3 teaspoons lime juice
- 2 tablespoons minced fresh cilantro
- 1 cup diced onion
- 1 minced jalapeno pepper
- 1 cup pureed tomato
- 1 teaspoon granulated garlic
- 2 deveined and chopped bell peppers

Directions

1. Put a skillet on medium-high heat and warm the lard.
2. Fry the chicken sausage until browned. Pour in the wine and cook for 3 minutes. Put to one side.
3. Make the salsa by mixing together the lime juice, cilantro, onion, jalapeno pepper, tomato, garlic and bell peppers.
4. Place the sausage on 4 plates and put the salsa on the side. Bon appétit!

Nutrition: Calories 156 ,Protein 16.2g ,Fat 4.2g ,Carbs 4.1g ,Sugar 2.4g

Bok Choy and Turkey Sausage

Servings 4
Preparation Time: 50 minutes

Ingredients

- 1 tablespoon butter
- 4 sliced mild turkey sausages, breakfast links
- 1 pound trimmed Bok Choy
- 2 chopped shallots
- Coarse salt and ground black pepper to taste
- 1/8 teaspoon freshly grated nutmeg
- 1 cup chicken stock
- ½ cup full-fat milk
- 6 ounces coarsely grated Gruyère

Directions

1. Preheat the oven to 3600F. In a saucepan melt the butter and brown the turkey sausages, turning every now and again. Put

to one side.
2. Add the Bok Choy, shallots, salt and pepper. Cook until soft. This should take 2 – 3 minutes.
3. Put the Bok Choy mixture in a greased baking dish and top with the turkey sausage.
4. Mix together the nutmeg, chicken stock and milk and pour over the Bok Choy and sausage.
5. Cover the baking dish with foil and cook for 40 minutes. Remove the foil and sprinkle the cheese on top.
6. Bake for a few minutes until the cheese bubbles.

Nutrition: Calories 189 ,Protein9.4g ,Fat 12g ,Carbs 2.6g ,Sugar 13g

252. SIMPLE TURKEY AND HERB DRUMSTICKS

Servings 2
Preparation Time: 1 hour

Ingredients

- 2 tablespoons apple cider vinegar
- 2 tablespoons olive oil
- 1 teaspoon granulated garlic
- 1 teaspoon dried basil
- 1 teaspoon dried marjoram
- 2 chopped thyme sprigs
- 2 chopped rosemary sprigs
- 2 turkey drumsticks
- Salt and black pepper, to taste
- 1/2 cup Taco bell sauce

Directions

1. Make the marinade first. Mix the apple cider vinegar with olive oil, garlic, basil, marjoram, thyme and rosemary.
2. Pour the marinade over the turkey drumsticks and put in the fridge for 3 hours.
3. Preheat the grill and cook the turkey drumsticks for 45 minutes – 1 hour. Season with as much salt and pepper you want.
4. Put the drumsticks on 2 plates and serve with Taco bell sauce. Bon appétit!

Nutrition: Calories 461 ,Protein 26.6g ,Fat 37.6g ,Carbs 4.2g ,Sugar 1g

253. CHICKEN DRUMSTICKS MEDITERRANEAN-STYLE WITH AIOLI

Servings 4
Preparation Time: 35 minutes

Ingredients

- 1 1/2 tablespoons ghee
- 4 chicken drumsticks
- Sea salt and crushed mixed peppercorns, to taste
- 6 pitted and halved Kalamata olives
- 1 tablespoon chopped fresh parsley
- 1 hard-boiled egg yolk
- 1 tablespoon finely minced garlic
- ¼ teaspoon sea salt
- 1 tablespoon lemon juice
- 1/2 cup extra-virgin olive oil
- 1 cup cubed Halloumi cheese1/4 teaspoon sea salt

Directions

1. Put your oven on at 3950F.
2. In a nonstick skillet melt the ghee.
3. Put the salt and peppercorns on the chicken and cook in the ghee until they are brown. This should take 3 – 4 minutes.
4. Put the drumsticks on a baking sheet and sprinkle the parsley and olives over them.
5. Make the Aioli by mixing together the egg yolk, garlic, sea salt, lemon juice and olive oil in a blender.
6. Spread the Aioli over the chicken and bake for around 25 minutes. Put the Halloumi on top and cook for another 3 – 4 minutes until the cheese starts to melt.

Nutrition: Calories 562 ,Protein 40.8g ,Fat 43.8g ,Carbs 2.1g ,Sugar 1g

254. CHEESY CHICKEN WITH PEPPERS

Servings 4
Preparation Time: 15 minutes

Ingredients

- 1 tablespoon olive oil
- 1 cup chopped shallots
- 1 teaspoon minced garlic
- 4 deveined and chopped bell peppers
- 1 deveined and chopped chili pepper
- 1 pound ground chicken,
- 1 teaspoon Italian seasonings
- 1/3 cup dry sherry
- Salt and black pepper, to taste
- 1/2 cup shredded Asiago cheese

Directions

1. Preheat a pan over a medium flame and heat the oil. Sauté the shallots and garlic until they are fragrant.
2. Put in the chicken and peppers and cook until the chicken has browned.
3. Add the Italian seasonings, sherry, pepper and salt and cook for 5 minutes until everything is hot.
4. Sprinkle the Asiago cheese on the top and allow to melt. Remove from the heat and serve straight away.

Nutrition: Calories 562 ,Protein 40.8g ,Fat 43.8g ,Carbs 2.1g ,Sugar 1g

255. THE TASTIEST CHICKEN TACOS EVER

Servings 4
Preparation Time: 20 minutes

Ingredients

- 2 teaspoons lard at room temperature
- 2 small peeled and finely chopped white onions
- 2 slices chopped bacon
- 1 clove minced garlic
- 1 pound ground chicken
- Coarse salt and freshly ground black pepper
- 1 tablespoon Mexican seasoning
- 2 ripe pureed tomatoes
- 1 ½ cups shredded Cotija cheese
- 1/2 cup sour cream
- 1/2 cup Pico de Gallo
- 1 head lettuce

Directions

1. Put a pan on medium heat and melt the lard. Cook the onions until soft.
2. Add the bacon, garlic and chicken and continue cooking until the chicken has browned. Add the black pepper, salt and Mexican seasoning.
3. Mix in the tomatoes and cook for another 5 minutes. Put to one side.
4. Put your oven on at 3600F. Line a baking tray with paper. Take the shredded cheese and form into 4 rounds.
5. Bake the cheese rounds in the middle of the oven for about 6 minutes.
6. Leave the cheese tacos to cool for 5 minutes. Then put on the chicken mixture, followed by Pico de Gallo, sour cream and lettuce leaves. Enjoy!

Nutrition: Calories 539.2 ,Protein 41.2g ,Fat 40.8g ,Carbs 1.8g ,Sugar 1g

256. TURKEY AND BABY BOK CHOY SOUP

Servings 8
Preparation Time: 40 minutes

Ingredients

- 1 tablespoon olive oil
- 1/2 pound sliced and quartered baby Bok Choy
- 1/2 halved onion
- 2 chopped stalks celery with leaves
- Salt and pepper to taste
- 2 pounds turkey carcass
- 1 tablespoon chili garlic sauce
- 2 teaspoons bouillon granules
- 6 cups water

Directions

1. Put a large pot on moderate-high heat and heat the oil. Sauté the baby Bok Choy, onion and celery until just soft. This should take about 5 minutes.
2. Add the salt and pepper, the turkey carcass, chili garlic sauce, bouillon granules and water. Bring to the boil.
3. Cover the pot and reduce the heat to medium-low.

4. Simmer for around 30 minutes and then serve. Bon appétit!

Nutrition: Calories 221.6 ,Protein 12.2g ,Fat 16.8g ,Carbs 5.4g ,Sugar 2.1g

257. TURKEY SOUP LIKE MOM USED TO MAKE

Servings 4
Preparation Time: 30 minutes

Ingredients

- 2 minced garlic cloves
- 1/2 stick butter
- 1/2 cup full fat Greek-style yogurt
- 1/3 cup heavy cream
- 1/4 teaspoon ground black pepper
- ½ teaspoon sea salt
- 1 ½ cups shredded leftover turkey

Directions

1. Put the garlic, butter and yogurt into a pot. Simmer over moderate-low heat.
2. Cook until it is hot and then add the cream, salt and pepper and turkey. Simmer for another 20 minutes and enjoy.

Nutrition: Calories 256 ,Protein 15.3g ,Fat 18.8g ,Carbs 5.4g ,Sugar 3.2g

258. DUCK FILLETS WITH VODKA AND SOUR CREAM

Servings 4
Preparation Time: 20 minutes

Ingredients

- 1 tablespoon lard, room temperature
- 4 duck fillets
- 1/2 teaspoon ground bay leaf
- 2 ounces vodka
- 3 tablespoons Worcestershire sauce
- 1 1/2 cups turkey stock
- 1 teaspoon mixed peppercorns
- Salt and cayenne pepper to taste
- 4 chopped green onion
- 1/2 cup sour cream

Directions

1. Preheat a skillet over a moderate-high heat and melt the lard. Sear the duck fillets turning once. This should take 4 – 6 minutes.
2. Add the bay leaf, vodka, Worcestershire sauce, turkey stock, peppercorns, salt, cayenne pepper and onion, partially cover and cook for another 7 minutes.
3. Garnish with sour cream and serve hot.

Nutrition: Calories351 ,Protein 22.1g ,Fat 24.7g ,Carbs 6.6g ,Sugar 13.6g

259. CHICKEN WITH SPICES AND BRUSSELS SPROUTS

Servings 4
Preparation Time: 20 minutes

Ingredients

- 2 tablespoons olive oil
- 1 ½ pounds trimmed and halved Brussels sprouts
- 1/4 teaspoon seasoned salt
- 3/4 pound chopped chicken breasts
- 2 minced cloves garlic
- 1/2 teaspoon whole black peppercorns
- 1/2 teaspoon chipotle chili powder
- 2 tablespoons Sauvignon wine
- 1 cup low-sodium bone broth
- 1/2 cup chopped white onions
- 2 tablespoons chopped fresh chives

Directions

1. Put a pan on a medium heat and heat 1 tablespoon of the oil. Sauté the Brussels sprouts until they are golden brown. This should take 2 – 4 minutes. Season with salt and put to one side.
2. Heat the other tablespoon of oil over medium heat and cook the chicken and garlic for 3 minutes.
3. Add the peppercorns, chipotle powder, wine, bone broth and onions and bring to the boil. Then simmer for 4 minutes.
4. Put the Brussels sprouts in the pan and heat everything through. Garnish with chopped chives and serve hot. Bon appétit!

260. CHICKEN SALAD WITH

TARRAGON

Servings 4
Preparation Time: 20 minutes

Ingredients

- 2 pitted, peeled and diced avocados
- 2 cups shredded skinless, boneless rotisserie chicken
- 1 tablespoon chopped fresh tarragon
- 1 thinly sliced red onion
- 1/4 cup mayonnaise
- 1/3 cup plain Greek yogurt
- 1 tablespoon Dijon mustard
- Salt and black pepper, to taste
- 3 quartered hard-boiled eggs

Directions

1. Mix together the avocado and chicken. Add the tarragon and the onion.
2. Stir in the mayonnaise, Greek yogurt and mustard. Season with pepper and salt to your liking and combine all the ingredients well.
3. Put the mixture in a salad bowl and garnish with the quartered hard-boiled eggs. Serve cool.

Nutrition: Calories353 ,Protein 27.8g ,Fat 23.5g ,Carbs 5.8g ,Sugar 2.2g

261. HER BY CHORIZO AND ASIAGO CHEESE

Servings 4
Preparation Time: 20 minutes

Ingredients

- 1 tablespoon extra-virgin olive oil
- 4 chopped spring onions
- 16 ounces crumbled smoked turkey and chicken chorizo
- 1 teaspoon garlic paste
- Sea salt and ground black pepper, to taste
- 1 teaspoon basil
- 1 teaspoon dried sage
- 3/4 teaspoon ground ginger
- 1 pureed tomato
- 2 tablespoons roughly chopped parsley
- 1 teaspoon chili powder
- 1 tablespoon dry sherry
- 2 tablespoons ketchup
- 1 ½ cups grated Asiago cheese

Directions

- Preheat the oven to 3700F.
- In a pot heat the oil over medium heat. Brown the chorizo and the onion, stirring all the time and crumbling the meat. This should take 5 – 6 minutes.
- Mix in the garlic paste, salt, pepper, basil, sage, ginger and pureed tomato. Cook for another 2 minutes till everything is heated through.
- Add the parsley, chili powder, dry sherry, ketchup and Asiago cheese. Cook for 8 minutes by which time the cheese should have completely melted.
- Serve with sour cream, avocado and cilantro. Enjoy!

Nutrition: Calories 330 ,Protein 3.4g ,Fat 17.2g ,Carbs 4.5g ,Sugar 1.5g

262. CHICKEN AND CAULIFLOWER CREAMY SOUP

Servings 6
Preparation Time: 30 minutes

Ingredients

- 1/2 stick butter
- 1 chopped celery
- 1/2 cup finely chopped shallots
- 1 finely minced spring garlic
- 1/2 teaspoon kosher salt
- 1/4 teaspoon ground black pepper
- 1/4 teaspoon ground white pepper, or more to taste
- 3 cups chicken stock
- 1 1/2 cups water
- 1 cup leftover shredded roast chicken
- 1 ¼ cups heavy cream
- 1 head cauliflower florets

Directions

1. In a stock pot melt the butter over a medium flame. Sauté the celery, shallots and spring garlic.Cook for 4 minutes or

until they are soft.

2. Mix in the salt, black pepper and white pepper and bring to the boil. Add the chicken stock, water, roast chicken, heavy cream and cauliflower florets. Turn the temperature to low and simmer for 25 minutes.
3. Put the soup in a blender and spritz it until it is smooth, Put in individual bowls and garnish with dill pickles.

Nutrition: Calories231 ,Protein 11.9g ,Fat 18.2g ,Carbs 5.9g ,Sugar 1.5g

263. TURKEY AND CHEESE DIP WITH FRESNO CHILES

Servings 4
Preparation Time: 25 minutes

Ingredients

- Nonstick cooking spray
- 1 tablespoon olive oil
- 1 minced garlic clove
- 1 chopped onion
- 1 pound ground turkey
- 1/4 cup Greek-style yogurt
- 1 1/2 cups creamed and softened Cottage cheese, 4% fat
- Salt and black pepper, to taste
- 1 teaspoon dried oregano
- 1 minced Fresno chili
- 1/2 cup shredded Gruyere cheese
- 1 /2 cups shredded Blue cheese

Directions

1. Put the oven on at 3600F. With nonstick cooking spray, lightly grease a baking pan.
2. In a skillet heat up the oil over a medium flame and sauté the garlic and onion until they are soft.
3. Put in the turkey and cook until it browns. Put this mixture to one side.
4. Mix the Greek yogurt and cottage cheese in a bowl until the mixture is creamy. Add the salt, pepper, oregano, Fresno chili and the turkey.
5. Put the mixture into the baking dish and sprinkle the Gruyere cheese and Blue cheese on top. Bake for about 18 minutes.
6. Serve with veggie sticks like peppers.

Nutrition: Calories 284 ,Protein 26.7g ,Fat 19g ,Carbs 3.2g ,Sugar 1g

264. TURKEY BACON AND HABANERO BALLS

Servings 4
Preparation Time: 5 minutes

Ingredients

- 4 ounces Cottage cheese
- 4 ounces chopped turkey bacon
- 1 deveined and minced Habanero pepper
- 1 tablespoon cold butter
- 1 minced teaspoon fresh sage
- 2 tablespoons finely chopped chives

Directions

1. Mix together the cottage cheese, turkey bacon, Habanero pepper, butter and sage.
2. Make 8 balls out of this mixture.
3. Put the chives on a plate and coat your balls in them. Serve straight away.

Nutrition: Calories 195 ,Protein 8.8g ,Fat 16.7g ,Carbs 2.2g ,Sugar 3.5g

265. CRISPY CHICKEN IN THE OVEN

Servings 4
Preparation Time: 50 minutes

Ingredients

- 1 tablespoon butter
- 4 chicken legs
- 1/4 teaspoon ground black pepper or to taste
- Salt, to your liking
- 1 teaspoon bouillon powder
- 1 teaspoon dried rosemary
- 1 teaspoon paprika
- 1 teaspoon dried basil

Directions

1. Put the oven on at 4200F. Line a baking sheet with parchment paper.
2. Air-dry the chicken legs and then put the butter on them. Sprinkle the pepper, salt,

bouillon powder, rosemary, paprika and basil on the legs.
3. Put the chicken legs on the baking sheet.
4. Bake the chicken legs for about 45 minutes. By this time the shin should be crispy. Serve with a spicy sauce.

Nutrition: Calories 345 ,Protein 50.8g ,Fat 14.1g ,Carbs 0.4g ,Sugar 0g

266. PROSCIUTTO WRAPPED HOLIDAY TURKEY

Servings 6
Preparation Time: 30 minutes

Ingredients

- 2 pounds marinated turkey breasts
- 1 1/2 tablespoons coconut butter, room temperature
- 1/2 teaspoon chili powder
- 1 teaspoon cayenne pepper
- 1 sprig finely chopped fresh thyme
- 2 sprigs finely chopped rosemary
- 2 tablespoons Cabernet Sauvignon
- 1 teaspoon sea salt
- 1/2 teaspoon freshly ground black pepper
- 1 teaspoon finely minced garlic
- 10 strips prosciutto

Directions

1. Chop the turkey into 10 slices of the same size.
2. In a skillet, melt the coconut butter over medium heat. Cook the turkey breasts on both sides for 2 – 3 minutes each side.
3. Sprinkle the chili powder, cayenne pepper, thyme, rosemary, salt, pepper and garlic. Drizzle a little wine over the turkey. Wrap each slice of turkey with a prosciutto strip.
4. Put your oven on at 4500F. Place the turkey and prosciutto in a roasting pan and cook for 25 minutes.
5. Garnish with fresh cilantro. Bon appétit!

Nutrition: Calories 286 ,Protein 39.9g ,Fat 9.7g ,Carbs 6.9g ,Sugar 4.4g

267. CHICKEN THIGHS WITH A RUM GLAZE

Servings 4
Preparation Time: 1 hour + marinating time

Ingredients

- 2 pounds chicken thighs
- 2 tablespoons olive oil
- Sea salt and ground black pepper, to taste
- 1 teaspoon dried marjoram
- 1 teaspoon paprika
- 1 teaspoon dried oregano
- 2 minced habanero chili peppers
- 1 tablespoon minced fresh ginger
- 1 teaspoon ground allspice
- 2 tablespoons Swerve
- 3 tablespoons soy sauce
- 3/4 cup dark rum
- 2 pureed ripe tomatoes
- 2 tablespoons fresh lime juice, plus wedges for serving

Directions

1. Put your oven on at 4200F.
2. Mix together the olive oil, salt, pepper, marjoram, paprika and oregano. Toss the chicken thighs in this mixture.
3. In another bowl mix together the habanero chili peppers, fresh ginger, allspice, Swerve, soy sauce, dark rum, tomatoes and lime juice.
4. Pour this mixture over the chicken thighs and marinate in the fridge for 2 hours. Make sure you cover the bowl.
5. Pour the marinade into a bowl and put the chicken thighs on a baking sheet. Cook for about 50 minutes.
6. While they are baking, heat the marinade over moderate heat. Cook until the liquid has reduced by half.
7. Pour the marinade over the chicken and cook under the broiler on high for 4 minutes. Serve hot.

Nutrition: Calories 307 ,Protein 33.6g ,Fat 12.1g, Carbs 2.7g ,Sugar 1g

268. OVEN BAKED CREAMY CHICKEN THIGHS

Servings: 6
Preparation Time: 10 minutes

Cooking Time: 40 minutes

Ingredients

- 3/4 cup mayonnaise
- 1/4 cup yellow mustard
- 1/2 cup Parmesan cheese freshly grated
- 1 tsp Italian seasoning
- 1/4 tsp of coriander
- 1/4 tsp of marjoram
- 2 lbs. chicken thighs (boneless and skinless)
- 1/2 tsp salt and ground black pepper

Directions:

1. Preheat oven to 400°F/200°C.
2. Oil one 8-inch square baking dish.
3. In a bowl combine the mayonnaise, mustard, Parmesan cheese, coriander, marjoram and Italian seasoning.
4. Season generously chicken thigh with salt and pepper and place in a prepared baking dish.
5. Spread with mayo-mustard sauce and bake for 35 - 40 minutes. Serve warm.

Nutrition:

Calories: 335 Carbohydrates: 7g Proteins: 34g Fat: 18g Fiber: 0.3g

269. ROASTED TURKEY MUSHROOM LOAF

Servings: 6
Preparation Time: 15 minutes
Cooking Time: 1 hour

Ingredients

- 1/2 cup ground almonds
- 1 Tbsp of dried parsley
- 1/4 tsp ground allspice
- 1/2 tsp dried thyme leaves
- 1/2 tsp salt and pepper to taste
- 1 1/2 lbs. ground turkey
- 8 oz turkey cut into 1/4-inch cubes
- 1/2 lbs. mushrooms coarsely chopped
- 1/2 cup spring onion chopped
- 2 cloves garlic minced
- 1 large egg beaten
- Olive oil cooking spray

Directions:

1. Preheat the oven to 350°F/175°C.
2. In large bowl combine ground almonds, parsley, allspice, thyme, salt and pepper.
3. Add ground turkey, turkey ham, mushrooms, spring onions, garlic and beaten egg; knead with your hands to get a compact mixture.
4. Coat one 9-inch pie plate with olive oil cooking spray, shape turkey mixture into round loaf.
5. Bake for 50 to 60 minutes or until inserted thermometer reaches 160 degrees F.
6. Serve hot.

Nutrition:

Calories: 310 Carbohydrates: 5.5g Proteins: 34g Fat: 18g Fiber: 2g

270. CHICKEN ARTICHOKE CASSEROLE

Servings: 4
Preparation Time: 10 minutes
Cooking Time: 25 minutes

Ingredients

- 2 Tbsp butter
- 1 can (11 oz) of artichoke hearts, drained
- 2 green onions, green and white parts included, chopped
- 1 chicken breast cut in cubes
- 1/2 cup dry white wine
- 1 Tbsp almond flour
- 1/2 cup bone broth (or water)
- 1/2 cup cream
- 1 tsp salt and ground black pepper
- 1/4 tsp tarragon leaves
- 2 Tbsp chopped parsley For serving

Directions:

1. Preheat oven to 350°F/175°C.
2. Grease one deep casserole dish with the butter.
3. Cut artichokes and place on the bottom of casserole dish.
4. Add the green onion, and the chicken cubes over the artichokes.
5. In a bowl, combine wine, bone broth, cream and almond flour; stir until almond

flour is completely dissolved.

6. Pour the mixture evenly in a casserole dish.
7. Place in the oven and bake for 20 - 25 minutes. Serve hot.

Nutrition:

Calories: 101 Carbohydrates: 8.5g Proteins: 22g Fat: 29g Fiber: 6g

271. CHICKEN LIVER AND PANCETTA CASSEROLE

Servings: 4
Preparation Time: 5 minutes
Cooking Time: 50 minutes

Ingredients

- 1/4 cup of olive oil
- 1 onion finely chopped
- 2 cloves of garlic
- 1 1/2 lbs. of chicken liver
- 1/2 tsp smoked red ground pepper
- 7 oz of pancetta (cut into strips)
- 1 tsp of dried thyme
- 1/2 cup of red wine
- 1 bunch of parsley finely chopped
- Salt and freshly ground black pepper

Directions:

1. Preheat oven to 350°F/175°C.
2. Grease a casserole with olive oil; set aside.
3. Heat the olive oil in a skillet over medium-high heat.
4. Sauté the onion and the garlic for 3 - 4 minutes.
5. Add chopped pancetta and stir for 1 - 2 minutes.
6. Add chicken liver, smoked pepper, thyme, salt and pepper and cook for 3-4 minutes.
7. Pour the red wine and add chopped parsley; stir.
8. Transfer the mixture in a prepared casserole dish.
9. Bake for 35 - 45 minutes. Serve hot.

Nutrition:

Calories: 340 Carbohydrates: 4g Proteins: 29g Fat: 22g Fiber: 1g

272. CHICKEN CASSEROLE

Servings: 6
Preparation Time: 15 minutes
Cooking Time: 35 minutes

Ingredients

- 1 Tbsp of chicken fat
- 2 lbs. of chicken, cubed
- Salt and ground pepper to taste
- 12 oz of frozen or fresh spinach
- 1/4 cup bacon crumbled
- 1 cup of cream cheese softened
- 1/2 cup of mayonnaise
- 1 tsp garlic powder
- 1 cup grated parmesan cheese

Directions:

1. Preheat oven to 350°F/ 175°C
2. Grease one 9 x13 baking dish with chicken fat.
3. Season the chicken generously with the salt and pepper, and place into baking dish.
4. Add the spinach over chicken, and sprinkle with crumbled bacon.
5. In a bowl, combine together the cream cheese, mayo, garlic, and grated parmesan cheese.
6. Pour the mixture in a casserole.
7. Place in oven and bake for 30 - 35 minutes.
8. Serve hot.

Nutrition:

Calories: 374 Carbohydrates: 8.5g Proteins: 15g Fat: 32g Fiber: 2g

273. CHICKEN WITH CURRY AND CORIANDER CASSEROLE

Servings: 4
Preparation Time: 10 minutes
Cooking Time: 25 minutes

Ingredients

- 1 lbs. of chicken breast cut in cubes
- 1 Tbsp of chicken fat
- 1 onion, finely sliced
- 1 carrot
- 2 tsp of curry powder
- 1 pinch of saffron

- 1/2 cup of wine
- 1/2 cup of bone broth
- 1 Tbsp of fresh coriander
- Salt to taste

Directions:

1. Cut the chicken breasts into large cubes.
2. Heat the chicken fat in a casserole and sauté the onion.
3. Add the chicken cubes and brown them on all sides; stir for 2 - 3 minutes.
4. Sprinkle with curry and saffron, stir in the carrots and stir well.
5. Pour the wine and bone broth and stir.
6. Season with the salt, cover and let simmer for 20 minutes.
7. Sprinkle with fresh chopped coriander leaves and serve.

Nutrition:

Calories: 186 Carbohydrates: 6g Proteins: 26g Fat: 8g Fiber: 2g

274. INSTANT POT ASIAGO CHICKEN WINGS

Servings: 6
Preparation Time: 10 minutes
Cooking Time: 20 minutes

Ingredients

- 2 Tbsp olive oil
- 20 frozen chicken wings
- 1 tsp salt
- 1/2 Tbsp garlic powder
- 2 tsp dried oregano
- 1 cup of grated Asiago cheese (or Parmesan)
- 1/2 can water

Directions:

1. Pour the oil to the inner stainless-steel pot in the Instant Pot.
2. Season frozen chicken legs with salt, garlic powder and oregano.
3. Place the seasoned chicken wings in your Instant Pot and pour water.
4. Lock lid into place and set on the POULTRY setting for 20 minutes.
5. Use Quick Release - turn the valve from sealing to venting to release the pressure.
6. Transfer chicken wings to serving platter and generously sprinkle with grated cheese.
7. Let rest for 10 minutes and serve.

Nutrition:

Calories: 438 Carbohydrates: 2g Proteins: 37g Fat: 35g Fiber: 0.5g

275. INSTANT POT CHICKEN CILANTRO WRAPS

Servings: 4
Preparation Time: 10 minutes
Cooking Time: 12 minutes

Ingredients

- 2 chicken breasts boneless, skinless
- 1 cup bone broth (or water)
- Juice of 1 lemon freshly squeezed
- 1 green onion finely chopped
- 1 cup cilantro, chopped
- 1 tsp chili powder
- 1 tsp cumin
- 1 tsp garlic powder
- Sea salt and pepper to taste
- 12 lettuce leaves of your choice but should be large enough to use as a wrap.

Directions:

1. Season chicken breast with the salt and pepper and place in your Instant Pot.
2. Add all remaining Ingredients (except lettuce leaves; lock lid into place and set on the POULTRY setting for 12 minutes.
3. When the timer beeps, press "Cancel" and carefully flip the Quick Release valve to let the pressure out.
4. Open lid and transfer chicken in a bowl; Shred chicken with two forks.
5. Combine shredded chicken with juices from Instant Pot.
6. Add one spoon of shredded chicken in each lettuce leaf and wrap. Serve immediately.

Nutrition:

Calories: 7163 Carbohydrates: 4g Proteins: 34g Fat: 5g Fiber: 1g

276. INSTANT POT PERFECT BRAISED TURKEY BREAST

Servings: 8
Preparation Time: 10 minutes
Cooking Time: 30 minutes

Ingredients

- 2 Tbsp butter softened on room temperature
- 4 lbs. turkey breast boneless
- 1 cup water
- 1/2 cup coconut aminos (from coconut sap)
- 1/2 tsp fresh rosemary, finely chopped
- 1/2 tsp fresh sage, finely chopped
- 1/2 tsp fresh rosemary finely chopped
- 1 tsp salt and ground red pepper to taste

Directions:

1. Season turkey breasts with salt and pepper.
2. Press SAUTÉ button on your Instant Pot.
3. When the word "hot" appears on the display, add butter and sear turkey breasts for 3 minutes.
4. Pour water and coconut aminos and stir for 2 minutes.
5. Sprinkle with herbs, and the salt and pepper and stir again. Turn off the SAUTÉ button.
6. Lock lid into place and set on the MANUAL high pressure setting for 28 - 30 minutes (turkey meat is ready when meat thermometer shows 161°F/80°C).
7. When the timer beeps, press "Cancel" and carefully flip the Natural Release for 15 minutes.
8. Remove turkey breast on a plate and allow it to cool for 10 minutes.
9. Slice and serve.

Nutrition:

Calories: 357 Carbohydrates: 1.5g Proteins: 62g Fat: 10g Fiber: 0.5g

277. INSTANT POT ROASTED WHOLE CHICKEN

Servings: 6
Preparation Time: 10 minutes
Cooking Time: 35 minutes

Ingredients

- 2 cups water
- 4 lbs. whole chicken
- 1/4 cup olive oil
- Seasoned salt and black ground pepper to taste
- 1/4 tsp dry thyme
- 1/4 tsp dry rosemary
- 1/4 tsp dry marjoram
- 1/4 tsp of dry sage

Directions:

1. Pour water to the inner stainless-steel pot in the Instant Pot and place the trivet inside (steam rack or a steamer basket).
2. Rinse well the turkey and pat dry. Rub with olive oil and season to taste with salt and pepper, thyme, rosemary, marjoram and sage.
3. Put the turkey on the trivet into Instant Pot.
4. Press MANUAL mode and set time for 35 minutes.
5. Use Natural Release - it takes 15 - 20 minutes to depressurize naturally.
6. Remove the chicken on a serving plate and allow cool for 15 minutes before serving.

Nutrition:

Calories: 589 Carbohydrates: 0.1g Proteins: 54g Fat: 47g Fiber: 1g

278. INSTANT POT SERRANO CHICKEN STIR FRY

Servings: 6
Preparation Time: 10 minutes
Cooking Time: 15 minutes

Ingredients

- 2 lbs. chicken breasts cut small pieces
- 1 tsp sea salt
- 1 Tbsp sesame oil
- 1 Tbsp ginger, minced
- 1 Tbsp lemon juice
- 2 Tbsp coconut oil

- 1 green onion, minced
- 2 cloves garlic, minced
- 8 Serrano peppers cut in half
- 1 cup water

Directions:

1. In a bowl, whisk the salt, sesame oil, ginger and lemon juice.
2. Season chicken breast with the mixture.
3. Turn on the Instant Pot and press SAUTÉ button.
4. When the word "hot" appears on the display, add the coconut oil and sauté the green onion and garlic about 3 minutes. Add halved peppers and sauté for about 2 minutes.
5. Turn off SAUTÉ button; add seasoned chicken, pour water and stir.
6. Lock lid into place and set on the POULTRY setting on HIGH pressure for 10 minutes.
7. When the timer beeps, press "Cancel" and carefully flip the Quick Release valve to let the pressure out. Serve hot.

Nutrition:

Calories: 359.55 Carbohydrates: 2.5g Proteins: 48g Fat: 17g Fiber: 1g

279. INSTANT POT TASTY CHICKEN CURRY

Servings: 4
Preparation Time: 10 minutes
Cooking Time: 10 minutes

Ingredients

- 2 Tbsp olive oil
- 1 lbs. chicken breast boneless, skinless, cut in small cubes
- Salt and ground black pepper
- 1/2 tsp onion powder
- 1/2 tsp garlic powder
- 1 tsp of curry powder
- 1 1/2 cup coconut cream
- 1/2 cup water
- 1 Tbsp of chopped parsley For serving

Directions:

1. Pour the oil to the inner stainless-steel pot in the Instant Pot.
2. Season salt and pepper the chicken breast and place in Instant Pot.
3. In a bowl, combine together all remaining Ingredients and pour over chicken.
4. Lock lid into place and set on the MANUAL setting for 10 minutes.
5. Use Natural Release for 15 minutes.
6. Serve hot with chopped parsley.

Nutrition:

Calories: 304 Carbohydrates: 2g Proteins: 25g Fat: 22g Fiber: 0.3g

280. SLOW COOKER CHICKEN THIGHS IN COCONUT SAUCE

Servings: 6
Preparation Time: 10 minutes
Cooking Time: 4 hours and 20 minutes

Ingredients

- 1 1/2 lbs. of chicken thighs, boneless and skinless
- 1 red bell pepper, finely chopped
- 1 green onion, chopped
- 1 chili pepper (cleaned and finely chopped)
- 2 cloves garlic (minced)
- 1 cup of bone broth
- 1/2 cup of coconut flakes
- 2 Tbsp of curry powder
- Salt and ground pepper to taste
- 1/4 tsp of ground cinnamon
- 1/2 cup of coconut milk (unsweetened)
- 1 Tbsp of coconut flour
- Fresh cilantro For serving

Directions:

1. Place the chicken thighs, bell pepper, onions, chili pepper and garlic in Crock Pot.
2. Pour broth, and add the coconut flakes, curry powder, salt and pepper, and cinnamon.
3. Cover and cook on LOW for 8 - 9 hours or HIGH for 4 hours.
4. In a small bowl, dissolve the coconut flour in coconut milk.
5. Open lid and pour the coconut mixture;

stir.

6. Cover again and cook on HIGH for further 20 minutes.
7. Serve hot with fresh chopped cilantro.

Nutrition:

Calories: 359 Carbohydrates: 5g Proteins: 24g Fat: 28g Fiber: 1.5g

281. DELICIOUS CHICKEN BREAST WITH TURMERIC

Servings: 4
Preparation Time: 15 minutes
Cooking Time: 4 hours

Ingredients

- 1/2 cup chicken fat
- 4 chicken breasts, boneless, skinless
- Table salt and ground white pepper to taste
- 4 cloves garlic, finely sliced
- 1 Tbsp ground turmeric
- 1 cup of bone broth

Directions:

1. Season the salt and pepper chicken breast and cut into pieces.
2. Add tallow in inner pot of your Slow Cooker and place the chicken breasts.
3. Add the turmeric, garlic and chicken broth.
4. Cover and cook on LOW for 3 - 4 hours.
5. Transfer the chicken breasts on a serving plate.
6. Serve hot with cooking juice.

Nutrition:

Calories: 488 Carbohydrates: 2.5g Proteins: 52g Fat: 32g Fiber: 0.5g

282. CHICKEN CUTLETS WITH SPINACH STIR-FRY

Servings: 4
Preparation Time: 5 minutes
Cooking Time: 15 minutes

Ingredients

- 2 Tbsp chicken fat
- 1 spring onion (only green parts), finely chopped
- 2 medium cloves garlic, thinly sliced
- 8 boneless, skinless, chicken breast cutlets cut in pieces
- Salt and freshly ground black pepper
- 3 Tbsp capers, rinsed and chopped
- 1 lbs. of fresh spinach, steamed
- 1/2 cup water
- 2 Tbsp fresh lemon juice

Directions:

1. Heat the chicken fat in a deep pot, and sauté spring onion and garlic for 3 - 4 minutes.
2. Add chicken cutlets and stir for 4 - 5 minutes.
3. Season with the salt and pepper,
4. Reduce the heat to medium and add the capers and spinach leaves. Cook stirring, until the spinach softens, about 3 minutes.
5. Pour water and lemon juice and cook for further 2 - 3 minutes.
6. Serve hot.

Nutrition:

Calories: 347 Carbohydrates: 5g Proteins: 57g Fat: 15g Fiber: 3g

283. CHICKEN AND ZOODLE STIR FRY

Servings: 4
Preparation Time: 15 minutes
Cooking Time: 7 - 10 minutes

Ingredients

- 1 lbs. chicken breasts, boneless, skinless, cut in slices
- 2 Tbsp of chicken fat
- 2 cups zucchini, spiralized (or made into ribbons with a vegetable peeler)
- Marinade
- 1 spring onion finely chopped
- 2 cloves garlic, minced
- 1 cup water
- 1 cup fresh lemon juice
- 1/3 cup coconut aminos
- 1/3 cup olive oil
- 4 green onion, sliced

- 1" piece of ginger, grated
- Salt and ground black pepper to taste

Directions:

1. Place the chicken slices in a container and season with the salt and pepper.
2. In a deep bowl, combine all Ingredients for marinade; stir until well combined.
3. Pour the marinade evenly over the chicken; cover and refrigerate for 2 hours.
4. Heat the chicken fat in a large and deep-frying skillet over medium-high heat.
5. Add the chicken to the skillet and stir-fry about 5 - 7 minutes. Toss in the zucchini ribbons and cook only for 2 minutes. Serve hot.

Nutrition:

Calories: 327 Carbohydrates: 6g Proteins: 27g Fat: 22g Fiber: 2g

284. HUNGARIAN CHICKEN FILLET STIR-FRY

Servings: 4
Preparation Time: 5 minutes
Cooking Time: 30 minutes

Ingredients

- 1 Tbsp of chicken fat
- 1 lbs. of chicken fillet cut in strips
- 2 - 3 spring onions, finely chopped
- 2 cloves garlic
- 1 green pepper, chopped
- 1 tomato grated
- Salt and black ground pepper to taste
- 1 Tbsp of fresh parsley, chopped
- 1 egg, beaten

Directions:

1. Heat the chicken fat in a large pan.
2. Sauté the onion and garlic with a pinch of salt for 4 - 5 minutes.
3. Add chicken strips and stir for 5 - 6 minutes.
4. Add chopped pepper and grated tomato; season with the salt and pepper.
5. Cover and cook for 12 - 15 minutes over low-medium heat.
6. Crack one egg in a pan and stir well.
7. Sprinkle with fresh parsley and serve hot.

Nutrition:

Calories: 67 Carbohydrates: 6.5g Proteins: 6g Fat: 3g Fiber: 2g

285. SPICY CHICKEN STIR-FRY

Servings: 4
Preparation Time: 10 minutes
Cooking Time: 20 minutes

Ingredients

- 2 lbs. chicken breasts, boneless skinless, cut in pieces
- 1 tsp sea salt
- 2 cloves garlic, minced
- 1 Tbsp almond flour
- 1 cup water
- 1 Tbsp sesame oil
- 1 Tbsp ginger, minced
- 4 - 5 Serrano peppers, sliced
- 3 Tbsp olive oil
- 2 green onions cut into thin slices

Directions:

1. Place chicken in a large container, and rub with the mixture of salt, garlic, sesame oil, ginger, almond flour and water.
2. Refrigerate for 1 hour.
3. Heat the olive oil in a large skillet over a high heat.
4. Add Serrano peppers and fry for about 2 minutes.
5. Add the chicken, stir, reduce the heat and stir-fry for 5 - 6 minutes.
6. Add chopped green onion, some water, and cook for further 6 - 7 minutes.
7. Adjust salt, stir and serve hot.

Nutrition:

Calories: 388 Carbohydrates: 2g Proteins: 48g Fat: 20g Fiber: 0.5g

286. SHREDDED TURKEY WITH ASPARAGUS STIR-FRY

Servings: 4
Preparation Time: 5 minutes
Cooking Time: 30 minutes

Ingredients

- 2 Tbsp of chicken fat
- 2 spring onions, diced
- 1 tsp minced garlic
- 1 red pepper finely chopped
- 1/4 lbs. button mushrooms sliced thin
- 1 cup cooked asparagus cut into small pieces
- 1/2 tsp dried rosemary
- Salt and ground black pepper to taste
- 1 1/2 lbs. turkey breast meat, boneless, shredded
- 1 cup bone broth

Directions:

1. In a large frying skillet heat the chicken fat over medium-high heat.
2. Sauté the onion, garlic and red pepper with a little salt for 4 to 5 minutes.
3. Add mushrooms and asparagus; sauté for 2 - 3 minutes.
4. Stir in rosemary, pepper, and season with the salt to taste.
5. Add shredded turkey meat and stir well.
6. Pour the bone broth, cover and cook for 13 -15 minutes over medium heat.
7. Taste and adjust seasonings. Serve hot.

Nutrition:

Calories: 240 Carbohydrates: 7g Proteins: 36g Fat: 8g Fiber: 2.5g

287. SQUASH SPAGHETTI AND GROUND CHICKEN STIR-FRY

Servings: 4
Preparation Time: 5 minutes
Cooking Time: 25 minutes

Ingredients

- 1/4 cup olive oil
- 1 1/4 lbs. squash, spiralized
- 1 lbs. ground chicken
- 1 Tbsp fresh lemon juice (about 2 lemons)
- 1/2 Tbsp fresh herbs mixture (tarragon, marjoram, oregano)
- Salt and freshly ground pepper to taste
- 1/2 cup shredded Mozzarella cheese for garnish

Directions:

1. Heat the olive oil in a skillet over medium-high heat.
2. Sauté the squash spaghetti with a pinch of salt for about 8 minutes.
3. Add the ground chicken, fresh lemon juice, fresh herbs and season salt and pepper to taste.
4. Stir, and stir-fry for 8 - 10 minutes over medium heat.
5. Taste and adjust seasonings; cook for further 5 minutes; gently stir.
6. Serve hot with shredded cheese.

Nutrition:

Calories: 358 Carbohydrates: 5g Proteins: 35.6g Fat: 22g Fiber:1.6g

288. GROUND TURKEY AND GREEN BEANS STIR-FRY

Servings: 4
Preparation Time: 5 minutes
Cooking Time: 15 minutes

Ingredients

- 1 Tbsp chicken fat
- 1 lbs. ground turkey
- 2 cloves garlic, minced
- 2 spring onions, sliced
- 1 piece ginger, finely grated
- 1/2 lbs. of green beans, boiled
- 2 zucchinis, cut into slices
- 2 Tbsp yellow mustard
- 1/2 cup fresh basil leaves
- Salt and ground black pepper

Directions:

1. Heat the chicken fat in a large frying pan.
2. Add turkey mince and stir-fry for 2 - 3 minutes,
3. Stir the garlic, spring onions and ginger; season with the salt and pepper and stir-fry for 3 -4 minutes.
4. Add green beans and zucchini, and stir-fry for 3 minutes; stir well.
5. At the end, add mustard and gently toss.
6. Serve hot with fresh basil leaves.

Nutrition:

Calories: 299 Carbohydrates: 9.8g Proteins: 34g

Fat: 16g Fiber: 3.7g

289. TURKEY CHILI WITH MONTEREY JACK CHEESE

Preparation Time: 40 minutes
Servings: 5

Nutrition: 390 Calories; 25.3g Fat; 4.8g Carbs; 33.7g Protein; 1.3g Fiber

Ingredients

- 1 ½ pounds ground turkey
- 1 onion, diced
- 1 cup spicy tomato sauce
- 5 ounces Monterey Jack cheese, shredded
- 2 medium Italian peppers, deveined and sliced

Directions

1. Preheat a Dutch oven over medium-high heat. Cook the ground turkey and onion for 5 to 6 minutes until no longer pink.
2. Add in a splash of red wine to scrape up the browned bits that stick to the bottom of the pan. Stir in Italian peppers and tomato sauce.
3. When your mixture starts to boil, turn the heat to simmer. Continue to simmer, partially covered, for 30 to 35 minutes.
4. Top with Monterey Jack cheese and place under preheated broil for 5 minutes until hot and bubbly. Enjoy!

290. SWISS TURKEY AND PEPPER TIMBALE

Preparation Time: 30 minutes
Servings: 5

Nutrition: 464 Calories; 28.5g Fat; 4.5g Carbs; 45.4g Protein; 0.3g Fiber

Ingredients

- 1 yellow onion, thinly sliced
- 1 cup bell peppers, sliced
- 1 ½ pounds turkey breast
- 1 cup double cream
- 1/2 cup Swiss cheese, shredded

Directions

1. In a saucepan, heat 2 teaspoons of the olive oil over medium-high heat. Sauté the onion and peppers until they have softened and reserve.
2. In the same saucepan, heat 1 teaspoon of olive oil; now, sear the turkey breasts until nicely browned on all sides.
3. Place the peppers and onions on the bottom of a lightly greased baking pan. Add the turkey breast on top.
4. Mix double cream with 1 cup of chicken bone broth and spoon the mixture over the turkey breasts.
5. Bake in the preheated oven at 360 degrees F for about 18 minutes.
6. Top with the Swiss cheese and continue to bake for a further 6 minutes or until bubbly and golden brown on top. Bon appétit!

291. CHICKEN AND VEGETABLE SOUVLAKI

Preparation Time: 20 minutes
Servings: 6

Nutrition: 200 Calories; 8.1g Fat; 7g Carbs; 24.3g Protein; 1.3g Fiber

Ingredients

- 2 tablespoons olive oil
- 1 tablespoon stone-ground mustard
- 1 ½ pounds chicken, skinless, boneless and cubed
- 2 red onions, cut into wedges
- 3 bell pepper, cut into 1-inch pieces

Directions

1. In a mixing bowl, combine the olive oil, mustard and chicken cubes. Drizzle with 4 tablespoons of dry sherry.
2. Alternate skewering the chicken and vegetables and season them with salt and black pepper.
3. Cook your souvlaki on the preheated grill, flipping a few times to ensure even cooking. Serve warm.

292. 10HUNGARIAN CHICKEN PAPRIKASH

Preparation Time: 35 minutes

Servings: 5

Nutrition: 358 Calories; 22.2g Fat; 4.4g Carbs; 33.3g Protein; 0.7g Fiber

Ingredients

- 2 pounds chicken drumsticks
- 1 cup marinara sauce, sugar-free
- 1 Hungarian wax pepper, chopped
- 1 bell pepper, deseeded and chopped
- 1/2 cup leeks, sliced

Directions

1. Heat 2 tablespoons of olive oil in a heavy-bottomed pot over medium-high flame. Then, brown the chicken drumsticks until no longer pink or about 8 minutes; shred the meat and discard the bones.
2. Then, cook the peppers and leeks in the pan drippings until they have softened or 4 to 5 minutes.
3. Add in the marinara sauce along with 4 cups of water or vegetable broth; season with salt and black pepper, if desired.
4. Fold in the reserved chicken and bring to a boil; turn the heat to simmer, let it simmer for 20 minutes more or until heated through. Enjoy!

293. SRI LANKAN CURRY

Preparation Time: 30 minutes
Servings: 5

Nutrition: 370 Calories; 16g Fat; 0.9g Carbs; 51g Protein; 0.2g Fiber

Ingredients

- 2 tablespoons coconut oil
- 1 ½ pounds chicken tenders, cut into chunks
- 1/2 cup coconut milk
- 1/2 cup chicken broth
- 1 tablespoon curry powder

Directions

1. Melt the coconut oil in a saucepan or wok over medium-high heat. Then, cook the chicken tenders for 6 to 7 minutes, stirring periodically to ensure even cooking.
2. Now, add in coconut milk, chicken broth and curry powder, bringing to a boil.
3. Turn the heat to medium-low and allow it to simmer for a further 20 minutes. Garnish with fresh cilantro just before serving, if desired. Enjoy!

294. TRADITIONAL JAPANESE RAMEN

Preparation Time: 35 minutes
Servings: 6

Nutrition: 199 Calories; 13.7g Fat; 2.4g Carbs; 14.7g Protein; 0.6g Fiber

Ingredients

- 1 tablespoon peanut oil
- 1 pound chicken thigs
- 4 ounces enokitake or enoki mushrooms
- 4 garlic cloves, chopped
- 2 tablespoons sake

Directions

1. Warm the peanut oil in a large soup pot over medium-high flame. Then, sear the chicken thighs for about 8 minutes, turning them over once or twice.
2. Add in 6 cups of dashi, enokitake, and garlic. When the soup reaches boiling, turn the heat to a simmer. Then, let it simmer for another 30 minutes.
3. Shred the chicken and return it to the pot. Pour in the sake and stir to combine well.
4. Taste, adjust the seasonings and serve warm.

295. SUMMER TURKEY DRUMSTICK

Preparation Time: 20 minutes + marinating time | 2

Nutrition: 388 Calories; 19.5g Fat; 6g Carbs; 42g Protein; 1.4g Fiber

Ingredients

- 1 turkey drumstick, skinless and boneless
- 1 tablespoon whiskey
- 1/4 cup chicken marinade, no sugar added
- 1 brown onion, peeled and chopped
- 1 teaspoon Mediterranean spice mix

Directions

1. Place the turkey, marinade, and whiskey in a ceramic dish; add in 1 tablespoon of stone ground mustard, if desired.
2. Cover and refrigerate for 2 hours.
3. Then, preheat your grill to the hottest setting.
4. Grill the turkey for 12 to 15 minutes per side. Season with Mediterranean spice and serve with brown onion. Bon appétit!

296. GREEK-STYLE ROASTED CHICKEN WITH HERBS

Preparation Time: 25 minutes
Servings: 5

Nutrition: 218 Calories; 9.1g Fat; 4.2g Carbs; 28.6g Protein; 0.7g Fiber

Ingredients

- 1 ½ pounds chicken drumettes
- 2 tablespoons olive oil
- 2 cloves garlic, minced
- 1 red onion, cut into wedges
- 1 tablespoon Mediterranean spice mix

Directions

1. Preheat your oven to 410 degrees F. Brush the sides and bottom a baking dish with 1 tablespoon of olive oil.
2. In a nonstick skillet, heat the remaining tablespoon of olive oil over medium heat. Sear the chicken drumettes for 10 to 12 minutes, turning them over periodically to ensure even cooking.
3. Place the chicken in a baking dish. Add in the garlic, spices, and red onion.
4. Roast in the preheated oven for about 15 minutes or until nicely browned on top. Serve and enjoy!

297. GARLICKY ROASTED CHICKEN DRUMSTICKS

Preparation Time: 50 minutes
Servings: 6

Nutrition: 343 Calories; 24.2g Fat; 1.6g Carbs; 28.2g Protein; 0.2g Fiber

Ingredients

- 4 cloves garlic, minced
- Sea salt and ground black pepper, to taste
- 1 tablespoon fresh thyme leaves
- 1 stick unsalted butter, softened
- 2 pounds chicken drumsticks

Directions

1. Start by preheating your oven to 395 degrees F.
2. Mix the garlic, salt, black pepper, thyme, and butter. Rub the mixture all over the chicken drumsticks.
3. Place the chicken drumsticks on a foil-lined baking dish. Bake in the preheated oven for 35 to 40 minutes.
4. Afterwards, place under the preheated broiler for 3 minutes to get nice, crisp skin. Bon appétit!

298. CHICKEN BREASTS IN CREAMY MUSHROOM SAUCE

Preparation Time: 15 minutes
Servings: 4

Nutrition: 335 Calories; 20.8g Fat; 4.3g Carbs; 30.9g Protein; 0.6g Fiber

Ingredients

- 2 chicken breast, skinless and boneless, cut into bite-sized pieces
- 2 garlic cloves, pressed
- 1 tablespoon olive oil
- 1 yellow onion, chopped
- 1/2 cup cream of mushroom soup

Directions

1. Heat the olive oil in a nonstick skillet over medium-high flame. Once hot, cook the onion for about 4 minutes or until caramelized and softened.
2. Then, cook the garlic for 30 seconds more.
3. Sear the chicken breast approximately 5 minutes, stirring continuously to ensure even cooking. Pour in the cream of mushroom soup.
4. Turn the heat to a simmer and continue to cook until the sauce has reduced and thickened about 8 minutes. Serve warm chicken topped with the sauce. Enjoy!

299. EASY COCKTAIL PARTY MEATBALLS

Preparation Time: 25 minutes
Servings: 4

Nutrition: 216 Calories; 11.2g Fat; 3.6g Carbs; 24.3g Protein; 0.5g Fiber

Ingredients

- 1 tablespoon Italian seasoning blend
- 1 egg, beaten
- 2 cloves garlic, minced
- 1/2 cup leeks, minced
- 1 pound ground turkey

Directions

1. Thoroughly combine all ingredients in a bowl.
2. Shape the mixture into small balls and transfer them to a foil-lined baking pan. Brush the meatballs with olive oil.
3. Bake in the preheated oven at 390 degrees F for about 20 minutes. Serve with toothpicks or cocktail sticks.

300. CHINESE DUCK WITH ONION

Preparation Time: 25 minutes
Servings: 4

Nutrition: 263 Calories; 11.3g Fat; 3.7g Carbs; 34.4g Protein; 0.5g Fiber

Ingredients

- 1 tablespoon sesame oil
- 1 ½ pounds duck breast
- 1 white onion, chopped
- 3 teaspoons soy sauce
- 1/4 cup rice wine

Directions

1. Preheat your oven to 395 degrees F.
2. Using a sharp knife, score the duck breast skin in a tight crosshatch pattern.
3. Heat the sesame oil in a wok over medium-high heat. Now, sauté the onion until softened and aromatic.
4. Add the duck breast to the wok and cook for about 15 minutes or until nicely brown on the top.
5. Pour in rice wine to scrape up the browned bits that stick to the bottom of the wok. Transfer duck breasts to a lightly greased baking pan; add the soy sauce to the baking pan.
6. Roast in the preheated oven for 10 minutes and serve warm. Enjoy!

301. CHICKEN DRUMSTICK SOUP

Preparation Time: 30 minutes
Servings: 2

Nutrition: 166 Calories; 4.9g Fat; 3.3g Carbs; 25.6g Protein; 0.7g Fiber

Ingredients

- 1 stalk celery, chopped
- 1/2 white onion, chopped
- 1 teaspoon poultry seasoning mix
- 1 tablespoon fresh cilantro, chopped
- 2 chicken drumsticks, skinless and boneless

Directions

1. Place the chicken in a medium-sized soup pot. Add enough water to cover the chicken by about two inches.
2. Now, add in celery, onion, and poultry seasoning mix. Bring to a boil; then, immediately reduce the heat to a simmer and continue cooking for about 40 minutes.
3. Serve with fresh cilantro. Enjoy!

302. OVEN-ROASTED BUFFALO CHICKEN

Preparation Time: 1 hour | 6

Nutrition: 288 Calories; 20.6g Fat; 1.4g Carbs; 23.5g Protein; 0.4g Fiber

Ingredients

- 1/2 cup melted butter
- 2 tablespoons white vinegar
- 1/2 cup hot sauce
- 1/4 teaspoon granulated garlic
- 2 pounds chicken drumettes

Directions

1. Preheat your oven to 330 degrees F. Lightly oil the sides and bottom of a baking pan. Place the chicken drumettes in the baking pan.
2. Whisk the melted butter, white vinegar, hot sauce, and garlic. Add in the salt and black pepper to taste and whisk until everything is well combined.
3. Pour the sauce over the chicken drumettes and bake for 50 to 55 minutes, flipping them once or twice to ensure even cooking. Bon appétit!

303. CHICKEN DRUMSTICKS WITH TOMATO

Preparation Time: 1 hour 15 minutes
Servings: 5

Nutrition: 352 Calories; 22.1g Fat; 2.5g Carbs; 33.3g Protein; 0.5g Fiber

Ingredients

- 2 pounds chicken drumsticks, boneless, skinless
- 2 garlic cloves, minced
- 1/2 cup tomato paste
- 1/2 cup chicken broth
- 2 fresh scallions, chopped

Directions

1. Spritz a baking pan with 1 tablespoon of olive oil.
2. Place the chicken drumsticks in the prepared baking pan. Drizzle 1 tablespoon of olive oil over chicken drumsticks.
3. Add the garlic, tomato paste, and chicken broth to the pan.
4. Bake in the preheated oven at 340 degrees F for about 65 minutes or until nicely brown and crisp on the top. Garnish with fresh scallions and enjoy!

304. CREAMED CHICKEN SALAD

Preparation Time: 20 minutes + chilling time | 4

Nutrition: 536 Calories; 49g Fat; 3.1g Carbs; 19g Protein; 0.5g Fiber

Ingredients

- 2 chicken breasts, skinless and boneless
- 1 teaspoon Dijon mustard
- 2 teaspoons freshly squeezed lemon juice
- 1 cup mayonnaise, preferably homemade
- 4 scallions, trimmed and thinly sliced

Directions

1. Place the chicken in a stockpot; cover with water by 1 inch and bring to a boil.
2. Then, continue to simmer for 13 to 16 minutes (a meat thermometer should read 165 degrees F).
3. When cool enough to handle, cut the chicken into strips and place them in a serving bowl. Toss the chicken with the remaining ingredients.
4. Serve with fresh coriander if desired. Bon appétit!

305. RUSTIC ITALIAN STUFFED TURKEY

Preparation Time: 1 hour | 6

Nutrition: 347 Calories; 22.2g Fat; 3g Carbs; 32g Protein; 0.5g Fiber

Ingredients

- 1 ½ pounds turkey breasts
- 6 ounces Asiago cheese, sliced
- 2 tablespoons extra-virgin olive oil
- 1 tablespoon Italian seasoning mix
- 2 bell peppers, thinly sliced

Directions

1. Start by preheating your oven to 370 degrees F. Brush the inside of a baking dish with 1 tablespoon of olive oil.
2. Sprinkle the turkey breast with the Italian seasoning mix; season with salt and black pepper to taste.
3. Create slits in turkey breasts to make a pocket; stuff them with Asiago cheese and bell peppers. You can add minced garlic if desired.
4. Drizzle the turkey breasts with the remaining tablespoon of olive oil.
5. Bake for 55 minutes or until thoroughly cooked. Let it stand for 10 minutes before slicing and serving.
6. Garnish with Italian parsley if desired and serve.

306. CHICKEN WITH TOMATO AND ROMANO CHEESE

Preparation Time: 15 minutes
Servings: 3

Nutrition: 359 Calories; 23.6g Fat; 5.8g Carbs; 30.4g Protein; 1.1g Fiber

Ingredients

- 1/2 pound chicken fillets
- 1 egg, whisked
- 3 ounces Romano cheese, grated
- 2 ounces pork rinds, crushed
- 1 large-sized Roma tomato, pureed

Directions

1. In a shallow dish, place the whisked egg.
2. In the second shallow dish, mix Romano cheese and crushed pork rinds; season with salt, black pepper, cayenne pepper, and dried parsley.
3. Dip the chicken fillets into the egg mixture; then, roll the chicken over the breading mixture until well coated.
4. In a frying pan, heat 2 tablespoons of olive oil over medium-high heat. Once hot, fry the chicken fillets for about 3 minutes per side.
5. Place the chicken in a lightly greased baking pan. Spread pureed tomato over the top. Bake for a further 3 minutes. Bon appétit!

307. INDIAN CHICKEN MASALA

Preparation Time: 30 minutes
Servings: 5

Nutrition: 294 Calories; 17.2g Fat; 4.6g Carbs; 29.3g Protein; 1.1g Fiber

Ingredients

- 1 ½ pounds chicken breasts, cut into bite-sized pieces
- 1 teaspoon garam masala
- 10 ounces tomato puree
- 1/2 cup heavy cream
- 1 onion, chopped

Directions

1. Spritz a saucepan with a nonstick cooking spray and preheat over medium-high heat. Now, sear the chicken breasts until nicely browned on both sides.
2. Remove the chicken to the sides of the saucepan and sauté the onions for about 3 minutes or until translucent and tender.
3. Stir in the garam masala and tomato puree. Cook for 9 to 10 minutes until the sauce is reduced by two-thirds.
4. Add in the heavy cream and stir for about 12 minutes or until thoroughly heated. Bon appétit!

308. AUTHENTIC ITALIAN PUTTANESCA

Preparation Time: 25 minutes
Servings: 5
Nutrition: 265 Calories; 11.4g Fat; 6.5g Carbs; 32.5g Protein; 1.4g Fiber
Ingredients

- 1 ½ pounds chicken wings, boneless
- 2 cups marinara sauce, no sugar added
- 1 bell pepper, chopped
- 1 red onion, chopped
- 1/4 cup parmesan cheese, preferably freshly grated

Directions

1. In a saucepan, heat 2 tablespoons of olive oil over a moderate flame. Once hot, sauté the peppers and onions until tender and translucent.
2. Stir in the chicken and marinara sauce; you can add garlic and capers, if desired; continue to simmer for 18 to 22 minutes.
3. Serve garnished with parmesan cheese. Bon appétit!

309. CHICKEN WITH WINE-MUSHROOM SAUCE

Preparation Time: 50 minutes
Servings: 4
Nutrition: 426 Calories; 29.2g Fat; 5.7g Carbs; 33.3g Protein; 1.1g Fiber
Ingredients

- 1 ½ pounds whole chicken, skinless and boneless
- 1 medium-sized leek, chopped
- 2 cups button mushrooms, sliced
- 1/4 cup dry red wine

- 1 cup marinara sauce, no sugar added

Directions

1. In a frying pan, heat 1 tablespoon of olive oil over medium-high heat. Sear the chicken until golden brown or about 9 minutes; reserve.
2. Then, cook the leek and mushrooms until they tender and aromatic or about 5 minutes. Pour in red wine to deglaze the pan.
3. Return the chicken to the frying pan. Season with salt and black pepper. Add in marinara sauce and stir to combine well.
4. Reduce the temperature to medium-low and let it cook for 25 to 30 minutes or until cooked through. Serve and enjoy!

310. 12GOURMET ITALIAN TURKEY FILLETS

Preparation Time: 20 minutes
Servings: 5
Nutrition: 335 Calories; 12.8g Fat; 5.3g Carbs; 47.7g Protein; 0.1g Fiber

Ingredients

- 2 eggs
- 1 cup sour cream
- 1 teaspoon Italian seasoning blend
- 1/2 cup grated parmesan cheese
- 2 pounds turkey fillets

Directions

1. Beat the eggs until frothy and light. Add in the sour cream and continue whisking until pale and well mixed.
2. In another bowl, mix the Italian seasoning blend and parmesan cheese; mix to combine well.
3. Dip the turkey fillets into the egg mixture; then, coat them with the parmesan mixture.
4. Fry turkey fillets in the greased sauté pan until golden brown and cooked through. Bon appétit!

311. MEDITERRANEAN CHICKEN WITH THYME AND OLIVES

Preparation Time: 1 hour 15 minutes
Servings: 5
Nutrition: 235 Calories; 7.5g Fat; 2.7g Carbs; 37.3g Protein; 1g Fiber

Ingredients

- 2 pounds whole chicken
- 1 teaspoon lemon zest, slivered
- 1 cup oil-cured black olives, pitted
- 4 cloves garlic
- 1 bunch fresh thyme, leaves picked

Directions

1. Begin by preheating your oven to 360 degrees F. Then, spritz the sides and bottom of a baking dish with nonstick cooking oil.
2. Sprinkle the chicken with paprika, lemon zest, salt, and black pepper. Bake for 60 minutes.
3. Scatter black olives, garlic, and thyme around the chicken and bake an additional 10 to 13 minutes; a meat thermometer should read 180 degrees F. Bon appétit!

312. DUCK WITH ZUCCHINI AND MARINARA SAUCE

Preparation Time: 30 minutes
Servings: 4
Nutrition: 274 Calories; 13.3g Fat; 3g Carbs; 34.3g Protein; 0.6g Fiber

Ingredients

- 1 ½ pounds duck breasts, chopped into small chunks
- 1/2 cup leeks, sliced
- 1 medium zucchini, sliced
- 1 bell pepper, sliced
- 1 cup marinara sauce, no sugar added

Directions

1. Melt 2 tablespoons of butter in a sauté pan over a moderate flame. Brown the duck breasts for about 7 minutes, stirring frequently.
2. Add in the leeks, zucchini, and pepper; continue to sauté for a further 3 to 4 minutes or until fragrant and tender.
3. Add in marinara sauce. Reduce the heat to a simmer and continue to cook for a further 11 minutes. Serve warm.

MEAT

313. GRILLED SKIRT STEAK

Servings: 4
Preparation Time: 15 minutes
Cooking Time: 8-9 minutes

Ingredients:

- 2 teaspoons fresh ginger herb, grated finely
- 2 teaspoons fresh lime zest, grated finely
- ¼ cup coconut sugar
- 2 teaspoons fish sauce
- 2 tablespoons fresh lime juice
- ½ cup coconut milk
- 1-pound beef skirt steak, trimmed and cut into 4-inch slices lengthwise
- Salt, to taste

Directions:

1. In a sizable sealable bag, mix together all ingredients except steak and salt.
2. Add steak and coat with marinade generously.
3. Seal the bag and refrigerate to marinate for about 4-12 hours.
4. Preheat the grill to high heat. Grease the grill grate.
5. Remove steak from refrigerator and discard the marinade.
6. With a paper towel, dry the steak and sprinkle with salt evenly.
7. Cook the steak for approximately 3½ minutes.
8. Flip the medial side and cook for around 2½-5 minutes or till desired doneness.
9. Remove from grill pan and keep side for approximately 5 minutes before slicing.
10. With a clear, crisp knife cut into desired slices and serve.

Nutrition:

Calories: 465, Fat: 10g, Carbohydrates: 22g, Fiber: 0g, Protein: 37g

314. SPICY LAMB CURRY

Servings: 6-8
Preparation Time: 15 minutes
Cooking Time: 2 hours 15 minutes

Ingredients:

For Spice Mixture:

- 4 teaspoons ground coriander
- 4 teaspoons ground coriander
- 4 teaspoons ground cumin
- ¾ teaspoon ground ginger
- 2 teaspoons ground cinnamon
- ½ teaspoon ground cloves
- ½ teaspoon ground cardamom
- 2 tablespoons sweet paprika
- ½ tablespoon cayenne pepper
- 2 teaspoons chili powder
- 2 teaspoons salt

For Curry:

- 1 tablespoon coconut oil
- 2 pounds boneless lamb, trimmed and cubed into 1-inch size
- Salt and freshly ground black pepper, to taste
- 2 cups onions, chopped
- 1¼ cups water
- 1 cup coconut milk

Directions:

1. For spice mixture in a bowl, mix together all spices. Keep aside.
2. Season the lamb with salt and black pepper.
3. In a large Dutch oven, heat oil on medium-high heat.
4. Add lamb and stir fry for around 5 minutes.
5. Add onion and cook approximately 4-5 minutes.
6. Stir in spice mixture and cook approximately 1 minute.
7. Add water and coconut milk and provide to some boil on high heat.
8. Reduce the heat to low and simmer, covered for approximately 1-120 minutes or till desired doneness of lamb.
9. Uncover and simmer for approximately 3-

4 minutes.
10. Serve hot.

Nutrition:

Calories: 466, Fat: 10g, Carbohydrates: 23g, Fiber: 9g, Protein: 36g

315. LAMB WITH PRUNES

Combo of lamb and prunes is really a wonderful meal for supper. Prunes create a perfect sweet and savory flavor in hearty lamb.
Servings: 4-6
Preparation Time: fifteen minutes
Cooking Time: a couple of hours 40 minutes

Ingredients:

- 3 tablespoons coconut oil
- 2 onions, chopped finely
- 1 (1-inch) piece fresh ginger, minced
- 3 garlic cloves, minced
- ½ teaspoon ground turmeric
- 2 ½ pound lamb shoulder, trimmed and cubed into 3-inch size
- Salt and freshly ground black pepper, to taste
- ½ teaspoon saffron threads, crumbled
- 1 cinnamon stick
- 3 cups water
- 1 cup runes, pitted and halved

Directions:

1. In a big pan, melt coconut oil on medium heat.
2. Add onions, ginger, garlic cloves and turmeric and sauté for about 3-5 minutes.
3. Sprinkle the lamb with salt and black pepper evenly.
4. In the pan, add lamb and saffron threads and cook for approximately 4-5 minutes.
5. Add cinnamon stick and water and produce to some boil on high heat.
6. Reduce the temperature to low and simmer, covered for around 1½-120 minutes or till desired doneness of lamb.
7. Stir in prunes and simmer for approximately 20-a half-hour.
8. Remove cinnamon stick and serve hot.

Nutrition:

Calories: 393, Fat: 12g, Carbohydrates: 10g, Fiber: 4g, Protein: 36g

316. LAMB WITH ZUCCHINI & COUSCOUS

One of fabulously delicious and healthy dish for whole family. This dish is chock filled with nutrient packed ingredients.
Servings: 2
Preparation Time: 15 minutes
Cooking Time: 8 minutes

Ingredients:

- ¾ cup couscous
- ¾ cup boiling water
- ¼ cup fresh cilantro, chopped
- 1 tbsp olive oil
- 5-ounces lamb leg steak, cubed into ¾-inch size
- 1 medium zucchini, sliced thinly
- 1 medium red onion, cut into wedges
- 1 teaspoon ground cumin
- 1 teaspoon ground coriander
- ¼ teaspoon red pepper flakes, crushed
- Salt, to taste
- ¼ cup plain Greek yogurt
- 1 garlic herb, minced

Directions:

1. In a bowl, add couscous and boiling water and stir to combine,
2. Cover whilst aside approximately 5 minutes.
3. Add cilantro and with a fork, fluff completely.
4. Meanwhile in a substantial skillet, heat oil on high heat.
5. Add lamb and stir fry for about 2-3 minutes.
6. Add zucchini and onion and stir fry for about 2 minutes.
7. Stir in spices and stir fry for about 1 minute
8. Add couscous and stir fry approximately 2 minutes.
9. In a bowl, mix together yogurt and garlic.
10. Divide lamb mixture in serving plates evenly.
11. Serve using the topping of yogurt.

Nutrition:

Calories: 392, Fat: 5g, Carbohydrates: 2g, Fiber: 12g, Protein: 35g

317. BAKED LAMB WITH SPINACH

A stunning main course meal to the holidays. This stunning meal isn't only mouth wateringly but super healthy too.
Servings: 6
Preparation Time: 15 minutes
Cooking Time: couple of hours 55 minutes

Ingredients:

- 2 tablespoons coconut oil
- 2-pound lamb necks, trimmed and cut into 2-inch pieces crosswise
- Salt, to taste
- 2 medium onions, chopped
- 3 tablespoons fresh ginger, minced
- 4 garlic cloves, minced
- 2 tablespoons ground coriander
- 1 tablespoon ground cumin
- 1 teaspoon ground turmeric
- ¼ cup coconut milk
- ½ cup tomatoes, chopped
- 2 cups boiling water
- 30-ounce frozen spinach, thawed and squeezed
- 1½ tablespoons garam masala
- 1 tablespoon fresh lemon juice
- Freshly ground black pepper, to taste

Directions:

1. Preheat the oven to 300 degrees F.
2. In a substantial Dutch oven, melt coconut oil on medium-high heat.
3. Add lamb necks and sprinkle with salt.
4. Stir fry approximately 4-5 minutes or till browned completely.
5. Transfer the lamb right into a plate and lower the heat to medium.
6. In exactly the same pan, add onion and sauté for about 10 minutes.
7. Add ginger, garlic and spices and sauté for around 1 minute.
8. Add coconut milk and tomatoes and cook approximately 3-4 minutes.
9. With an immersion blender, blend the mix till smooth.
10. Add lamb, boiling water and salt and convey to some boil.
11. Cover the pan and transfer into the oven.
12. Bake approximately 2½ hours.
13. Now, take away the pan from oven and place on medium heat.
14. Stir in spinach and garam masala and cook for about 3-5 minutes.
15. Stir in fresh lemon juice, salt and black pepper and take off from heat.
16. Serve hot.

Nutrition:

Calories: 423, Fat: 15g, Carbohydrates: 26g, Fiber: 11g, Protein: 33g

318. GROUND LAMB WITH HARISSA

A delicious full meal for your table at dinnertime. Ground lamb, harissa and spices are combined very nicely on this delicious recipe.
Servings: 4
Preparation Time: 15 minutes
Cooking Time: one hour 11 minutes

Ingredients:

- 1 tablespoon extra-virgin olive oil
- 2 red peppers, seeded and chopped finely
- 1 yellow onion, chopped finely
- 2 garlic cloves, chopped finely
- 1 teaspoon ground cumin
- ½ teaspoon ground turmeric
- ¼ teaspoon ground cinnamon
- ¼ teaspoon ground ginger
- 1½ pound lean ground lamb
- Salt, to taste
- 1 (14½-ounce) can diced tomatoes
- 2 tablespoons harissa
- 1 cup water
- Chopped fresh cilantro, for garnishing

Directions:

In a sizable pan, heat oil on medium-high heat.

1. Add bell pepper, onion and garlic and sauté for around 5 minutes.
2. Add spices and sauté for around 1 minute.
3. Add lamb and salt and cook

approximately 5 minutes, getting into pieces.

4. Stir in tomatoes, harissa and water and provide with a boil.
5. Reduce the warmth to low and simmer, covered for about 1 hour.
6. Serve hot while using garnishing of harissa.

Nutrition:

Calories: 441, Fat: 12g, Carbohydrates: 24g, Fiber: 10g, Protein: 36g

319. GROUND LAMB WITH PEAS

A best tasting spiced ground lamb recipe for supper. Surely all so want to eat this spiced dish of lamb and veggies.
Servings: 4
Preparation Time: 15 minutes
Cooking Time: 55 minutes

Ingredients:

- 1 tablespoon coconut oil
- 3 dried red chilies
- 1 (2-inch) cinnamon stick
- 3 green cardamom pods
- ½ teaspoon cumin seeds
- 1 medium red onion, chopped
- 1 (¾-inch) piece fresh ginger, minced
- 4 garlic cloves, minced
- 1½ teaspoons ground coriander
- ½ teaspoon garam masala
- ½ teaspoon ground cumin
- ½ teaspoon ground turmeric
- ¼ teaspoon ground nutmeg
- 2 bay leaves
- 1-pound lean ground lamb
- ½ cup Roma tomatoes, chopped
- 1-1½ cups water
- 1 cup fresh green peas, shelled
- 2 tablespoons plain Greek yogurt, whipped
- ¼ cup fresh cilantro, chopped
- Salt and freshly ground black pepper, to taste

Directions:

- In a Dutch oven, melt coconut oil medium-high heat.
- Add red chilies, cinnamon stick, cardamom pods and cumin seeds and sauté for around thirty seconds.
- Add onion and sauté for about 3-4 minutes.
- Add ginger, garlic cloves and spices and sauté for around thirty seconds.
- Add lamb and cook approximately 5 minutes.
- Add tomatoes and cook approximately 10 min.
- Stir in water and green peas and cook, covered approximately 25-thirty minutes.
- Stir in yogurt, cilantro, salt and black pepper and cook for around 4-5 minutes.
- Serve hot.

Nutrition:

Calories: 430, Fat: 10g, Carbohydrates: 22g, Fiber: 6g, Protein: 26g

320. ROASTED LEG OF LAMB

One of best dish for weeknight dinners. Slow roasting gives leg of lamb a great perfection of flavoring.
Servings: 8
Preparation Time: 15 minutes
Cooking Time: 75-100 minutes

Ingredients:

- 1/3 cup fresh parsley, minced
- 4 garlic cloves, minced
- 1 teaspoon fresh lemon zest, grated finely
- 1 tablespoon ground coriander
- 1 tablespoon ground cumin
- 1 teaspoon ground cinnamon
- 1 teaspoon ground turmeric
- 1 tablespoon sweet paprika
- ½ teaspoon allspice
- 20 saffron threads, crushed
- 1/3 cup essential olive oil
- 1 (5-pound) leg of lamb, trimmed

Directions:

1. In a bowl, mix together all ingredients except lamb.
2. Coat the leg of lamb with marinade

mixture generously.

3. With a plastic wrap, cover the leg of lamb and refrigerate to marinate for about 4-8 hours.
4. Remove from refrigerator and keep in room temperature for about a half-hour before roasting.
5. Preheat the oven to 350 degrees F. Arrange the rack inside the center of the oven.
6. Lightly, grease a roasting pan make a rack inside roasting pan.
7. Place the lower limb of lamb in the rack in prepared roasting pan.
8. Roast for approximately 75-100 minutes or till desired doneness, rotating once inside the middle way.

Nutrition:

Calories: 392, Fat: 12g, Carbohydrates: 20g, Fiber: 4g, Protein: 37g

321. BROILED LAMB SHOULDER

A super-healthy and flavorful dish for supper table. This healthy and delicious dish is prepared with no fuss in less time.
Servings: 10
Preparation Time: 10 minutes
Cooking Time: 8-10 minutes

Ingredients:

- 2 tablespoons fresh ginger, minced
- 2 tablespoons garlic, minced
- ¼ cup fresh lemongrass stalk, minced
- ¼ cup fresh orange juice
- ¼ cup coconut aminos
- Freshly ground black pepper, to taste
- 2-pound lamb shoulder, trimmed

Directions:

1. In a bowl, mix together all ingredients except lamb shoulder.
2. In a baking dish, squeeze lamb shoulder and coat the lamb with half in the marinade mixture generously.
3. Reserve remaining mixture.
4. Refrigerate to marinate for overnight.
5. Preheat the broiler of oven. Place a rack inside a broiler pan and arrange about 4-5-inches from heating unit.
6. Remove lamb shoulder from refrigerator and remove excess marinade.
7. Broil approximately 4-5 minutes from both sides.
8. Serve with all the reserved marinade like a sauce.

Nutrition:

Calories: 250, Fat: 19g, Carbohydrates: 2g. Fiber: 0g, Protein: 15g

322. PAN-SEARED LAMB CHOPS

A hearty lamb chops recipe using the flavorful touch of warm spices. This recipe will probably be perfect for dinner and launch too.
Servings: 4
Preparation Time: 10 minutes
Cooking Time: 4-6 minutes

Ingredients:

- 4 garlic cloves, peeled
- Salt, to taste
- 1 teaspoon black mustard seeds, crushed finely
- 2 teaspoons ground cumin
- 1 teaspoon ground ginger
- 1 teaspoon ground coriander
- ½ teaspoon ground cinnamon
- Freshly ground black pepper, to taste
- 1 tablespoon coconut oil
- 8 medium lamb chops, trimmed

Directions:

1. Place garlic cloves onto a cutting board and sprinkle with salt.
2. With a knife, crush the garlic till a paste forms.
3. In a bowl, mix together garlic paste and spices.
4. With a clear, crisp knife, make 3-4 cuts on both side in the chops.
5. Rub the chops with garlic mixture generously.
6. In a large skillet, melt butter on medium heat.
7. Add chops and cook for approximately 2-3 minutes per side or till desired doneness.

Nutrition:

Calories: 443, Fat: 11g, Carbohydrates: 27g, Fiber:

4g, Protein: 40g

323. ROASTED LAMB CHOPS WITH RELISH

Entertain all your family members with these satisfying roasted lamb chops. These delicious roasted lamb chops are infused using the taste of spices, yogurt fresh lime.
Servings: 4
Preparation Time: 15 minutes
Cooking Time: half an hour

Ingredients:

For Lamb Marinade:

- 4 garlic cloves, chopped
- 1 (2-inch) piece fresh ginger, chopped
- 2 green chilies, seeded and chopped
- 1 teaspoon fresh lime zest
- 2 teaspoons garam masala
- 1 teaspoon ground coriander
- 1 teaspoon ground cumin
- ½ teaspoon ground cinnamon
- 1 teaspoon coconut oil, melted
- 2 tablespoons fresh lime juice
- 6-7 tablespoons plain Greek yogurt
- 1 (8-bone) rack of lamb, trimmed
- 2 onions, sliced

For Relish:

- ½ of garlic herb, chopped
- 1 (1-inch) piece fresh ginger, chopped
- ¼ cup fresh cilantro, chopped
- ¼ cup fresh mint, chopped
- 1 green chili, seeded and chopped
- 1 teaspoon fresh lime zest
- 1 teaspoon organic honey
- 2 tablespoons fresh apple juice
- 2 tablespoons fresh lime juice

Directions:

1. For chops in a very mixer, add all ingredients except yogurt, chops and onions and pulse till smooth.
2. Transfer the mixture in a large bowl with yogurt and stir to combine well.
3. Add chops and coat with mixture generously.
4. Refrigerate to marinate for approximately 24 hours.
5. Preheat the oven to 375 degrees F. Linea roasting pan with a foil paper.
6. Place the onion wedges in the bottom of prepared roasting pan.
7. Arrange rack of lamb over onion wedges.
8. Roast approximately half an hour.
9. Meanwhile for relish in the blender, add all ingredients and pulse till smooth.
10. Serve chops and onions alongside relish.

Nutrition:

Calories: 439, Fat: 17g, Carbohydrates: 26g, Fiber: 10g, Protein: 41g

324. GRILLED LAMB CHOPS

A really simple and easy to organize grilled lamb chops which might be rich in flavors. This recipe is a great option for barbecue parties.
Servings: 4
Preparation Time: 10 min
Cooking Time: 6 minutes

Ingredients:

- 1 tablespoon fresh ginger, grated
- 4 garlic cloves, chopped roughly
- 1 teaspoon ground cumin
- ½ teaspoon red chili powder
- Salt and freshly ground black pepper, to taste
- 1 tbsp essential olive oil
- 1 tablespoon fresh lemon juice
- 8 lamb chops, trimmed

Directions:

1. In a bowl, mix together all ingredients except chops.
2. With a hand blender, blend till a smooth mixture forms.
3. Add chops and coat with mixture generously.
4. Refrigerate to marinate for overnight.
5. Preheat the barbecue grill till hot. Grease the grill grate.
6. Grill the chops for approximately 3 minutes per side.

Nutrition:

Calories: 227, Fat: 12g, Carbohydrates: 1g, Fiber: 0g, Protein: 30g

325. LAMB BURGERS WITH AVOCADO DIP

A winner and delicious burger recipe for whole family. These burgers are wonderful when with smooth and silky textured avocado dip.
Servings: 4-6
Preparation Time: 20 minutes
Cooking Time: 10 minutes

Ingredients:

For Burgers:

- 1 (2-inch) piece fresh ginger, grated
- 1-pound lean ground lamb
- 1 medium onion, grated
- 2 minced garlic cloves
- 1 bunch fresh mint leaves, chopped finely
- 2 teaspoons ground coriander
- 2 teaspoons ground cumin
- ½ teaspoon ground allspice
- ½ teaspoon ground cinnamon
- Salt and freshly ground black pepper, to taste
- 1 tbsp essential olive oil

For Dip:

- 3 small cucumbers, peeled and grated
- 1 avocado, peeled, pitted and chopped
- ½ of garlic oil, crushed
- 2 tablespoons fresh lemon juice
- 2 tablespoons olive oil
- 2 tablespoons fresh dill, chopped finely
- 2 tablespoons chives, chopped finely
- Salt and freshly ground black pepper, to taste

Directions:

1. Preheat the broiler of oven. Lightly, grease a broiler pan.
2. For burgers in a big bowl, squeeze the juice of ginger.
3. Add remaining ingredients and mix till well combined.
4. Make equal sized burgers from your mixture.
5. Arrange the burgers in broiler pan and broil approximately 5 minutes per side.
6. Meanwhile for dip squeeze the cucumbers juice in a bowl.
7. In a blender, add avocado, garlic, lemon juice and oil and pulse till smooth.
8. Transfer the avocado mixture in a bowl.
9. Add remaining ingredients and stir to mix.
10. Serve the burgers with avocado dip.

Nutrition:

Calories: 462, Fat: 15g, Carbohydrates: 23g, Fiber: 9g, Protein: 39g

326. LAMB & PINEAPPLE KEBABS

One from the delicious recipe of lamb and pineapple kebabs using a tasty layer of char. Fresh mint provides a refreshing touch to those kebabs.
Servings: 4-6
Preparation Time: 15 minutes
Cooking Time: 10 minutes

Ingredients:

- 1 large pineapple, cubed into 1½-inch size, divided
- 1 (½-inch) piece fresh ginger, chopped
- 2 garlic cloves, chopped
- Salt, to taste
- 16-24-ounce lamb shoulder steak, trimmed and cubed into 1½-inch size
- Fresh mint leaves coming from a bunch
- Ground cinnamon, to taste

Directions:

1. In a blender, add about 1½ of pineapple, ginger, garlic and salt and pulse till smooth.
2. Transfer the amalgamation right into a large bowl.
3. Add chops and coat with mixture generously.
4. Refrigerate to marinate for about 1-2 hours.
5. Preheat the grill to medium heat. Grease the grill grate.
6. Thread lam, remaining pineapple and mint leaves onto pre-soaked wooden skewers.
7. Grill the kebabs approximately 10 min, turning occasionally.

Nutrition:

Calories: 482, Fat: 16g, Carbohydrates: 22g, Fiber: 5g, Protein: 377g

327. BAKED MEATBALLS & SCALLIONS

A recipe of lamb meatballs that is filled with flavor and aroma. Baked meatballs pair nicely with all the crispy tips of braised scallions.
Servings: 4-6
Preparation Time: 20 min
Cooking Time: 35 minutes

Ingredients:

For Meatballs:

- 1 lemongrass stalk, outer skin peeled and chopped
- 1 (1½-inch) piece fresh ginger, sliced
- 3 garlic cloves, chopped
- 1 cup fresh cilantro leaves, chopped roughly
- ½ cup fresh basil leaves, chopped roughly
- 2 tablespoons plus 1 teaspoon fish sauce
- 2 tablespoons water
- 2 tablespoons fresh lime juice
- ½ pound lean ground pork
- 1-pound lean ground lamb
- 1 carrot, peeled and grated
- 1 organic egg, beaten

For Scallions:

- 16 stalks scallions, trimmed
- 2 tablespoons coconut oil, melted
- Salt, to taste
- ½ cup water

Directions:

1. Preheat the oven to 375 degrees F. Grease a baking dish.
2. In a blender, add lemongrass, ginger, garlic, fresh herbs, fish sauce, water and lime juice and pulse till chopped finely.
3. Transfer the amalgamation in a bowl with remaining ingredients and mix till well combined.
4. Make about 1-inch balls from mixture.
5. Arrange the balls into prepared baking dish in a single layer.
6. In another rimmed baking dish, arrange scallion stalks in a very single layer.
7. Drizzle with coconut oil and sprinkle with salt.
8. Pour water in the baking dish 1nd with a foil paper cover it tightly.
9. Bake the scallion for around a half-hour.
10. Bake the meatballs for approximately 30-35 minutes.

Nutrition:

Calories: 432, Fat: 13g, Carbohydrates: 25g, Fiber: 8g, Protein: 40g

328. PORK WITH BELL PEPPER

This stir fry not simply tastes wonderful but additionally is packed with nutritious benefits. Fresh lime juice intensifies the taste with this stir fry.
Servings: 4
Preparation Time: 15 minutes
Cooking Time: 13 minutes

Ingredients:

- 1 tablespoon fresh ginger, chopped finely
- 4 garlic cloves, chopped finely
- 1 cup fresh cilantro, chopped and divided
- ¼ cup plus 1 tbsp olive oil, divided
- 1-pound tender pork, trimmed, sliced thinly
- 2 onions, sliced thinly
- 1 green bell pepper, seeded and sliced thinly
- 1 tablespoon fresh lime juice

Directions:

1. In a substantial bowl, mix together ginger, garlic, ½ cup of cilantro and ¼ cup of oil.
2. Add pork and coat with mixture generously.
3. Refrigerate to marinate approximately a couple of hours.
4. Heat a big skillet on medium-high heat.
5. Add pork mixture and stir fry for approximately 4-5 minutes.
6. Transfer the pork right into a bowl.
7. In the same skillet, heat remaining oil on medium heat.
8. Add onion and sauté for approximately 3 minutes.
9. Stir in bell pepper and stir fry for about 3 minutes.
10. Stir in pork, lime juice and remaining cilantro and cook for about 2 minutes.

11. Serve hot.

Nutrition:

Calories: 429, Fat: 19g, Carbohydrates: 26g, Fiber: 9g, Protein: 35g

329. PORK WITH PINEAPPLE

A wonderfully delicious recipe which will surely impress a meat lover. Pineapple compliments pork tenderloin in the wonderful way.
Servings: 4
Preparation Time: 15 minutes
Cooking Time: 14 minutes

Ingredients:

- 2 tablespoons coconut oil
- 1½ pound pork tenderloin, trimmed and cut into bite-sized pieces
- 1 onion, chopped
- 2 minced garlic cloves
- 1 (1-inch) piece fresh ginger, minced
- 20-ounce pineapple, cut into chunks
- 1 large red bell pepper, seeded and chopped
- ¼ cup fresh pineapple juice
- ¼ cup coconut aminos
- Salt and freshly ground black pepper, to taste

Directions:

1. In a substantial skillet, melt coconut oil on high heat.
2. Add pork and stir fry approximately 4-5 minutes.
3. Transfer the pork right into a bowl.
4. In exactly the same skillet, heat remaining oil on medium heat.
5. Add onion, garlic and ginger and sauté for around 2 minutes.
6. Stir in pineapple and bell pepper and stir fry for around 3 minutes.
7. Stir in pork, pineapple juice and coconut aminos and cook for around 3-4 minutes.
8. Serve hot.

Nutrition:

Calories: 431, Fat: 10g, Carbohydrates: 22g, Fiber: 8g, Protein: 33g

330. SPICED PORK

One from the absolute delicious dish of spiced pork. Slow cooking helps you to infuse the spice flavors in pork very nicely.
Servings: 6
Preparation Time: fifteen minutes
Cooking Time: 1 hour 52 minutes

Ingredients:

- 1 (2-inch) piece fresh ginger, chopped
- 5-10 garlic cloves, chopped
- 1 teaspoon ground cumin
- ½ teaspoon ground turmeric
- 1 tablespoon hot paprika
- 1 tablespoon red pepper flakes
- Salt, to taste
- 2 tablespoons cider vinegar
- 2-pounds pork shoulder, trimmed and cubed into 1½-inch size
- 2 cups domestic hot water, divided
- 1 (1-inch wide) ball tamarind pulp
- ¼ cup olive oil
- 1 teaspoon black mustard seeds, crushed
- 4 green cardamoms
- 5 whole cloves
- 1 (3-inch) cinnamon stick
- 1 cup onion, chopped finely
- 1 large red bell pepper, seeded and chopped

Directions:

1. In a food processor, add ginger, garlic, cumin, turmeric, paprika, red pepper flakes, salt and cider vinegar and pulse till smooth.
2. Transfer the amalgamation in to a large bowl.
3. Add pork and coat with mixture generously.
4. Keep aside, covered for around an hour at room temperature.
5. In a bowl, add 1 cup of warm water and tamarind and make aside till water becomes cool.
6. With the hands, crush the tamarind to extract the pulp.
7. Add remaining cup of hot water and mix till well combined.
8. Through a fine sieve, strain the tamarind

juice inside a bowl.

9. In a sizable skillet, heat oil on medium-high heat.
10. Add mustard seeds, green cardamoms, cloves and cinnamon stick and sauté for about 4 minutes.
11. Add onion and sauté for approximately 5 minutes.
12. Add pork and stir fry for approximately 6 minutes.
13. Stir in tamarind juice and convey with a boil.
14. Reduce the heat to medium-low and simmer 1½ hours.
15. Stir in bell pepper and cook for about 7 minutes.

Nutrition:

Calories: 435, Fat: 16g, Carbohydrates: 27g, Fiber: 3g, Protein: 39g

331. PORK CHILI

A great bowl of healthy chili with the amazing addition of Bok choy. This healthy chili is tasty, spicy and refreshing on the same time.
Servings: 8
Preparation Time: 15 minutes
Cooking Time: 1 hour

Ingredients:

- 2 tablespoons extra-virgin organic olive oil
- 2-pound ground pork
- 1 medium red bell pepper, seeded and chopped
- 1 medium onion, chopped
- 5 garlic cloves, chopped finely
- 1 (2-inch) part of hot pepper, minced
- 1 tablespoon ground cumin
- 1 teaspoon ground turmeric
- 3 tablespoon chili powder
- ½ teaspoon chipotle chili powder
- Salt and freshly ground black pepper, to taste
- 1 cup chicken broth
- 1 (28-ounce) can fire-roasted crushed tomatoes
- 2 medium Bok choy heads, sliced
- 1 avocado, peeled, pitted and chopped

Directions:

1. In a sizable pan, heat oil on medium heat.
2. Add pork and stir fry for about 5 minutes.
3. Add bell pepper, onion, garlic, hot pepper and spices and stir fry for approximately 5 minutes.
4. Add broth and tomatoes and convey with a boil.
5. Stir in Bok choy and cook, covered for approximately twenty minutes.
6. Uncover and cook approximately 20-half an hour.
7. Serve hot while using topping of avocado.

Nutrition:

Calories: 402, Fat: 9g, Carbohydrates: 18g, Fiber: 6g, Protein: 32g

332. GROUND PORK WITH WATER CHESTNUTS

This recipe is an easy way to prepare weeknight meal which has a healthy touch. This recipe prepares a flavor packed meal.
Servings: 4
Preparation Time: fifteen minutes
Cooking Time: 12 minutes

Ingredients:

- 1 tablespoon plus 1 teaspoon coconut oil
- 1 tablespoon fresh ginger, minced
- 1 bunch scallion (white and green parts separated), chopped
- 1-pound lean ground pork
- Salt, to taste
- 1 tablespoon 5-spice powder
- 1 (18-ounce) can water chestnuts, drained and chopped
- 1 tablespoon organic honey
- 2 tablespoons fresh lime juice

Directions:

1. In a big heavy bottomed skillet, heat oil on high heat.
2. Add ginger and scallion whites and sauté for approximately ½-1½ minutes.
3. Add pork and cook for approximately 4-5 minutes.
4. Drain the extra Fat from skillet.
5. Add salt and 5-spice powder and cook for

approximately 2-3 minutes.

6. Add scallion greens and remaining ingredients and cook, stirring continuously for about 1-2 minutes.

Nutrition:

Calories: 520, Fat: 30g, Carbohydrates: 37g, Fiber: 4g, Protein: 25g

333. GLAZED PORK CHOPS WITH PEACH

One associated with an easy and impressive strategy to enjoy pork and fresh peach in the delicious glaze. This sweet and spicy glaze makes pork super delicious.
Servings: 2
Preparation Time: 15 minutes
Cooking Time: 16 minutes

Ingredients:

- 2 boneless pork chops
- Salt and freshly ground black pepper, to taste
- 1 ripe yellow peach, peeled, pitted, chopped and divided
- 1 tbsp organic olive oil
- 2 tablespoons shallot, minced
- 2 tablespoons garlic, minced
- 2 tablespoons fresh ginger, minced
- 1 tablespoon organic honey
- 1 tablespoon balsamic vinegar
- 1 tablespoon coconut aminos
- ¼ teaspoon red pepper flakes, crushed
- ¼ cup water

Directions:

1. Sprinkle the pork chops with salt and black pepper generously.
2. In a blender, add 1 / 2 of peach and pulse till a puree forms.
3. Reserve remaining peach.
4. In a skillet, heat oil on medium heat.
5. Add shallots and sauté approximately 1-2 minutes.
6. Add garlic and ginger and sauté approximately 1 minute.
7. Add remaining ingredients and lower heat to medium-low.
8. Bring to your boil and simmer for approximately 4-5 minutes or till a sticky glaze forms.
9. Remove from heat and reserve 1/3 with the glaze and keep aside.
10. Coat the chops with remaining glaze.
11. Heat a nonstick skillet on medium-high heat.
12. Add chops and sear for around 4 minutes from both sides.
13. Transfer the chops in a plate and coat with all the remaining glaze evenly.
14. Top with reserved chopped peach and serve.

Nutrition:

Calories: 446, Fat: 20g, Carbohydrates: 26g, Fiber: 5g, Protein: 38g

334. PORK CHOPS IN CREAMY SAUCE

Pork chops with extra twist of delish flavors. This special and straightforward strategy of coconut sauce gives extra flavor and texture to pork chops.
Servings: 4
Preparation Time: fifteen minutes
Cooking Time: 14 minutes

Ingredients:

- 2 garlic cloves, chopped
- 1 small jalapeño pepper, chopped
- ¼ cup fresh cilantro leaves
- 1½ teaspoons ground turmeric, divided
- 1 tablespoon fish sauce
- 2 tablespoons fresh lime juice
- 1 (13½-ounce) can coconut milk
- 4 (½-inch thick) pork chops
- Salt, to taste
- 1 tablespoon coconut oil
- 1 shallot, chopped finely

Directions:

1. In a blender, add garlic, jalapeño pepper, cilantro, 1 teaspoon of ground turmeric, fish sauce, lime juice and coconut milk and pulse till smooth.
2. Sprinkle the pork with salt and remaining turmeric evenly.
3. In a skillet, melt butter on medium-high heat.

4. Add shallots and sauté approximately 1 minute.
5. Add chops and cook for approximately 2 minutes per side.
6. Transfer the chops inside a bowl.
7. Add coconut mixture and convey to your boil.
8. Reduce heat to medium and simmer, stirring occasionally for approximately 5 minutes.
9. Stir in pork chops and cook for about 3-4 minutes.
10. Serve hot.

Nutrition:

Calories: 437, Fat: 9g, Carbohydrates: 21g, Fiber: 4g, Protein: 38g

335. BAKED PORK & MUSHROOM MEATBALLS

Servings: 6
Preparation Time: 15 minutes
Cooking Time: fifteen minutes

Ingredients:

- 1-pound lean ground pork
- 1 organic egg white, beaten
- 4 fresh shiitake mushrooms, stemmed and minced
- 1 tablespoon fresh parsley, minced
- 1 tablespoon fresh basil leaves, minced
- 1 tablespoon fresh mint leaves, minced
- 2 teaspoons fresh lemon zest, grated finely
- 1½ teaspoons fresh ginger, grated finely
- Salt and freshly ground black pepper, to taste

Directions:

1. Preheat the oven to 425 degrees F. Arrange the rack inside center of oven.
2. Line a baking sheet with a parchment paper.
3. In a sizable bowl, add all ingredients and mix till well combined.
4. Make small equal-sized balls from mixture.
5. Arrange the balls onto prepared baking sheet in a single layer.
6. Bake for approximately 12-15 minutes or till done completely.

Nutrition:

Calories: 411, Fat: 19g, Carbohydrates: 27g, Fiber: 11g, Protein: 35g

336. BUTTERNUT SQUASH, KALE AND GROUND BEEF BREAKFAST BOWL

Preparation Time: 10 minutes
Cooking Time: 20 minutes
Serving: 3

Ingredients:

- ¼ cup coconut milk
- 1 to 2 tbsp coconut shavings
- ¼ tsp ground cinnamon
- ¼ tsp ground ginger
- ½ tsp spicy curry
- 1 tsp garam masala
- ¼ large butternut squash, cook and peeled
- 5 kale leaves, chopped
- Salt and pepper to taste
- ¼-lb lean grass-fed beef
- 1 to 2 chopped button mushrooms
- ½ of small onion, diced
- Coconut oil

Directions:

1. In a skillet, heat a small amount of coconut oil over medium high heat. Sauté the mushroom and onions. Add the salt and pepper. Continue cooking for three minutes.
2. Add the ground beef, curry, garam masala, cinnamon and ginger. Continue to cook until the beef turns brown.
3. Add the chopped kale and cook until the leaves wilt.
4. Stir in the coconut milk and add the cooked squash. Continue cooking until the squash breaks down.
5. Transfer in a bowl and garnish with coconut shavings. Serve warm.

Nutrition Facts Per Serving

Calories 225, Total Fat 14g, Saturated Fat 3g, Total Carbs 17g, Net Carbs 13g, Protein 10g, Sugar: 6g, Fiber 4g, Sodium 43mg, Potassium 469mg

337. LIGHT BEEF SOUP

Preparation Time: 10 minutes
Cooking Time: 1 hour and 10 minutes
Serving: 8

Ingredients:

- 1 tablespoon olive oil
- 1 large onion, chopped
- 2 cloves of garlic, minced
- 2 stalks celery, sliced
- 1-pound beef chuck, bones removed and cut into cubes
- salt and pepper to taste
- 2 carrots, peeled and diced
- 8 ounces mushrooms, sliced
- ½ teaspoon dried thyme
- 2 cups beef broth
- 2 cups chicken broth
- 2 cups water
- 1 bay leaf

Directions:

1. Heat the oil in a pot and sauté the onion, garlic, and celery until fragrant.
2. Stir in the beef chuck and season with salt and pepper.
3. Add the rest of the ingredients.
4. Close the lid and bring to a boil.
5. Allow to simmer for 60 minutes until the beef is soft.
6. Serve and enjoy.

Nutrition Facts Per Serving

Calories 117, Total Fat 5g, Saturated Fat 1g, Total Carbs 5g, Net Carbs 4g, Protein 13g, Sugar: 2g, Fiber 1g, Sodium 546mg, Potassium 409mg

338. BEEF NOODLE SOUP

Preparation Time: 20 minutes
Cooking Time: 25 minutes
Serving: 4

Ingredients:

- 4 cups zucchini, spiral
- 1 cup carrots, spiral
- 1 cup jicama, spiral
- 2 pcs Beef Knorr Cubes
- 8 cups water
- freshly ground pepper to taste
- 3 stalks green onions, chopped
- ¼ lb beef, thinly sliced
- 4 tbsp ground pork rinds (chicharon), divided
- 2 hardboiled eggs, halved
- 1 tsp salt

Directions:

1. In a pot, bring water to a boil. Add Knorr cubes and fish sauce.
2. With a strainer, dip into the boiling water the zucchini noodles and cook for 3 minutes. Remove from water, drain and arrange into 4 bowls. If needed, you can cook zucchini noodles in batches.
3. Next, cook the carrots in the boiling pot of water using a strainer still. Around 2-3 minutes, drain and arrange on top of the zucchini noodles.
4. Do the same with jicama, cook in the pot, drain and arrange equally into the bowls.
5. Do the same for the thinly sliced beef. Cook for 5-10 minutes in the boiling pot of soup, swirling the strainer occasionally to ensure uniform cooking for the beef. Arrange equally on the 4 bowls.
6. Sprinkle 1 tbsp of ground pork rinds on each bowl, topped by chopped green onions, ½ hardboiled egg and freshly ground pepper.
7. Taste the boiling pot of soup and adjust to your taste. It should be slightly saltier than the usual so that the noodles will absorb the excess salt once you pour it into the bowls. Add more fish sauce to make it salty or add water to make the pot less salty. Keep soup on a rolling boil before pouring 1-2 cups of soup on each bowl. Serve right away.

Nutrition Facts Per Serving

Calories 101, Total Fat 4g, Saturated Fat 1g, Total Carbs 7g, Net Carbs g, Protein 10g, Sugar: 3g, Fiber 3g, Sodium 1100mg, Potassium 353mg

339. SPANISH RICE CASSEROLE WITH BEEF

Preparation Time: 10 minutes

Cooking Time: 25 minutes
Serving: 2

Ingredients:

- 2 tablespoons chopped green bell pepper
- 1/4 teaspoon Worcestershire sauce
- 1/4 teaspoon ground cumin
- 1/4 cup finely chopped onion
- 1/4 cup chile sauce
- 1/3 cup uncooked long grain, brown rice
- 1/2-pound lean ground beef
- 1/2 teaspoon salt
- 1/2 teaspoon brown sugar
- 1/2 pinch ground black pepper
- 1/2 cup water
- 1/2 (14.5 ounce) can canned tomatoes
- 1 tablespoon chopped fresh cilantro

Directions:

1. Place a nonstick saucepan on medium fire and brown beef for 10 minutes while crumbling beef. Discard fat.
2. Stir in pepper, Worcestershire sauce, cumin, brown sugar, salt, chile sauce, rice, water, tomatoes, green bell pepper, and onion. Mix well and cook for 10 minutes until blended and a bit tender.
3. Transfer to an ovenproof casserole and press down firmly. Broil for 3 minutes until top is lightly browned.
4. Serve and enjoy with chopped cilantro.

Nutrition Facts Per Serving

Calories 437, Total Fat 16g, Saturated Fat 2.5g, Total Carbs 38g, Net Carbs 30g, Protein 38g, Sugar: 12g, Fiber 8g, Sodium 1144mg, Potassium 1235mg

340. KEFTA STYLED BEEF PATTIES WITH CUCUMBER SALAD

Preparation Time: 10 minutes
Cooking Time: 10 minutes
Serving: 4

Ingredients:

- 2 pcs of 6-inch pita, quartered
- ½ tsp freshly ground black pepper
- 1 tbsp fresh lemon juice
- ½ cup plain Greek yogurt, fat free
- 2 cups thinly sliced English cucumber
- ½ tsp ground cinnamon
- ½ tsp salt
- 1 tsp ground cumin
- 2 tsp ground coriander
- 1 tbsp peeled and chopped ginger
- ¼ cup cilantro, fresh
- ¼ cup plus 2 tbsp fresh parsley, chopped and divided
- 1 lb. ground sirloin

Directions:

1. On medium high fire, preheat a grill pan coated with cooking spray.
2. In a medium bowl, mix together cinnamon, salt, cumin, coriander, ginger, cilantro, parsley and beef. Then divide the mixture equally into four parts and shaping each portion into a patty ½ inch thick.
3. Then place patties on pan cooking each side for three minutes or until desired doneness is achieved.
4. In a separate bowl, toss together vinegar and cucumber.
5. In a small bowl, whisk together pepper, juice, 2 tbsp parsley and yogurt.
6. Serve each patty on a plate with ½ cup cucumber mixture and 2 tbsp of the yogurt sauce.

Nutrition Facts Per Serving

Calories 306, Total Fat 13g, Saturated Fat 2g, Total Carbs 11g, Net Carbs 9g, Protein 34g, Sugar: 2g, Fiber 2g, Sodium 433mg, Potassium 507mg

341. BROILED LAMB CHOPS

Preparation Time: 10 minutes
Cooking Time: 10 minutes
Serving: 4

Ingredients:

- Cooking spray
- 8 pcs of lamb loin chops, around 4 oz
- ¼ tsp black pepper
- ½ tsp salt

- 1 tbsp bottled minced garlic
- 2 tbsps lemon juice
- 1 tbsp dried oregano

Directions:

1. Preheat broiler.
2. In a big bowl or dish, combine the black pepper, salt, minced garlic, lemon juice and oregano. Then rub it equally on all sides of the lamb chops.
3. Then coat a broiler pan with the cooking spray before placing the lamb chops on the pan and broiling until desired doneness is reached or for five minutes per side.

Nutrition Facts Per Serving

Calories 332, Total Fat 16g, Saturated Fat 2.3g, Total Carbs 3g, Net Carbs 2.7g, Protein 46g, Sugar: 0.6g, Fiber 0.3g, Sodium 466mg, Potassium 780mg

342. MUSTARD CHOPS WITH APRICOT-BASIL RELISH

Preparation Time: 20 minutes
Cooking Time: 12 minutes
Serving: 4

Ingredients:

- 1 tsp ground cardamom
- 2 tbsp olive oil
- 3 tbsp raspberry vinegar
- ¼ cup basil, finely shredded
- 1 shallot, diced small
- ¾ lb. fresh apricots, stone removed, and fruit diced
- ½ cup mustard
- Pepper and salt
- 4 pork chops

Directions:

1. Make sure that pork chops are defrosted well. Season with pepper and salt. Slather both sides of each pork chop with mustard. Preheat grill to medium-high fire.
2. In a medium bowl, mix cardamom, olive oil, vinegar, basil, shallot, and apricots. Toss to combine and season with pepper and salt, mixing once again.
3. Grill chops for 5 to 6 minutes per side. As you flip, baste with mustard.
4. Serve pork chops with the Apricot-Basil relish and enjoy.

Nutrition Facts Per Serving

Calories 488, Total Fat 25g, Saturated Fat 3.5g, Total Carbs 22g, Net Carbs 19g, Protein 42g, Sugar: 18g, Fiber 3g, Sodium 478mg, Potassium 763mg

343. SIRLOIN ROLLS WITH BRUSSELS SPROUTS & FENNEL

Preparation Time: 10 minutes
Cooking Time: 50 minutes
Serving: 4

Ingredients:

- 3 fennel fronds
- 1 tsp olive oil
- ½ fennel bulb cut into thick slices
- 2 cups Brussels sprouts, bottoms trimmed off and quartered
- Pepper and salt to taste
- 2 pieces of ½ lb. each sirloin steak

Filling Ingredients:

- 1 tsp oregano
- 1 tsp sage
- 1 tsp rosemary
- 2 garlic cloves
- ½ cup Brussels sprouts, bottoms trimmed off and halved
- ½ fennel bulb, roughly chopped

Directions:

1. Preheat oven to 375oF.
2. In a blender, puree all filling ingredients.
3. With a mallet, pound steaks until ½-inch thick. Divide into two the pureed filling ingredients and spread on each steak. Roll steak and secure ends with a toothpick.
4. In a large roasting pan, place fennel and Brussels sprouts slices. Season with pepper, salt, and olive oil. Toss well to coat. Arrange sprouts and fennel on the side of pan.
5. Place steaks in middle of roasting pan and season with pepper and salt.
6. Roast for 35 to 40 minutes. Remove steak

if desired doneness is reached and let it rest as you continue to roast veggies for another 5 to 10 minutes.

Nutrition Facts Per Serving

Calories 342, Total Fat 21g, Saturated Fat 4g, Total Carbs 12g, Net Carbs 7.5g, Protein 28g, Sugar: 4.4g, Fiber 4.5g, Sodium 168mg, Potassium 952mg

344. STONE FRUIT SLAW TOPPED GRILLED CHOPS

Preparation Time: 10 minutes
Cooking Time: 20 minutes
Serving: 4

Ingredients:

- 1 tsp ground paprika
- 1 tsp ground cumin
- 1 tsp ground coriander
- 1 tsp sea salt
- 4 bone-in pork chops, around 1 – 1 ½ inches thick

Slaw Ingredients:

- A pinch of salt
- 1 tsp lime juice
- 1 tsp lime zest
- ¼ tsp ground chipotle powder
- 1 lb. assorted firm stone fruit (apricots, plums, and peaches preferably)

Directions:

1. Grease grate and preheat grill to medium high fire.
2. In a small bowl, mix well paprika, coriander, cumin and salt. Rub spice evenly on all sides of pork chops.
3. Grill pork chops per side for five minutes. Remove from grill, transfer to a plate and loosely tent with foil and let it stand for at least 10 minutes.
4. Meanwhile, slice the firm stone fruits thin strips and place in a bowl.
5. Add salt, lime juice, lime zest, and chipotle powder into bowl, and toss well to coat.
6. To serve, place one pork chop per plate and top with ¼ of the fruit slaw mixture.

Nutrition Facts Per Serving

Calories 426, Total Fat 18g, Saturated Fat 2g, Total Carbs 25g, Net Carbs 23g, Protein 41g, Sugar: 23g, Fiber 2g, Sodium 674mg, Potassium 725mg

345. LAMB STEW

Preparation Time: 10 minutes
Cooking Time: 180 minutes
Serving: 4

Ingredients:

- Pepper and salt to taste
- 1 tbsp olive oil
- 1 tbsp fresh coriander, roughly chopped
- 1 tbsp honey, optional
- 1 tbsp Ras el Hanout
- 2 cups beef stock or lamb stock
- ½ cup golden raisins
- 1 cup dates, cut in half
- 1 cup dried figs, cut in half
- 2 cloves garlic, minced
- 1 onion, minced
- 1 lb. lamb shoulder, trimmed of fat and cut into 2-inch cubes

Spice Mixture:

- ¼ tsp ground cloves
- ½ tsp anise seeds'1/2 tsp ground cayenne pepper
- ½ tsp ground black pepper
- 1 tsp ground turmeric
- 1 tsp ground nutmeg
- 1 tsp ground allspice
- 1 tsp ground cinnamon
- 2 tsp ground mace
- 2 tsp ground cardamom
- 2 tsp ground ginger

Directions:

1. Preheat oven to 300oF.
2. In small bowl, add all Ras el Hanout ingredients and mix thoroughly. Just get what the ingredients need and store remaining in a tightly lidded spice jar.
3. On high fire, place a heavy bottomed medium pot and heat olive oil. Once hot, brown lamb pieces on each side for around 3 to 4 minutes.
4. Lower fire to medium high and add

remaining ingredients, except for the coriander.

5. Mix well. Season with pepper and salt to taste. Cover pot and bring to a boil.
6. Once boiling, turn off fire, and pop pot into oven.
7. Bake uncovered for 2 to 2.5 hours or until meat is fork tender.
8. Once meat is tender, remove from oven.
9. To serve, sprinkle fresh coriander, and enjoy.

Nutrition Facts Per Serving

Calories 566, Total Fat 16g, Saturated Fat 2g, Total Carbs 85g, Net Carbs 75g, Protein 28g, Sugar: 60g, Fiber 10g, Sodium 606mg, Potassium 1243mg

346. LAMB WITH SPINACH SAUCE

Preparation Time: 10 minutes
Cooking Time: 3 hours
Serving: 8

Ingredients:

- Juice from ½ of a lemon
- Freshly ground black pepper
- 1 ½ tbsp garam masala
- 30-oz frozen spinach, defrosted and squeezed dry
- ¼ cup full fat coconut milk
- ½ cup diced tomatoes
- 1 tsp ground turmeric
- 2 tbsp ground coriander
- 1 tbsp ground cumin
- 3 tbsp minced ginger
- 4 cloves of garlic, minced
- 2 medium onions, thinly sliced
- 3 tsp kosher salt, divided
- 2 lbs. boneless lamb meat
- 2 tbsp olive oil

Directions:

1. Preheat oven to 300oF.
2. On medium high fire, place a large Dutch oven and heat ghee.
3. With paper towels, dry lamb meat. Season with 1 tsp salt.
4. Once ghee is hot, sear lamb meat on all sides in batches. Transfer seared lamb into a plate with a slotted spoon.
5. Once all meat is done searing, lower fire to medium and sauté onions until soft and translucent.
6. Add turmeric, coriander, cumin, ginger, and garlic. Sauté until fragrant around a minute.
7. Add tomatoes, cook for 3 minutes.
8. Add coconut milk and simmer until sauce is thickened.
9. Puree sauce with a stick blender. Return lamb meat.
10. Add 2 cups water and 2 tsp salt. Bring to a boil.
11. Once boiling, mix and scrape bottom of pot, cover, and pop in the oven.
12. Bake until meat is tender, around 2 ½ hours.
13. Serve and enjoy while still hot.

Nutrition Facts Per Serving

Calories 246, Total Fat 12g, Saturated Fat 2.7g, Total Carbs 7g, Net Carbs 3g, Protein 28g, Sugar: 1.4g, Fiber 4g, Sodium 1045mg, Potassium 826mg

347. PEPPER STEAK TACO

Preparation Time: 10 minutes
Cooking Time: 20 minutes
Serving: 8

Ingredients:

- 2 tbsp sliced pickled jalapenos
- 2 tbsp chopped fresh cilantro
- ½ avocado, sliced
- 8 small whole wheat tortillas, warmed
- ½ cup fresh frozen corn kernels
- 3 bell pepper, 1 each red, yellow and orange, sliced thinly
- ½ red onion, sliced
- 3 tsp vegetable oil
- ½ tsp mild chili powder
- 2 garlic cloves, crushed
- 1 tsp salt
- Juice of 1 lime, plus lime wedges for serving
- 1 lb. flank or hanger steak

Directions:

1. In a re-sealable plastic bag, mix chili powder, garlic, salt and lime juice until salt is dissolved. Add steak and marinate for at least 30 minutes while making sure to flip over or toss around steak halfway through the marinating time.
2. On high fire, place a large saucepan and heat 2 tsp oil. Once hot, sauté bell peppers and red onion for 5 minutes. Add corn and continue sautéing for another 3 to 5 minutes. Transfer veggies to a bowl and keep warm.
3. With paper towel, wipe skillet and return to medium high fire. Heat remaining teaspoon of oil. Once hot add steak in pan in a single layer and cook 4 minutes per side for medium rare. Remove from fire and let it rest for 5minutes on a chopping board before cutting into thin slices.
4. To make tortilla, layer jalapenos, cilantro, avocado, steak and veggies. Best serve with a dollop of sour cream.

Nutrition Facts Per Serving

Calories 268, Total Fat 11g, Saturated Fat 2g, Total Carbs 26g, Net Carbs 23g, Protein 17g, Sugar: 3g, Fiber 6g, Sodium 539mg, Potassium 514mg

348. TENDERLOIN STEAKS WITH CARAMELIZED ONIONS

Preparation Time: 10 minutes
Cooking Time: 20 minutes
Serving: 4

Ingredients:

- 4 pcs of 4-oz beef tenderloin steaks, trimmed
- ¼ tsp ground black pepper
- 1 tsp dried thyme
- ½ tsp salt, divided
- 2 tbsp honey
- 2 tbsp red wine vinegar
- 1 large red onion, sliced into rings and separated

Directions:

1. On medium high fire, place a large nonstick fry pan and grease with cooking spray.
2. Add onion, cover and cook for three minutes.
3. Add ¼ tsp salt, honey and vinegar. Stir to mix and reduce fire to medium low.
4. Simmer until sauce has thickened around 8 minutes. Stir constantly. Turn off fire.
5. In an oven safe pan, grease with cooking spray add beef. Season with pepper, thyme and remaining salt.
6. Pop into a preheated broiler on high and broil for 4 minutes. Remove from oven and turnover tenderloin pieces. Return to oven and broil for another 4 minutes or until desired doneness is achieved.
7. Transfer to a serving plate and pour onion sauce over.
8. Serve and enjoy.

Nutrition Facts Per Serving

Calories 285, Total Fat 10g, Saturated Fat 4g, Total Carbs 12g, Net Carbs g, Protein 35g, Sugar: g, Fiber 0.6g, Sodium 358mg, Potassium 456mg

349. LAMB BURGER ON ARUGULA

Preparation Time: 10 minutes
Cooking Time: 6 minutes
Serving: 6

Ingredients:

- 2 tbsp shelled and salted Pistachio nuts
- ½ oz fresh mint, divided
- 1 tbsp salt
- 3 oz dried apricots, diced
- 2 lbs. ground lamb
- 4 cups arugula

Directions:

1. In a bowl, with your hands blend salt, ½ of fresh mint (diced), apricots and ground lamb.
2. Then form into balls or patties with an ice cream scooper. Press ball in between palm of hands to flatten to half an inch. Do the same for remaining patties.
3. In a nonstick thick pan on medium fire, place patties without oil and cook for 3 minutes per side or until lightly browned.

Flip over once and cook the other side.

4. Meanwhile, arrange 1 cup of arugula per plate. Total of 4 plates.
5. Divide evenly and place cooked patties on top of arugula.
6. In a food processor, process until finely chopped the remaining mint leaves and nuts.
7. Sprinkle on top of patties, serve and enjoy.

Nutrition Facts Per Serving

Calories 332, Total Fat 20g, Saturated Fat 4g, Total Carbs 6g, Net Carbs 5g, Protein 32g, Sugar: 5g, Fiber 1g, Sodium 1264mg, Potassium 520mg

350. ROASTED LEG OF LAMB

Preparation Time: 10 minutes
Cooking Time: 120 minutes
Serving: 8

Ingredients:

- ¼ cup + 1 tbsp olive oil, divided
- Pepper and salt to taste
- ½ tbsp garlic powder
- 1 tbsp fresh rosemary, chopped
- 1 tbsp fresh parsley, chopped
- 2 tbsp fresh tarragon, chopped
- 2 tbsp fresh thyme, chopped
- 1 cup almond flour
- 5 tbsp Dijon mustard
- 1 large red onion, roughly chopped
- 2 apples, cored and sliced
- 2 sweet potatoes, diced
- 2 heads of garlic, ¼ inch of top end removed to show individual cloves
- 4 lbs. leg of lamb, bone in

Directions:

1. Let leg of lamb sit in room temperature for an hour. Then pat dry with a paper towel.
2. Grease a roasting pan and preheat oven to 400oF.
3. Mix well the pepper, salt, ¼ cup olive oil, garlic powder, all the chopped herbs and almond flour in a medium bowl.
4. With mustard, coat leg of lamb. Then with a basting brush, coat leg of lamb with the herb mixture all around.
5. Pop in the oven and roast for 30 minutes. Then reduce oven temperature to 350oF and remove lamb.
6. Add veggies and apple. Season with pepper, salt and remaining olive oil and return to oven.
7. Bake for 1 ½ hours for a medium rare meat around 130oF when thermometer is inserted into lamb.
8. Remove from oven and let lamb rest for 20 minutes before carving.

Nutrition Facts Per Serving

Calories 408, Total Fat 16g, Saturated Fat 5g, Total Carbs 17g, Net Carbs 14g, Protein 47g, Sugar: 8g, Fiber 3g, Sodium 268mg, Potassium 874mg

351. CASHEW BEEF STIR FRY

Preparation Time: 10 minutes
Cooking Time: 15 minutes
Serving: 8

Ingredients:

- Salt and pepper to taste
- 1 small can water chestnut, sliced
- 1 small onion, sliced
- 1 red bell pepper, julienned
- 1 green bell pepper, julienned
- ¼ cup coconut aminos
- 1 tablespoon garlic, minced
- 2 tablespoon ginger, grated
- 1 ½ pound ground beef
- 2 teaspoon coconut oil
- 1 cup raw cashews

Directions:

1. Heat a skillet over medium heat then add raw cashews. Toast for a couple of minutes or until slightly brown. Set aside.
2. In the same skillet, add the coconut oil and sauté the ground beef for 5 minutes or until brown.
3. Add the garlic, ginger and season with coconut aminos. Stir for one minute before adding the onions, bell peppers and water chestnuts. Cook until the vegetables are almost soft.
4. Season with salt and pepper to taste.

5. Add the toasted cashews last.

Nutrition Facts Per Serving

Calories 259, Total Fat 15g, Saturated Fat 3g, Total Carbs 5g, Net Carbs 4g, Protein 26g, Sugar: 2g, Fiber 1g, Sodium 85mg, Potassium 513mg

352. LAMB CURRY STEW WITH ARTICHOKE HEARTS

Preparation Time: 10 minutes
Cooking Time: 80 minutes
Serving: 4

Ingredients:

- ½ teaspoon black pepper
- ½ teaspoon curry powder
- ½ teaspoon ground cinnamon
- 1 clove garlic, minced
- 2 cups beef broth
- 2 cups water
- 2 tablespoons onion powder
- 1 tablespoon curry powder
- 1 tablespoon fresh lemon juice
- 1 tablespoon olive oil
- 1 teaspoon garam masala
- 1 teaspoon salt
- 1/3 cup manzanilla olives
- 14 ½ ounce fire roasted diced tomatoes
- 14-ounces artichoke hearts, quartered
- 2 teaspoon ginger root, grated
- 2-pounds lamb leg, trimmed from fat and cut into chunks

Directions:

1. In a bowl, combine the lamb meat with salt, pepper and ½ tablespoon of curry.
2. Place a heavy bottomed pot on medium high fire and heat for 2 minutes.
3. Add oil and heat for 2 minutes.
4. Add lamb meat and sauté until all sides are brown. Remove from the pot and set aside.
5. Sauté garlic and ginger for a minute or two. Pour the broth and scrape the sides or bottoms from the browning. Add the lamb back and place the rest of the ingredients except for the lemon juice.
6. Cover and bring to a boil. Boil for 10 minutes. Lower fire to a simmer and simmer until fork tender, around 60 minutes.
7. Add the lemon juice and let it rest for 5 minutes before serving.

Nutrition Facts Per Serving

Calories 436, Total Fat 18g, Saturated Fat 2g, Total Carbs 19g, Net Carbs 10.8g, Protein 51g, Sugar: 1.7g, Fiber 8.2g, Sodium 1417mg, Potassium 1357mg

353. BEEFY CABBAGE BOWLS

Preparation Time: 10 minutes
Cooking Time: 80 minutes
Serving: 4

Ingredients:

- ½ teaspoon paprika
- 2 cups beef broth
- 1 cup cauliflower rice
- 1 garlic clove, minced
- 1 medium head cabbage, cored and chopped
- 1 tablespoon dried marjoram
- 1-pound lean ground beef
- 2 tablespoon raisins
- 8-ounces tomato sauce
- 1 tbsp oil
- Salt and pepper to taste

Directions:

1. Place a heavy bottomed pot on medium high fire and heat pot for 2 minutes.
2. Add oil and heat for 2 minutes.
3. Add the beef. Season with salt and pepper. Cook the beef until it is browned. Add the garlic and marjoram. Cook for a few minutes.
4. Add the tomato sauce, beef broth, paprika and raisins.
5. Bring to a boil and boil for 5 minutes. Lower fire to a simmer and simmer until beef is fork tender, around 60 minutes.
6. Adjust seasoning. Stir in rice and cabbage and boil for 5 minutes.
7. Turn off fire and let it rest for 10 minutes.
8. Serve and enjoy.

Nutrition Facts Per Serving

Calories 345, Total Fat 17g, Saturated Fat 3g, Total Carbs 16g, Net Carbs 14g, Protein 34g, Sugar: 7.1g, Fiber 4g, Sodium 613mg, Potassium 975mg

354. MEXICAN PORK CARNITAS

Preparation Time: 10 minutes
Cooking Time: 70 minutes
Serving: 6

Ingredients:

- ¼ teaspoon adobo seasoning
- ¼ teaspoon dry oregano
- ½ teaspoon garlic powder
- ¾ cup chicken broth
- 1 ½ teaspoon cumin
- 2 pounds pork loin
- 2 bay leaves
- 3 chipotle peppers
- 6 cloves garlic, slivered
- Salt and pepper to taste

Directions:

1. Season the pork with salt and pepper.
2. Place a heavy bottomed pot on high fire and heat pot for 2 minutes.
3. Add oil and heat for 2 minutes.
4. Place the pork inside the pot and sear each side until brown, around 3 minutes per side.
5. Lower fire to medium. Add the garlic, cumin, oregano, adobo sauce and garlic powder.
6. Mix well then pour the chicken broth and chipotle peppers.
7. Add the bay leaves and continue stirring.
8. Cover with the lid and bring to a boil and boil for 5 minutes. Lower fire to a simmer and simmer for 45 minutes or until fork tender.
9. Shred the pork using two forks.
10. Place the pork back and let it simmer for another 10 minutes.

Nutrition Facts Per Serving

Calories 264, Total Fat 8.4g, Saturated Fat 2.5g, Total Carbs 4g, Net Carbs 3g, Protein 41g, Sugar: 1g, Fiber 1g, Sodium 287mg, Potassium 708mg

355. SLOW COOKED BEEF POT ROAST

Preparation Time: 10 minutes
Cooking Time: 7 hours
Serving: 8

Ingredients:

- ½ teaspoon black pepper
- ½ teaspoon dried oregano
- 1 tablespoon dried thyme
- 1 teaspoon salt
- 1 whole bay leaf
- 1 medium onion, sliced
- 2 pounds beef pot roast cut
- 1 tablespoon olive oil
- 3 cups water

Directions:

1. In a bowl, mix together thyme, black pepper, oregano and salt.
2. Rub the mixture all over the pot roast cut.
3. Heat a skillet and add oil. Place the marinated pot roast and sear all sides.
4. Meanwhile, put remaining ingredients in slow cooker.
5. Add the seared pot roast and cook for 7 hours.

Nutrition Facts Per Serving

Calories 181, Total Fat 9g, Saturated Fat 3.3g, Total Carbs 1g, Net Carbs 0.9g, Protein 24g, Sugar: 0g, Fiber 0.1g, Sodium 383mg, Potassium 416mg

356. BEEF RAGU

Preparation Time: 10 minutes
Cooking Time: 10 minutes
Serving: 2

Ingredients:

- ¼ cup packaged pesto
- 1 teaspoon salt
- 2 large zucchinis, cut into noodle strips
- 1 tablespoon olive oil
- 1/4-pound ground beef
- 4 tablespoons fresh parsley, chopped

Directions:

1. Heat the oil in a skillet under medium flame and cook the ground beef until

thoroughly cooked, around 5 minutes. Discard excess fat.

2. Add the packaged pesto sauce and season with salt. Add t
3. he chopped parsley and cook for three more minutes. Set aside.
4. In the same saucepan, place the zucchini noodles and cook for five minutes. Turn off the heat then add the cooked meat. Mix well.
5. Serve and enjoy.

Nutrition Facts Per Serving

Calories 353, Total Fat 30g, Saturated Fat 6g, Total Carbs 2g, Net Carbs 1.3g, Protein 19g, Sugar: 0.3g, Fiber 0.7g, Sodium 1481mg, Potassium 341mg

357. ASIAN-INSPIRED PORKCHOPS

Preparation Time: 10 minutes
Cooking Time: 15 minutes
Serving: 4

Ingredients:

- ½ tbsp chili paste
- ½ tbsp sugar-free ketchup
- ½ tsp five spice powder
- ½ tsp pepper corn
- 1 ½ tsp soy sauce
- 1 medium star anise
- 1 stalk lemongrass, peeled and diced
- 1 tbsp almond flour
- ½ tsp salt
- 1 tsp Sesame oil
- 4 boneless pork chops
- 4 halved garlic cloves, crushed

Directions:

1. Place the pork chops on a stable working surface. With a rolling pin wrapped in wax paper, pound the pork chop to ½ inch thickness.
2. Ground the star anise and peppercorns using a mortar and pestle. Add the lemon grass and garlic and continue pounding until they form a puree.
3. Add soy sauce, salt, five spice powder and sesame oil. Mix well. This will be the marinade.
4. Put the pork chops on a baking tray and add marinade. Toss or massage the marinade to the pork chops. Let it sit for 2 hours at room temperature.
5. Using a skillet, heat the pan and put a little amount oil for frying.
6. Separately, coat the pork chops with almond flour. Put the pork chops to the pan and sear both sides.
7. Cook for two minutes for each side until it becomes golden brown in color.
8. Meanwhile, make the sauce by mixing the sugar-free ketchup and chili paste.
9. Let it cool. Evenly divide into suggested, and place in meal prep containers with sauce on the side.

Nutrition Facts Per Serving

Calories 266, Total Fat 8g, Saturated Fat 2.4g, Total Carbs 4g, Net Carbs 3.4g, Protein 43g, Sugar: 0.1g, Fiber 0.6g, Sodium 483mg, Potassium 860mg

358. ASIAN BEEF SHORT RIBS

Preparation Time: 10 minutes
Cooking Time: 10 hours
Serving: 4

Ingredients:

- 1 cup water
- 1 onion, diced
- 1 tablespoon Szechuan peppercorns
- 2 pounds beef short ribs
- 2 tablespoons curry powder
- 3 tablespoons coconut aminos
- 6-pieces star anise
- 1 tablespoon sesame oil
- Salt and pepper to taste

Directions:

1. Add all ingredients in slow cooker and mix well.
2. Cook on low settings for 10 hours.
3. Serve and enjoy.

Nutrition Facts Per Serving

Calories 442, Total Fat 26g, Saturated Fat 4g, Total Carbs 6g, Net Carbs 4g, Protein 47g, Sugar: 2g, Fiber 2g, Sodium 264mg, Potassium 836mg

359. STIR-FRIED GROUND BEEF

Preparation Time: 10 minutes
Cooking Time: 15 minutes
Serving: 4

Ingredients:

- ½ cup broccoli, chopped
- ½ of medium-sized onions, chopped
- ½ of medium-sized red bell pepper, chopped
- 1 tbsp cayenne pepper (optional)
- 1 tbsp Chinese five spices
- 1 tbsp coconut oil
- 1-lb ground beef
- 2 kale leaves, chopped
- 5 medium-sized mushrooms, sliced

Directions:

1. In a skillet, heat the coconut oil over medium high heat.
2. Sauté the onions for one minute and add the vegetables while stirring constantly.
3. Add the ground beef and the spices.
4. Cook for two minutes and reduce the heat to medium.
5. Cover the skillet and continue to cook the beef and vegetables for another 10 minutes.
6. Serve and enjoy.

Nutrition Facts Per Serving

Calories 304, Total Fat 17g, Saturated Fat 3g, Total Carbs 6g, Net Carbs 4g, Protein 32g, Sugar: 2g, Fiber 2g, Sodium 86mg, Potassium 624mg

360. TRADITIONAL SCOTCH EGGS RECIPE

Preparation Time: 20 minutes
Cooking Time: 20 minutes
Serving: 5

Ingredients:

- ½ teaspoon paprika powder
- 1 ½ pounds ground pork
- 1 egg, beaten
- 1 garlic clove minced
- 5 eggs, hardboiled and peeled

Directions:

1. Combine the beaten egg, ground pork, garlic, and paprika in a mixing bowl. Season with salt and pepper to taste.
2. Divide the meat mixture into 5 balls.
3. Flatten the balls with your hands and place an egg at the center. Cover the egg with the meat mixture. Do the same thing with the other balls.
4. Place a nonstick pan on medium fire and cook ground pork coating for 4 minutes per side.
5. Serve and enjoy.

Nutrition Facts Per Serving

Calories 481, Total Fat 33g, Saturated Fat 4g, Total Carbs 0.7g, Net Carbs 0.6g, Protein 42g, Sugar: 0.2g, Fiber 0.1g, Sodium 175mg, Potassium 573mg

361. BURRITO BREAKFAST BOWL

Preparation Time: 10 minutes
Cooking Time: 20 minutes
Serving: 2

Ingredients:

- 1 tbsp keto taco seasoning
- 1 tsp olive oil
- 1/2-pound lean ground beef
- 1/3 head cauliflower riced
- 2 tbsp cilantro chopped
- 3 eggs beaten
- 3/4 cup water
- sea salt & pepper to taste

Directions:

1. Place a large nonstick skillet on medium high fire.
2. Sauté ground beef for 3 minutes. Season with taco seasoning and continue cooking until liquid has evaporated, around 8 minutes. Discard any fat dripping. Transfer to a large bowl.
3. In same pan, sauté cauliflower.Season with salt and cilantro. Continue sautéing for 4 minutes or until tender. Transfer to same bowl with ground beef.
4. In same pan, heat oil. Pour in eggs and scramble for 3 minutes.
5. Return ground beef and cauliflower in pan and continue stirring and cooking for a

minute or two.

6. Let it cool. Evenly divide into suggested and place in meal prep containers.

Nutrition Facts Per Serving

Calories 382, Total Fat 21g, Saturated Fat 5g, Total Carbs 5g, Net Carbs 3.5g, Protein 40g, Sugar: 1.6g, Fiber 1.5g, Sodium 721mg, Potassium 610mg

362. STIR-FRIED MUSHROOMS AND BEEF

Preparation Time: 10 minutes
Cooking Time: 25 minutes
Serving: 4

Ingredients:

- 2 tablespoons olive oil
- 2 cloves of garlic, minced
- 1-lb 4 beef steaks, cut into strips
- ¼ cup water
- salt and pepper to taste
- 2 cups mushrooms, sliced
- ½ tsp salt

Directions:

1. Heat oil and butter in a skillet and sauté the garlic until fragrant.
2. Stir in the beef strips for 3 minutes until lightly golden.
3. Pour in water and season with salt and pepper to taste.
4. Close the lid and allow to simmer for 15 minutes.
5. Stir in the mushrooms and salt.
6. Cook for another 5 more minutes.
7. Serve and enjoy.

Nutrition Facts Per Serving

Calories 226, Total Fat 13g, Saturated Fat 3g, Total Carbs 1.7, Net Carbs 1.5g, Protein 24g, Sugar: g, Fiber 0.2g, Sodium 358mg, Potassium 474mg

363. MALAYSIAN BEEF STEW

Preparation Time: 10 minutes
Cooking Time: 1 hour and 10 minutes
Serving: 8

Ingredients:

- 1 tablespoon olive oil
- 6 cloves of garlic, minced
- 1 onion, chopped
- 1 thumb-size ginger, grated
- 1 teaspoon ground cumin
- 1 teaspoon turmeric powder
- 6 dried chilies, chopped
- 1 stalk of lemon grass, chopped
- 1-pound beef sirloin, cut into strips
- 1 cup coconut milk
- ¼ cup water
- Salt and pepper to taste
- ½ cup desiccated coconut
- 6 kaffir lime leaves

Directions:

1. In a saucepan, heat the oil and sauté the garlic, onion, onion, ginger, cumin, turmeric powder, chilies, and lemon grass.
2. Stir in the beef for 3 minutes. Add the coconut milk and water. Season with salt and pepper to taste.
3. Allow to simmer for 60 minutes until the meat is tender.
4. Open the lid until the sauce reduces.
5. Add the desiccated coconut and kaffir lime leaves and cook for another 3 more minutes.
6. Serve and enjoy.

Nutrition Facts Per Serving

Calories 162, Total Fat 9g, Saturated Fat 3.4g, Total Carbs 6g, Net Carbs 5g, Protein 13g, Sugar: 3g, Fiber 1g, Sodium 81mg, Potassium 360mg

364. HOMEMADE MEATBALLS

Preparation Time: 10 minutes
Cooking Time: 15 minutes
Serving: 6

Ingredients:

- 1 tablespoon olive oil
- 2 pounds ground beef
- 1 teaspoon paprika
- 4 eggs, beaten
- ½ cup almond flour
- 3 cloves of garlic, minced
- 1 tablespoon dried parsley

- Salt and pepper to taste

Directions:

1. Preheat oven to 350oF.
2. Place all ingredients except for the coconut oil in a mixing bowl. Use your hands to mix everything.
3. Use your hands to form small balls.
4. Lightly grease a cookie sheet with cooking spray and evenly spread meatballs in sheet.
5. Bake for 20 minutes.
6. Serve and enjoy with your favorite sauce.

Nutrition Facts Per Serving

Calories 390, Total Fat 22g, Saturated Fat 4g, Total Carbs 1g, Net Carbs 0.8g, Protein 44g, Sugar: 0.1g, Fiber 0.2g, Sodium 238mg, Potassium 513mg

365. GOAT CURRY

Preparation Time: 10 minutes
Cooking Time: 1 hour and 10 minutes
Serving: 8

Ingredients:

- 1 tablespoon avocado oil
- 1 tablespoon coriander powder
- 1 teaspoon cumin powder
- 1 teaspoon garam masala
- 1 teaspoon chili powder
- 1 teaspoon paprika
- 2 onions, chopped
- 3 cloves of garlic, chopped
- 4 cloves
- 4 cardamom pods
- 2 pounds goat meat
- ½ cup water
- Salt and pepper to taste

Directions:

1. In a deep pan, heat avocado oil. Sauté the coriander, cumin, garam masala, chili powder, and paprika for a minute.
2. Stir in the onion and garlic until fragrant. Add the cloves and cardamom pods.
3. Add the goat meat and stir for 3 minutes. Pour in water and season with salt and pepper to taste.
4. Close the lid and allow to simmer for 60 minutes on medium flame.
5. Serve and enjoy.

Nutrition Facts Per Serving

Calories 157, Total Fat 5g, Saturated Fat 1g, Total Carbs 4g, Net Carbs 3g, Protein 24g, Sugar: 2g, Fiber 1g, Sodium 105mg, Potassium 519mg

366. PORK BREAKFAST MUFFINS

Servings 6
Preparation Time: 25 minutes

Ingredients

- 1 tablespoon olive oil
- 1 1/2 cups ground pork
- 1/2 teaspoon dried oregano
- 1/2 teaspoon ground cloves
- 2 tablespoons full-fat milk
- 1/2 teaspoon baking soda
- 1/2 teaspoon baking powder
- 3 large eggs, lightly beaten
- 3 1/2 cups almond flour
- 1 stick butter
- Salt and cayenne pepper to taste

Directions

1. In a frying pan heat the oil over moderate heat. Cook the ground pork for 4 – 5 minutes or until the juices run clear.
2. Put your oven on to 3600F.
3. Combine all the other ingredients.
4. Put the mixture into 12 muffin cups and bake for 15 - 18 minutes.
5. Let the muffins cool down before removing them from the tin. Serve with sour cream. Bon appétit!

Nutrition: Calories 479 ,Protein 17.9g ,Fat 42g ,Carbs 5.8g ,Sugar 0.5g

367. PORK GUMBO FOR ENTERTAINING

Servings 6
Preparation Time: 35 minutes

Ingredients

- 2 tablespoons olive oil
- 1 pound cubed pork shoulder
- 8 ounces sliced pork sausage

- 2 roughly chopped shallots
- 4 cups bone broth
- 1 tablespoon Cajun spice
- 1 teaspoon crushed red pepper
- 1 teaspoon gumbo file
- 1 teaspoon beef bouillon granules
- Salt and freshly cracked black pepper
- 1 cup water
- 2 chopped celery stalks
- 2 deveined and thinly sliced bell peppers
- 1/4 cup flaxseed meal
- 3/4 pound okra

Directions

1. Preheat a pot over a medium-high flame and heat the oil. Cook the pork until it is brown. Put to one side.
2. Put in the sausage and cook for 5 minutes. Put to one side.
3. Put in the shallots and cook until they are translucent. Add the bone broth, Cajun spice, red pepper, gumbo file, beef bouillon granules, salt and pepper. Bring to the boil.
4. Add the water, celery and bell pepper. Reduce the heat to moderate-low and cook for around 20 minutes.
5. Put in the flaxseed and okra and cook for another 5 minutes.

Nutrition: Calories 427 ,Protein 35.2g ,Fat 26.2g ,Carbs 3.6g ,Sugar 1.3g

368. PORK MEATLOAF WITH TOMATO SAUCE

Servings 6
Preparation Time: 45 minutes

Ingredients

- Nonstick cooking spray
- 1 1/2 pounds ground pork
- 1/4 cup crushed pork rinds
- 1 teaspoon mustard powder
- 3 finely minced cloves of garlic
- 2 chopped shallots
- 1 large egg
- 1/3 cup flaxseed meal
- Sea salt and ground black pepper
- For the Sauce:
- 2 pureed ripe plum tomatoes
- 1 teaspoon fresh parsley
- 1/2 teaspoon dried thyme
- 1/2 tablespoons Swerve
- 2 tablespoons ketchup
- 1 tablespoon cider vinegar

Directions

1. Put your oven on at 3600F. Spray a loaf pan with nonstick cooking oil.
2. In a mixing dish, combine the ground pork, pork rinds, mustard, garlic, shallots, egg, flaxseed meal, salt and pepper. Make sure that it is thoroughly combined.
3. Put the meatloaf mixture into the loaf pan.
4. Put all the sauce ingredients in a saucepan and cook over medium heat. Pour this over the meatloaf. Put it in the oven and bake for 40 minutes.
5. When cooked, let it cool for a couple of minutes and then cut into slices. Serve hot.

Nutrition: Calories 251 ,Protein 34.6g Fat 7.9g ,Carbs 4.5g ,Sugar 1g

369. PORK SHOULDER A CHEESY SAUCE

Servings 6
Preparation Time: 30 minutes

Ingredients

- 1 1/2 pounds boneless pork shoulder, cut into 6 pieces
- 1 teaspoon dried thyme
- Salt and freshly cracked black peppercorns, to taste
- 1 tablespoon butter
- 2 chopped garlic cloves
- 1 chopped onion
- 1/3 cup homemade broth
- 1/3 cup dry sherry wine
- 1 tablespoon soy sauce
- 1 teaspoon dried hot chili flakes
- 1/3 cup double cream
- 6 ounces blue cheese

Directions

1. Rub the pieces of pork shoulder with thyme, salt and black peppercorns.
2. Put a pan on medium-high heat and warm the butter. Then cook the pork for 18 minutes, making sure it is browned all over. Put to one side.
3. Sauté the garlic and onions until the onions become caramelized. Add the broth and the wine and stir, scraping any brown bits from the bottom of the pan.
4. Lower the heat to medium and add the soy sauce, chili flakes, double cream and blue cheese. Simmer until it is thick.
5. Put the pork onto individual plates and serve the sauce over them. Bon appétit!

Nutrition: Calories 495 ,Protein 33.4g ,Fat 36.9g ,Carbs3.6g ,Sugar 1.1g

370. MEATLOAF MUFFINS

Servings 6
Preparation Time: 35 minutes

Ingredients

- 1 pound ground turkey
- 1/2 pound ground pork
- 2 pureed ripe tomatoes
- 1 tablespoon Worcestershire sauce
- 1 ounce envelope onion soup mix
- 1 tablespoon Dijon mustard
- 1 teaspoon dry oregano
- 1/2 teaspoon dry basil
- 2 cloves of minced garlic
- Kosher salt and ground black pepper, to taste
- 1 cup shredded mozzarella cheese
- 1 whisked egg

Directions

1. Put your oven on at 3500F.
2. Mix together all the ingredients until they are combined well.
3. Spray a muffin tin with nonstick cooking spray and put it in the mixture.
4. Cook them in the oven for half an hour. Let them cool a little before removing from the tin. Bon appétit!
5. Nutrition: Calories 220 ,Protein 33.8g ,Fat 6.3g ,Carbs 2.9g Sugar 1g

371. A MUG OF BREAKFAST PORK

Servings 2
Preparation Time: 10 minutes

Ingredients

- 1/2 pound ground pork
- 1/2 cup tomato sauce
- 1/2 cup shredded Asiago cheese
- 1/2 teaspoon cayenne pepper
- 1/2 teaspoon onion powder
- 1 teaspoon garlic paste
- Salt and ground black pepper to your liking

Directions

1. Mix together the pork, tomato sauce, cheese, cayenne pepper, onion powder, garlic paste, salt and pepper.
2. Split the mixture in two and put it in 2 microwave-safe mugs.
3. Put in the microwave on high and cook for 7 minutes. It tastes good hot and served with pickles. Bon appétit!

Nutrition: Calories 327 ,Protein 40g ,Fat 16.6g ,Carbs 5.8g ,Sugar 2.6g

372. SPICY AND CREAMY PORK SOUP

Servings 4
Preparation Time: 25 minutes

Ingredients

- 2 tablespoons olive oil
- 1 chopped shallot
- 1 chopped celery stalk
- 3/4 pound bone-in pork chops
- 1 tablespoon chicken bouillon granules
- 3 cups water
- 1/2 teaspoon Tabasco sauce
- 2 pureed tomatoes
- Seasoned salt and freshly cracked black pepper, to taste
- 1/2 teaspoon red pepper flakes
- 1 cup double cream
- 1/2 cup avocado, pitted, peeled and diced

Directions

1. Preheat a pot over a moderate-high flame and heat 1 tablespoon of oil. Cook the shallots until they are just tender.
2. Stir in the celery and cook until they have softened. Put to one side.
3. Heat another tablespoon of olive oil and cook the pork chops for 4 minutes until they are brown. Stir every now and then.
4. When the pork chops have cooled down, get rid of any bones and then cut the pork into small chunks. Put the pork and vegetables in the pot.
5. Add the bouillon granules, water, pureed tomatoes, red pepper flakes, salt and pepper. Partially cover the pot and simmer for 10 minutes more.
6. Pour in the double cream and cook until hot. Stir all the time. Drizzle Tabasco sauce on the mixture and when plated, garnish with avocado.

Nutrition: Calories490 ,Protein 24.3g ,Fat 44g ,Carbs 6.1g ,Sugar 2.6g

373. LETTUCE WRAPS WITH PORK

Servings 4
Preparation Time: 15 minutes

Ingredients

- 2 tablespoons apple cider vinegar
- 2 sliced spring onions
- 1 grated celery
- 1/4 teaspoon kosher salt
- 1/2 pound ground pork
- 1 deveined and finely minced jalapeno pepper
- 2 finely minced garlic cloves
- 1 1/2 teaspoons Dijon mustard
- 1/2 teaspoon salt
- 1/3 teaspoon freshly cracked mixed peppercorns
- 1 tablespoon Worcestershire sauce1
- 1 head lettuce
- 1 tablespoon sunflower seeds

Directions

1. Whisk the vinegar together with spring onions, celery and kosher salt.
2. In a pan, cook the ground pork until brown, together with the jalapeno pepper and garlic. This should take 7 minutes over a medium flame.
3. Add the Dijon mustard, salt, peppercorns, and Worcestershire sauce to the pan and mix well.
4. Then make your wraps. Put the lettuce leaves on individual plates and divide the pork mixture among them and put the celery mixture on top. Sprinkle on sunflower seeds and roll the lettuce leaves to make wraps.

374. PORK STEAKS

Servings 4
Preparation Time: 30 minutes

Ingredients

- 4 pork butt steaks
- 2 tablespoons lard at room temperature
- 1/4 cup dry red wine
- 1/2 teaspoon freshly ground black pepper
- 1/2 teaspoon salt
- 1 teaspoon celery seeds
- 1/2 teaspoon cayenne pepper
- 1 peeled and chopped red onion
- 1 minced garlic clove

Directions

1. In a skillet that has been heated over medium heat, melt 1 tablespoon of the lard. Sear the steaks for 10 minutes with the skillet covered.
2. Deglaze the pot with a splash of wine. Put in pepper, salt, celery seeds and cayenne pepper. Cook for between 8 – 12 minutes. Put to one side.
3. Heat the rest of the lard and cook the garlic and onions until they are soft and fragrant. Serve with the pork butt steaks. Bon appétit!

Nutrition: Calories 305 ,Protein 22.5g ,Fat 20.6g ,Carbs 3.7g ,Sugar 1.3g

375. PORK AND VEGGIE SKEWERS

Servings 6
Preparation Time: 20 minutes + marinating time

Ingredients

- 2 cloves crushed garlic
- 1 tablespoon Italian spice mix
- 2 tablespoons fresh lime juice
- 3 tablespoons tamari sauce
- 3 tablespoons olive oil
- 1 ½ pounds cubed pork shoulder
- 1 thickly sliced red bell pepper
- 1 thickly sliced green bell pepper
- 1 pound small button mushrooms
- 1 onion, cut into wedges
- 1 cubed zucchini1
- Wooden skewers, soaked in cold water for 30 minutes

Directions

1. First make the marinade. Combine the garlic, Italian spice mix, fresh lime juice, tamari sauce and olive oil.
2. Pour the marinade over the pork and marinate for 2 hours. Then thread the pork cubes, peppers, mushrooms, onions and zucchini onto skewers.
3. Preheat your grill and cook the skewers for about 13 minutes, turning often. Enjoy!

Nutrition: Calories 428 ,Protein 28.9g ,Fat 31.6g ,Carbs 7.7g ,Sugar 4.2g

376. PORK WITH BAMBOO SHOOTS AND CAULIFLOWER

Servings 6
Preparation Time: 20 minutes

Ingredients

- 1 ½ pounds boneless pork loin
- 1 1/2 tablespoons olive oil
- 1/2 cup vodka
- 2 tablespoons oyster sauce
- 1/2 teaspoon dried marjoram
- 1/2 teaspoon garlic powder
- 1/4 teaspoon dried thyme
- Celery salt and ground black pepper to your liking
- 1 chopped yellow onion
- 1 head cauliflower florets
- 1 8-ounce can bamboo shoots

Directions

1. Put the pork loin in a bowl. Add the olive oil, vodka, oyster sauce, marjoram, garlic powder, thyme, salt and ground pepper. Combine thoroughly. Add the pork loin to a mixing dish.
2. In a skillet heat 1 tablespoon of olive oil over a moderate-high heat. Sauté the onion until soft.
3. Put in the cauliflower florets and cook for 3 – 4 minutes until they are tender. Put this to one side.
4. Put another tablespoon of olive oil in the pan and heat with a high flame. Put the marinade to one side and brown the pork for 3 minutes on each side.
5. Put in the marinade, the cauliflower and bamboo shoots.
6. Cook for another 4 minutes until the sauce has thickened. Serve hot. Enjoy!

Nutrition: Calories 356 ,Protein 33.1g ,Fat 19.5g ,Carbs 6.4g ,Sugar 3g

377. EASY FRAGRANT PORK CHOPS

Servings 4
Preparation Time: 30 minutes

Ingredients

- 2 tablespoons lard, melted
- 3 minced cloves of garlic
- 1/2 cup thinly sliced
- 4 pork chops
- 1/2 teaspoon grated fresh ginger
- 4 lightly crushed allspice berries
- 2 tablespoons Worcestershire sauce
- 1 teaspoon dried thyme
- 1/4 cup dry white wine

Directions

1. Take a saucepan and melt the lard over moderate heat. Sauté the garlic and onions until they have lightly browned and are fragrant.

2. Add the pork to the saucepan and cook for 15 – 20 minutes, turning occasionally. Pour in the white wine with the ginger, allspice berries, Worcestershire sauce and thyme.
3. Cook for another 8 minutes when everything should be thoroughly heated. Bon appétit!

Nutrition: Calories 335 ,Protein 18.3g ,Fat 26.3g ,Carbs 2.5g ,Sugar 0.8g

378. CRISPY PORK SHOULDER

Servings 4
Preparation Time: 25 minutes

Ingredients

- 1 pound pork shoulder, cut into 1-inch-thick pieces
- Salt and cayenne pepper, to your liking
- 2 tablespoons lard
- 2 smashed garlic cloves
- 2 sliced shallots
- 1 cup bone broth
- 2 tablespoons rice vinegar
- 2 tablespoons pitted and sliced Kalamata olives
- 1 tablespoon fish sauce
- 1 tablespoon tamarind paste
- 1 thyme sprig
- 1 rosemary sprig
- 1/2 cup freshly grated Asiago cheese

Directions

1. Preheat your broiler. Sprinkle the pork all over with cayenne pepper and salt.
2. Preheat a pan over a medium-high flame and melt the lard. Cook the garlic and shallots for 5 minutes. Put to one side.
3. Heat the remaining tablespoon of lard and sear the pork for 8 minutes. Turn over once and then put it to one side.
4. Put the rice vinegar, olives, fish sauce, tamarind paste, thyme, and rosemary in the pan and cook until the sauce reduces by half. Put in an oven dish.
5. Add in the pork and shallot mix and sprinkle with the Asiago cheese. Broil for about 5 minutes. Serve hot and enjoy!

Nutrition: Calories 476 ,Protein 31.1g ,Fat 35.3g ,Carbs 6.2g ,Sugar 1.2g

379. FRITTATA WITH SPICY SAUSAGE

Servings 4
Preparation Time: 35 minutes

Ingredients

- 3 tablespoons olive oil
- 2 minced garlic cloves
- 1 cup chopped onion
- 1 teaspoon finely minced jalapeno pepper
- 1/4 teaspoon cayenne pepper
- 1 teaspoon salt
- 1/2 teaspoon ground black pepper
- 1/2 pound thinly sliced pork sausage
- 8 beaten eggs
- 1 teaspoon crushed dried sage

Directions

1. Preheat a skillet over a moderate-high flame and heat the oil. Sauté the garlic, onion and jalapeno pepper until the onion is translucent.
2. Sprinkle in the cayenne pepper, salt and black pepper. Then add the sausage and cook until it has slightly browned. Stir often.
3. Put the mixture into a greased baking dish. Beat the eggs and pour over the sausage mixture. Scatter the dried sage on top.
4. Preheat the oven to 4200F and cook for 25 minutes. Bon appétit!

Nutrition: Calories 423 ,Protein 22.6g ,Fat 35.4g ,Carbs 4.1g ,Sugar 2g

380. PORK STIR-FRY CHINESE-STYLE WITH MUENSTER CHEESE

Servings 6
Preparation Time: 20 minutes

Ingredients

- 1 tablespoon softened lard
- 1 1/2 pounds pork butt, cut into strips
- 1/2 teaspoon red pepper flakes
- Celery salt and freshly ground black pepper, to taste

- 2 sliced bell peppers
- A bunch of roughly chopped scallions
- 2 tablespoons Sauvignon wine
- 1 tablespoon soy sauce
- 1/2 teaspoon Chinese hot sauce
- 1 tablespoon peanut butter
- 1/4 cup bone broth
- 3 ounces small pieces of Muenster cheese

Directions

1. Preheat a skillet over medium-high heat and melt the lard. Mix the pork strips with red pepper flakes, salt and black pepper.
2. Stir-fry the pork strips for around 4 minutes. Then add the bell peppers and scallions and cook for another 3 minutes.
3. Add the Sauvignon, soy sauce, Chinese hot sauce, peanut butter and bone broth. Stir-fry for another 2 minutes.
4. Put the pieces of Muenster cheese on top of this mixture and cook until the cheese melts. Bon appétit!

Nutrition: Calories 320 ,Protein 39.8g ,Fat 15.4g ,Carbs 2.7g Sugar 1.3g

381. SLOW COOKER HUNGARIAN GOULASH

Servings 4
Preparation Time: 10 hours

Ingredients

- 1 1/2 tablespoons butter
- 1 pound chopped pork shoulder off the bone
- 3 crushed garlic cloves
- 1 cup chopped yellow onions
- 2 deveined and finely chopped chili peppers
- 2 1/2 cups tomato puree
- 4 cups chicken stock
- 2 teaspoons cayenne pepper
- 1 teaspoon sweet Hungarian paprika
- 1 teaspoon ground caraway seeds
- For the Sour Cream Sauce:
- 1 cup sour cream
- 1 teaspoon lemon zest
- 1 chopped bunch parsley

Directions

1. Preheat a pan over medium heat and melt the butter. Cook the pork until it has browned. Put to one side.
2. Sauté the garlic and onions until they are soft and aromatic.
3. Put the pork into the slow cooker with the onions and garlic. Add the chili peppers, tomato puree, chicken stock, cayenne pepper, paprika and caraway seeds.
4. Put the lid on the slow cooker and cook on a low setting for 8 – 10 hours.
5. While this is cooking, make the sour cream sauce by whisking together the sour cream, lemon zest and parsley. Serve the goulash in individual bowls topped by a spoonful of sour cream sauce. Enjoy!

Nutrition: Calories 517 ,Protein 38.2g ,Fat 35.7g ,Carbs 5.7 ,Sugar 3g

382. PORK AND BELL PEPPER QUICHE

Servings 6
Preparation Time: 50 minutes

Ingredients

- 6 lightly beaten eggs
- 1 stick melted butter
- 2 1/2 cups almond flour
- 1 1/4 pounds ground pork
- Salt and pepper, to the taste
- 1 thinly sliced red bell pepper
- 1 thinly sliced green bell pepper
- 1 cup heavy cream
- 1/2 teaspoon dried dill weed
- 1/2 teaspoon mustard seeds

Directions

1. Put your oven on at 3500F.
2. Combine an egg, butter and almond flour in a mixing bowl.
3. Grease a baking pan with nonstick cooking spray, roll the dough and put in the pan.
4. Brown the ground pork for 3 – 5 minutes. Crumble with a spatula. Season with salt and pepper to your liking.
5. In a bowl, combine the other 5 eggs with

the bell peppers, cream, dill weed and mustard seeds. Put in the pork.

6. Put this mixture in the crust and bake for 35 – 43 minutes. Eat warm and enjoy!

Nutrition: Calories 478 ,Protein 36g ,Fat 4.9g ,Carbs 33.5g , Sugar 1.4g

383. GRILLED SUMMER BABY BACK RIBS

Servings 6
Preparation Time: 1 hour 40 minutes + marinating time

Ingredients

- 1 ½ pounds baby back ribs
- 1 teaspoon dried marjoram
- Salt and ground black pepper, to your liking
- 1 lime, halved
- 1 minced garlic clove

Directions

1. Rub the marjoram, salt and pepper into the baby back ribs. Then rub in the lime.
2. Put the minced garlic on the ribs. Cover and put the ribs in your fridge for 6 hours.
3. Put the ribs on the grill for 1 and a half hours, turning twice. This is good served with your favorite Keto salads and mustard.

Nutrition: Calories 255 ,Protein 29.9g ,Fat 13.9g ,Carbs 0.8g ,Sugar 0.1g

384. SKILLET OF PORK AND SWISS CHARD

Servings 4
Preparation Time: 25 minutes

Ingredients

- 2 tablespoons olive oil
- 1 sliced Serrano pepper
- 2 cloves pressed garlic
- 1 cup sliced leeks
- 1 chopped bell pepper
- 1 1/2 pounds ground pork
- 1 cup beef bone broth
- 1 teaspoon sea salt
- 1/4teaspoon lemon pepper
- 1/4 cup tomato puree
- 1 bunch trimmed and roughly chopped Swiss chard
- 1/4 cup dry sherry wine

Directions

1. Put a pan on a medium-high heat and heat 1 tablespoon of the olive oil. Sauté the peppers, leeks and garlic until they are tender. Put to one side.
2. Add the rest of the olive oil and brown the ground pork, stirring all the time. This should take 3 – 4 minutes.
3. Add the bone broth, sea salt, lemon pepper, tomato puree, Swiss chard and sherry wine as well as the sautéed vegetables and cook, covered for 10 minutes.
4. Take the lid off and cook for another 5 minutes. Serve hot.

Nutrition: Calories349 ,Protein 45.3g ,Fat 13g ,Carbs 4.4g ,Sugar 1.5g

385. ROASTED PEPPERS WITH PORK RIBS

Servings 4
Preparation Time: 2 hours

Ingredients

- 2 tablespoons olive oil
- 1 pound baby back ribs
- Salt and pepper, to taste
- 1 tablespoon crushed sage
- 2 rosemary sprigs
- 1 tablespoon garlic paste
- 1 chopped red onion
- 2 chopped roasted chili peppers
- 2 chopped roasted red bell peppers
- 1/2 cup soy sauce
- 1/2 cup dry sherry
- 1 tablespoon tamarind paste
- 1 cup beef broth

Directions

1. Put your oven on at 3400F. Spray a roasting pan with nonstick cooking spray.
2. In a pan heat the oil over a medium-high

flame and brown the baby back ribs. This should take 10 minutes. Scatter salt and pepper over the ribs.

3. Add the sage, rosemary, garlic paste and onion and cook for another 4 minutes. Mix in the peppers, soy sauce, sherry, tamarind paste and beef broth.
4. Put the mixture in the roasting pan and cook for 1 hour and 30 minutes in the middle of the oven. Serve hot.

386. MEATLOAF FOR THE HOLIDAYS

Servings 6
Preparation Time: 1 hour 10 minutes

Ingredients

- 1 teaspoon melted lard
- 1 teaspoon finely minced garlic
- 1 chopped yellow onion
- 1 1/4 pounds ground pork
- 1 bunch roughly chopped cilantro
- 1/2 pound broken up pork sausage
- 1/4 teaspoon cayenne pepper
- Salt and ground black pepper, to taste
- beaten egg
- 2 ounces half-and-half
- 1 teaspoon celery seeds
- 6 strips bacon

Directions

1. Put your oven on at 3950F. Grease a baking dish.
2. In a cast-iron skillet heat the lard over a moderate heat. Sauté the garlic and onions until they are soft and aromatic. This should take 2 – 4 minutes.
3. Put in the ground pork and brown. This should take 2 minutes.
4. In a bowl combine the cilantro, pork sausage, cayenne pepper, salt, pepper, egg, half-and-half and celery seeds.
5. Put the ground pork mixture into the bowl and combine well. Shape into a loaf.
6. Place the strips of bacon on top of the meatloaf and bake for an hour. Place the bacon on the top of your meatloaf. Bake about 1 hour. Cool a little before serving. Bon appétit!

Nutrition: Calories 405 ,Protein 40.6g ,Fat 24.6g ,Carbs 2.8g ,Sugar 0.9g

387. PORK GUMBO FOR A SPECIAL DINNER

Servings 6
Ready in about 35 minutes

Ingredients

- 2 tablespoons olive oil
- 1 pound cubed pork shoulder
- 8 ounces sliced pork sausage
- 2 roughly chopped shallots
- 4 cups bone broth
- 1 tablespoon Cajun spice
- 1 teaspoon crushed red pepper
- 1 teaspoon gumbo file
- Sea salt and freshly cracked black pepper
- 1 teaspoon beef bouillon granules
- 2 chopped celery stalks
- 2 deveined and sliced bell peppers
- 1 cup water
- 3/4 pound okra
- 1/4 cup flaxseed meal

Directions

1. Preheat a pan over a medium-high flame and warm the oil. Cook the pork until it is brown. Put to one side.
2. Cook the pork sausage in the pan drippings for 5 minutes and put to one side.
3. Put the shallots in the pan and cook until they are tender. Add the bone broth, Cajun spice, red pepper, gumbo, salt and pepper and the beef bouillon granules. Bring this to the boil.
4. Mix in the pork, sausage, celery, bell peppers and water and reduce the heat to medium-low. Simmer for 20 minutes.
5. Mix in the okra and flaxseed meal and cook for another 5 minutes. Serve hot and enjoy!

Nutrition: 427 Calories;35.2g Protein; 26.2g Fat; 7.6g Carbs; 3.3g Sugar

388. MEATLOAF WITH GRUYERE

Servings: 6

Preparation Time: 15 minutes
Cooking Time: 40 minutes

Ingredients

- 1 1/2 lbs. ground beef
- 1 cup ground almonds
- 1 large egg from free-range chickens
- 1/2 cup grated Gruyere cheese
- 1 tsp fresh parsley finely chopped
- 1 scallion finely chopped
- 1/2 tsp ground cumin
- 3 eggs boiled
- 2 Tbsp of butter, melted

Directions:

1. Preheat oven to 350°F/175°C.
2. Combine all Ingredients (except eggs and butter) in a large bowl.
3. Using your hands, combine well the mixture.
4. Shape the mixture into a roll and place in the middle sliced hard-boiled eggs.
5. Transfer the meatloaf to a 5x9 inch loaf pan greased with melted butter.
6. Place in oven and bake for 40 minutes or until internal temperature of 160 degrees F.
7. Remove from the oven and allow rest for 10 minutes.
8. Slice and serve.

Nutrition:

Calories: 598 Carbohydrates: 5,3g Proteins: 28g Fat: 63g Fiber: 2.6g

389. ROASTED FILLET MIGNON IN FOIL

Servings: 6
Preparation Time: 15 minutes
Cooking Time: 45 minutes

Ingredients

- 3 lbs. fillet mignon in one piece
- Salt to taste and ground black pepper
- 1 tsp of garlic powder
- 1 tsp of onion powder
- 1 tsp of cumin
- 4 Tbsp of olive oil

Directions:

1. Preheat the oven to 425°F/210°C.
2. Rinse and clean the filet mignon, removing all fats, or ask your butcher to do it for you.
3. Season with the salt and pepper, garlic powder, onion powder and cumin.
4. Wrap filet mignon in foil and place in a roasting pan; drizzle with the olive oil.
5. Roast for 15 minutes per pound for medium-rare or to desired doneness.
6. Remove from the oven and allow to rest for 10 -15 minutes before serving.

Nutrition:

Calories: 350 Carbohydrates: 0.8g Proteins: 52.5g Fat: 12.2g Fiber: 0.2g

390. STEWED BEEF WITH GREEN BEANS

Servings: 6
Preparation Time: 10 minutes
Cooking Time: 50 minutes

Ingredients

- 1/2 cup olive oil
- 1 1/2 lbs. beef cut into cubes
- 2 scallions, finely chopped
- 2 cups water
- 1 lbs. fresh green beans - trimmed and cut diagonally in half
- 1 bay leaf
- 1 grated tomato
- 1/2 cup fresh mint leaves, finely chopped
- 1 tsp fresh or dry rosemary
- Salt and freshly ground pepper to taste

Directions:

1. Chop the beef into 1-inch thick cubes.
2. Heat the olive oil in a large pot at high heat. Sauté the beef for about 4 - 5 minutes; sprinkle with a pinch of salt and pepper.
3. Add the scallions and stir and sauté for about another 3 - 4 minutes until softened. Pour water and cook for 2-3 minutes.
4. Add the bay leaf and grated tomato. Cook for about 5 minutes; lower the heat at

medium low. Cover and simmer for about 15 minutes.

5. Add the green beans, rosemary, salt, fresh ground pepper and water enough to cover all Ingredients. Gently simmer for 15 - 20 minutes until the green beans are tender.
6. Sprinkle with the mint and rosemary, gently mix and remove from the heat. Serve hot.

Nutrition:

Calories: 354 Carbohydrates: 6g Proteins: 23g Fat: 26.5g Fiber: 2.7g

391. BEEF AND CHICKEN MEATBALLS WITH CURRY SAUCE

Servings: 8
Preparation Time: 15 minutes
Cooking Time: 30 minutes

Ingredients

- 1 lbs. of ground beef
- 3/4 lbs. of ground chicken
- 1 hot pepper, finely chopped
- 2 fresh onions, finely chopped
- 1 tsp of fresh grated ginger
- 3 Tbsp of fresh coriander, chopped
- Ground almonds
- Salt and ground black pepper
- For curry sauce
- 3 Tbsp of sesame oil
- 2 spring onions, finely chopped
- 2 cloves garlic minced
- 1 Tbsp of curry paste
- 1 Tbsp of cumin
- 1 grated tomato
- 2 cups of canned coconut milk
- 2 Tbsp of fresh coriander

Directions:

1. Combine all the Ingredients in a bowl; with your hand knead until combine well.
2. Form from the mixture fine meatballs.
3. Heat the oil in a large wok or in a frying skillet.
4. Fry the meatballs for about 10 minutes in total.
5. Remove the meatballs on a plate lined with absorbent paper.
6. Curry sauce
7. In the wok or frying skillet, sauté the green onions for 3 - 4 minutes; add the garlic, ginger and curry paste and stir.
8. Add the ground cumin and grated tomato, and cook for 5 minutes, stirring occasionally.
9. Add the coconut milk, season with the salt and bring to boil.
10. Cook, stirring, for 4 - 5 minutes.
11. Add the meatballs and cook for 5 minutes at medium-low heat.
12. Add fresh coriander and stir well.
13. Adjust salt and pepper, stir and serve.

Nutrition:

Calories: 389 Carbohydrates: 7.1g Proteins: 19g Fat: 32g Fiber: 2.7g

392. CREAMY AND PEPPERY BEEF FILLETS

Servings: 6
Preparation Time: 10 minutes
Cooking Time: 15 minutes

Ingredients

- 4 beef fillets (about 2 lbs.)
- 1 small red bell pepper, thinly chopped
- 1 red hot chili pepper, finely chopped
- 2 cloves garlic, finely sliced
- 2 Tbsp olive oil
- 1/3 cup of brandy
- 2 Tbsp of butter
- 1 cup of fresh cream
- 1/2 cup of bone broth
- Salt and ground black pepper

Directions:

1. Sprinkle the beef fillets with the chopped bell pepper, garlic and red hot chili pepper; press deep into the meat. Wrap fillets with a foil and refrigerate for 30 minutes.
2. Heat the oil in a wok or in a large frying pan and fry the fillets for 6 minutes in total for medium-rare.
3. Transfer them on a plate lined with absorbent paper; sprinkle with a pinch of

the salt and pepper.
4. In the same wok or the frying pan add brandy, butter, cream and bone broth; stir and cook for 5 minutes, stirring periodically.
5. Return your fillets in a work or skillet and cover with the sauce. Serve.

Nutrition:

Calories: 587 Carbohydrates: 2.7g Proteins: 31g Fat: 55g Fiber: 0.7g

393. PERFECT OVEN ROASTED SPARERIBS

Servings: 6
Preparation Time: 10 minutes
Cooking Time: 1 hour 25 minutes

Ingredients

- 3 lbs. beef spareribs with the bone
- 1 Tbsp fresh butter
- 2 Tbsp of olive oil
- 2 green onions, finely chopped
- 2 cloves garlic
- 3 Tbsp of fresh celery, chopped
- 1 Tbsp of grated tomato
- 2 Tbsp of fresh thyme, chopped
- 1 cup of dry white wine
- 1/2 cup of bone broth
- Salt and freshly ground black pepper

Directions:

1. Preheat the oven to 360°F/180°C.
2. Grease one large baking dish with the butter.
3. Season beef spareribs with the salt and pepper.
4. Place meat in a baking dish with the fat side down.
5. Heat the oil in a frying pan and sauté the onions, garlic for 3 - 4 minutes.
6. Add fresh celery, grated tomato and fresh thyme; stir well and cook for 2 - 3 minutes.
7. Pour the wine and bone broth and stir for 3 minutes.
8. Pour the sauce over the meat.
9. Cover with aluminum foil and bake for 1 1/2 hours.
10. 1Uncover and baste meat with the sauce and roast for further 30 minutes.
11. 1Allow the meat to cool for 10 - 15 minutes and serve.

Nutrition:

Calories: 554 Carbohydrates: 2g Proteins: 33.5g Fat: 88g Fiber: 0.8g

394. BAKED GROUND BEEF AND EGGPLANT CASSEROLE

Servings: 6
Preparation Time: 15 minutes
Cooking Time: 35 minutes

Ingredients

- 1 Tbsp of beef tallow
- 1 lbs. ground beef
- 1 spring onion, finely chopped
- 1 eggplant, diced
- 1 grated tomato
- 1/2 tsp dried parsley flakes
- 1/2 tsp dried celery flakes
- 1 tsp seasoned salt
- 1/2 cup water
- 1 cup cheddar cheese, grated

Directions:

1. Preheat oven to 350°F/286°C.
2. In a large casserole dish, heat the tallow and sauté the ground beef, chopped onion for two minutes; stir.
3. Add eggplant and stir for two minutes.
4. Add all remaining Ingredients and give a good stir.
5. Sprinkle with grated cheese and bake for 15 minutes. Serve hot.

Nutrition:

Calories: 477 Carbohydrates: 8g Proteins: 29g Fat: 36g Fiber: 4.5g

395. FESTIVE ROSEMARY BEEF FILLET

Servings: 6
Preparation Time: 15 minutes
Cooking Time: 15 minutes

Ingredients

- 1/4 cup olive oil
- 3 1/2 lbs. center-cut beef tenderloin roast
- Kosher salt and ground black pepper to taste
- 2 cloves garlic finely chopped
- 2 - 3 Tbsp fresh rosemary (chopped)

Directions:

1. Preheat oven to 350ºF/175ºC.
2. Grease one roasting pan with olive oil; set aside.
3. Pat beef roast dry, and generously coat with the salt, pepper, garlic and rosemary.
4. Place meat in a prepared roasting pan.
5. Bake for 25 - 30 minutes per pound or until inserted thermometer for internal temperature reaches 175º F/85º C.
6. Remove from oven and allow to rest for 10 -15 minutes.
7. Slice and serve.

Nutrition:

Calories: 549 Carbohydrates: 0.3g Proteins: 40g Fat: 42g Fiber: 0.3g

396. GRILLED FILLET MIGNON WITH BLACK PEPPERCORN

Servings: 6
Preparation Time: 10 minutes
Cooking Time: 15 minutes

Ingredients

- 8 beef filet mignon steaks 1-inch cut
- Sea salt to taste
- 2 Tbsp of olive oil
- Cracked black peppercorn, to taste

Directions:

1. Preheat your grill (pellet, gas, charcoal) to HIGH according to manufacturer Instructions.
2. Season each fillet with the sea salt.
3. Brush each filet with oil and press some peppercorns in the top side of each steak.
4. Place your fillets in a grill racks, close the lid, and grill for 10 to 12 minutes for medium-rare turning once.
5. Serve hot.

Nutrition:

Calories: 569 Carbohydrates: 0 g Proteins: 43g Fat: 46g Fiber: 0 g

397. KETO BEEF SATAY

Servings: 4
Preparation Time: 15 minutes
Cooking Time: 5 minutes

Ingredients

- 1 lbs beef strips, sliced
- 1 tsp turmeric
- 1/2 tsp dried chili flakes
- 1 Tbsp of coconut aminos
- 1 tsp of stevia granulated sweetener
- 1/2 tsp salt
- 1/2 cup coconut milk
- 1 Tbsp of beef tallow

Directions:

1. Cut beef in strips about 1/4" thick. In a container, combine all remaining Ingredients, add the beef strips and marinate for 2 hours.
2. Remove the beef strips from fridge and drain on a kitchen paper towel: reserve marinade.
3. Heat the tallow in a skillet and fry the beef strips for 5 minutes in total over medium heat.
4. Pour the marinade over the pork and simmer for two minutes.
5. Serve hot.

Nutrition:

Calories: 579 Carbohydrates: 2g Proteins: 64g Fat: 34g Fiber: 0.2g

398. KETO BEEF STROGANOFF

Servings: 6
Preparation Time: 10 minutes
Cooking Time: 30 minutes

Ingredients

- 2 Tbsp of butter
- 1/2 cup green onions (scallions) finely chopped
- 1/2 cup cream cheese, at room temperature
- 1/2 tsp of ground garlic

- 1/2 tsp dried sage
- 1 tsp celery
- 2 lbs. of beef tenderloin cut into 2-inch strips
- 1 cup sliced mushrooms
- Salt and ground pepper to taste

Directions:

1. Melt butter in medium skillet over medium heat; add green onion and sauté for 3 minutes. Add cream cheese, ground garlic, sage and celery; stir until combined well. Remove skillet from heat; set aside.
2. Place beef strips with mushrooms in a large frying skillet. Cover and cook for 3 minutes on high heat. Uncover; add the cream cheese mixture and stir well.
3. Cover and cook for 20 -25 minutes over low heat.
4. Remove from the heat and let sit for 10 minutes before serving.

Nutrition:

Calories: 506 Carbohydrates: 2g Proteins: 29g Fat: 42g Fiber: 0.4g

399. TASTY VEAL ROAST WITH HERB CRUST

Servings: 6
Preparation Time: 12 minutes
Cooking Time: 2 hours and 15 minutes

Ingredients

- 3 lbs. veal leg round roast, boneless
- 1/4 cup ground almonds
- 2 Tbsp water
- 1 Tbsp mustard (Dijon, English, or whole grain)
- 1 Tbsp lemon juice
- 1/2 tsp ground pepper
- 1 tsp dried thyme
- 1 tsp dried basil
- 1 cup bone broth (or water)
- 2 Tbsp almond flour
- 1/4 cup sour cream

Directions:

1. Heat the oven to 350°F/175°C.
2. Place meat in a roasting pan.
3. In a bowl, stir together ground almonds, water, mustard, lemon juice, basil, thyme, and pepper.
4. Generously spread mixture over the meat.
5. Place a pan in oven and bake for 2-1/2 hours or until inserted thermometer reaches 160 F/ 80 C.
6. Transfer meat to a platter; cover and set aside.
7. In a saucepan stir bone broth or water with the flour. Cook and stir until thickened and bubbly, about two minutes.
8. Stir in the sour cream and just heat through.
9. Serve meat with the sauce, and Bon appetite!

Nutrition:

Calories: 515 Carbohydrates: 2g Proteins: 83g Fat: 15g Fiber: 1g

400. BEEF PROSCIUTTO CASSEROLE

Servings: 8
Preparation Time: 35 minutes
Cooking Time: 10 minutes

Ingredients

- 8 beef steaks
- 1 cup of white wine
- 8 slices prosciutto
- 8 leaves of sage
- 2 Tbsp of capers
- Salt and freshly ground black pepper
- 2 Tbsp of butter

Directions:

1. Put the steaks in the container; season generously with the salt and pepper and pour in the wine; marinate for 30 minutes; drain and reserve the wine.
2. Preheat the oven to 350° F/ 175° C.
3. Place the prosciutto slice and sage leave on each beef steak and fasten with a toothpick or slice into a roll, and then fasten.
4. Grease the casserole dish with the butter and place the steaks.
5. Sprinkle with capers, little fresh pepper, and pour with reserved wine.

6. Bake for 7 - 10 minutes per side.
7. Remove from the oven, and let the meat rest before serving.

Nutrition:

Calories: 432 Carbohydrates: 1.5g Proteins: 34g Fat: 53g Fiber: 0.2g

401. GROUND BEEF AND BABY SPINACH CASSEROLE

Servings: 4
Preparation Time: 10 minutes
Cooking Time: 45 minutes

Ingredients

- 1 lbs. of ground beef (or turkey, beef, lamb, bison)
- Salt and freshly ground black pepper
- 1 grated tomato or small dice
- 2 cups of baby spinach
- 1 cup sliced black olives
- 1 Tbsp of fresh cilantro, finely chopped
- 8 eggs
- 1/2 cup grated cheese (Cheddar or Parmesan)

Directions:

1. Preheat oven to 350°F/175°C.
2. Place the ground beef in a greased casserole and sprinkle with a pinch of salt and pepper.
3. Add grated tomato, olives and baby spinach over the meat; sprinkle with the little salt and fresh cilantro.
4. In a bowl, whisk the eggs until frothy; add grated cheese and stir. Season it with the salt and pepper and stir.
5. Pour the egg mixture in casserole.
6. Place in the oven and bake for 40 - 45 minutes. Serve hot.

Nutrition:

Calories: 484 Carbohydrates: 3.5g Proteins: 35g Fat: 36g Fiber: 2g

402. INSTANT POT TANGY BEEF CHUCK ROAST

Servings: 6
Preparation Time: 10 minutes
Cooking Time: 1 hour and 5 minutes

Ingredients

- 2 Tbsp olive oil
- 3 lbs. beef chuck roast, boneless
- Seasoned salt and ground black pepper to taste
- 1 pinch garlic powder
- 2 spring onions, finely chopped
- 1 carrot, sliced
- 1 1/2 cup bone broth
- 1 1/2 Tbsp Worcestershire sauce

Directions:

1. Season generously the beef roast with seasoned salt and ground black pepper and garlic powder.
2. Press SAUTÉ button on your Instant Pot
3. When the word "hot" appears on the display, add beef and sear from all sides.
4. Add onions and sliced carrot, turn-off the SAUTÉ button.
5. Pour bone broth and Worcestershire sauce
6. Lock lid into place and set on the MANUAL setting for 60 minutes.
7. Naturally release pressure for 5 minutes and quick release remaining pressure.
8. Remove lid, transfer roast to the large plate and shred the roast. Serve hot.

Nutrition:

Calories: 654 Carbohydrates: 5g Proteins: 49g Fat: 60g Fiber: 1g

403. BEEF ROAST WITH HERBS AND MUSTARD

Servings: 6
Preparation Time: 10 minutes
Cooking Time: 8 hours

Ingredients

- 2 Tbsp beef tallow
- 2 lbs. beef roast
- Salt and black ground pepper to taste
- 2 Tbsp yellow ground mustard seeds
- 1 Tbsp fresh parsley, finely chopped
- 1 tsp fresh thyme, finely chopped
- 1 tsp fresh cilantro chopped

- 1 Tbsp butter
- 1 1/2 cup water

Directions:

1. Grease the inner steel pot in the Slow Cooker.
2. Season the beef with the salt and pepper from all sides.
3. Place the beef roast in Slow Cooker and sprinkle with mustard seeds and fresh herbs.
4. Pour the water, add the mustard and sprinkle with parsley-cilantro mix; stir.
5. Cover and cook on LOW for 6 - 8 hours.
6. Remove roast from Slow Cooker on a platter; allow to cool, slice and serve.

Nutrition:

Calories: 466 Carbohydrates: 0.5g Proteins: 27g Fat: 38g Fiber: 0.3g

404. GROUND BEEF WITH SWISS CHARD STIR-FRY

Servings: 4
Preparation Time: 10 minutes
Cooking Time: 20 minutes

Ingredients

- 1 Tbsp lard or butter
- 2 green onions (only green parts finely chopped)
- 1 lbs. ground beef
- 1 tsp garlic powder
- 1 tsp ground cumin
- 1 tsp oregano
- Salt and ground pepper to taste
- 1 lbs. Swiss chard, tender stems and leaves finely chopped

Directions:

1. In a large pot boil water and cook Swiss Chard for 5 - 7 minutes or until soft; transfer in colander to drain.
2. Heat the lard in a large and deep-frying pan.
3. Add the green onions with a pinch of salt, and sauté for 3 - 4 minutes over medium heat.
4. Add ground beef and stir for 4 -5 minutes.
5. Season with the garlic powder, cumin and oregano; stir well.
6. Add steamed Swish Card and gently stir to combine all Ingredients; cover and cook for further 2 - 3 minutes. Serve hot.

Nutrition:

Calories: 351 Carbohydrates: 5g Proteins: 23g Fat: 21g Fiber: 3g

405. GROUND BEEF KALE STEW WITH ALMONDS

Servings: 4
Preparation Time: 5 minutes
Cooking Time: 25 minutes

Ingredients

- 1 lbs. kale (chopped, tough stems discarded)
- 2 Tbsp olive oil
- 1 lbs. of ground beef
- 1/4 tsp of cinnamon
- 1 tsp cumin
- 1 tsp oregano
- 1 tsp garlic powder
- Salt and freshly ground black pepper, to taste
- 1 cup almonds, finely chopped or ground

Directions:

1. Boil water in a large pot; submerge kale and boil for 5 - 6 minutes; transfer kale in a colander to drain.
2. Heat the oil in a large and deep-frying and sauté ground meat for 6 - 7 minutes.
3. Season with the cinnamon, cumin, oregano, garlic powder, and the ground pepper and salt; stir well.
4. Add streamed kale, stir gently, cover and cook for 3 - 4 minutes over low heat.
5. Taste and adjust seasonings. Sprinkle with ground almonds and serve hot.

Nutrition:

Calories: 481 Carbohydrates: 8g Proteins: 28g Fat: 38g Fiber: 3.5g

406. PERFECT KETO BEEF AND BROCCOLI STIR-FRY

Servings: 4
Preparation Time: 10 minutes
Cooking Time: 15 minutes

Ingredients

- 1 lbs. pre-cut beef strips or beef for stir-fry
- 2 Tbsp almond flour
- 1/2 cup water
- 1/2 tsp garlic powder
- 2 Tbsp olive oil, divided
- 4 cups broccoli florets
- 1 small onion, cut into wedges
- 1 tsp ground of fresh ginger

Directions:

1. In a bowl, combine 2 tablespoons of almond flour, 2 tablespoons water and garlic powder until smooth.
2. Pour the mixture over the beef and toss to combine well.
3. In a large skillet heat the oil over medium-high heat, stir-fry the beef strips for 4 - 5 minutes, or l until beef reaches desired doneness. Remove the beef on a plate.
4. Heat some more oil in the same skillet and sauté the onion for 3 - 4 minutes.
5. Add the broccoli; season with the salt and pepper and sauté for about 2 - 3 minutes.
6. Add the chicken again in a skillet, stir and cook along with remaining Ingredients for 2 minutes. Serve hot.

Nutrition:

Calories: 228 Carbohydrates: 1.5g Proteins: 29g Fat: 11g Fiber: 0.5g

407. GRILLED LAMB SKEWERS

Servings: 6
Preparation Time: 15 minutes
Cooking Time: 10 minutes

Ingredients

- 2 lbs. of lamb fillet cut in cubes
- Salt to taste
- 1/2 cup of olive oil
- 1 Tbsp of grated ginger
- 1 cup of white wine
- 2 Tbsp of wine vinegar
- 1/4 tsp of freshly ground black pepper

Directions:

1. Rinse and trim your lamb fillet; cut lamb fillet into 1 1/2-inch cubes. Season the lamb meat generously with salt.
2. In a bowl, whisk the olive oil, ginger, wine, vinegar, and pepper to make the marinade.
3. Add the lamb cube and combine with marinade. Cover and refrigerate for 2-3 hours or overnight.
4. Preheat your grill (pellet, gas, charcoal) to HIGH according to manufacturer Instructions.
5. Remove the lamb from the fridge and pat dry on kitchen paper towel. Thread the meat onto skewers and place on grill.
6. Grill for about 10 minutes in total for medium-rare, turning every 1-2 minutes, until lamb is cooked to desired doneness.
7. Remove skewers from the grill and let sit for 5 minutes. Serve.

Nutrition:

Calories: 487 Carbohydrates: 1.3g Proteins: 28g Fat: 38.5g Fiber: 0.05g

408. GRILLED LAMB PATTIES

Servings: 6
Preparation Time: 15 minutes
Cooking Time: 10 minutes

Ingredients

- 1 3/4 lbs. of ground lamb meat
- 1/4 cup ground almonds
- 1 tsp dried oregano
- 1 large egg at room temperature
- 1/2 tsp garlic powder
- 1/2 tsp of onion powder
- 1 tsp cumin
- 2 tsp chopped fresh rosemary
- Cayenne pepper (to taste)
- Sea salt to taste

Directions:

1. Combine all Ingredients in a large bowl.
2. Using your hands, combine and knead the mixture until combine well.
3. Wet your hands and form mixture into 6 patties, and place on a plate lined with

parchment paper.

4. Place the lamb patties in a fridge for one hour.
5. Preheat your grill (pellet, gas, charcoal) to HIGH according to manufacturer Instructions.
6. Arrange lamb patties on grill rack and cook for about 4 - 5 minutes per side for medium-rare.
7. Transfer lamb patties to serving plate and let rest for 10 minutes.
8. Serve.

Nutrition:

Calories: 270 Carbohydrates: 4g Proteins: 39g Fat: 10g Fiber: 1g

409. ROASTED LAMB LOIN WITH YOGURT SAUCE

Servings: 6
Preparation Time: 15 minutes
Cooking Time: 35 minutes

Ingredients

- 2 Tbsp olive oil
- 1 cup of yogurt
- 1 Tbsp of tomato paste
- 2 Tbsp of fresh thyme, chopped
- 3 cloves garlic finely chopped
- 2 lbs. lamb loin
- Salt and black pepper freshly ground
- 1 bunch of parsley, chopped

Directions:

1. Preheat the oven at 325°F/160°C.
2. Combine olive oil, yogurt, tomato paste, thyme and garlic in a bowl and pour in a large baking pan.
3. Season the lamb loin with the salt and pepper and place in a baking pan.
4. Baste the lamb with sauce.
5. Cover with aluminum foil and place in oven.
6. Bake for 1 hour, and then uncover and bake for additional 40 minutes.
7. Sprinkle with chopped parsley and remove from the oven.
8. Before serving, allow to cool for 10 minutes.

Nutrition:

Calories: 389 Carbohydrates: 4.8g Proteins: 30g Fat: 27g Fiber: 0.8g

410. GRILLED LAMB CHOPS

Servings: 4
Preparation Time: 20 minutes
Cooking Time: 10 minutes

Ingredients

- 16 lamb chops
- Roasted red peppers
- 1 garlic clove, minced
- 1 tsp parsley, chopped
- 3 Tbsp Spanish extra virgin olive oil
- Pinch of salt
- Black pepper

Directions:

1. Preheat your grill (pellet, gas, charcoal) to HIGH according to manufacturer Instructions.
2. Season the lamb chops with the salt and pepper, and drizzle with the olive oil.
3. Place the lamb chops on grill and cook for 3 – 4 minutes per side for medium-rare.
4. Meanwhile cut the red peppers into strips and add the garlic clove, parsley, Spanish olive oil, salt and black pepper.
5. Season the lamb chops with salt and serve immediately along with the peppers.

Nutrition:

Calories: 285 Carbohydrates: 1g Proteins: 38g Fat: 13g Fiber: 0.4g

411. GRILLED LAMB CHOPS WITH SWEET MARINADE

Servings: 4
Preparation Time: 15 minutes
Cooking Time: 15 minutes

Ingredients

- 3 Tbsp of olive oil
- 1/4 cup stevia granulate sweetener
- 1 tsp garlic powder
- 2 tsp ground ginger
- 2 tsp dried tarragon
- 1 tsp ground cinnamon

- Salt and ground black pepper to taste
- 4 lamb chops

Instructions.

1. In a bowl, combine the olive oil, stevia, garlic, ginger, tarragon, cinnamon and salt and pepper. Rub lamb chops with mixture, and place in a deep container. Cover, and refrigerate for 2 hours (preferable overnight).
2. Preheat your grill (pellet, gas, charcoal) to HIGH (on 450°F) according to manufacturer Instructions.
3. Remove the lamb chops from marinade and place directly on grill grate.
4. Grill for 4 to 6 minutes per side or until inserted thermometer reaches135°F internal temperature. Serve hot.

Nutrition:

Calories: 407 Carbohydrates: 0.3g Proteins: 28g Fat: 32g Fiber: 0.5g

412. INSTANT POT LAMB CHOPS WITH GREENS

Servings: 8
Preparation Time: 10 minutes
Cooking Time: 35 minutes

Ingredients

- 1/4 cup olive oil
- 2 spring onions finely chopped
- 2 cloves of garlic, minced
- 3 lbs. lamb chops
- 2 lbs. wild greens such, Dandelions, ramps, mustard etc.
- 1 tsp dry rosemary
- 1 cup water
- Salt and ground pepper to taste
- Lemon wedges For serving

Directions:

1. Rinse and clean wild greens from any dirt.
2. Press SAUTÉ button on your Instant Pot.
3. When the word "hot" appears on the display, add the oil and sauté green onions and garlic for about 2 - 3 minutes.
4. Add lamb meat and sear for 2 - 3 minutes.
5. Lock lid into place and set on the MANUAL setting for 25 minutes.
6. Use Quick Release - turn the valve from sealing to venting to release the pressure.
7. Add greens, season with the salt and pepper and sprinkle with rosemary. Pour one cup of water and cover.
8. Lock lid into place and set on the MANUAL setting for 3 minutes.
9. When the timer beeps, press "Cancel" and carefully flip the Quick Release valve to let the pressure out.
10. 1Serve hot with lemon wedges.

Nutrition:

Calories: 322 Carbohydrates: 8g Proteins: 35g Fat: 16g Fiber: 5g

VEGETABLES

413. COLLARD GREEN WRAP

Preparation Time: 10 minutes
Cooking Time: 0 minutes
Serving: 4

Ingredients:

- ½ block feta, cut into 4 (1-inch thick) strips (4-oz)
- ½ cup purple onion, diced
- ½ medium red bell pepper, julienned
- 1 medium cucumber, julienned
- 4 large cherry tomatoes, halved
- 4 large collard green leaves, washed
- 8 whole kalamata olives, halved

Sauce Ingredients:

- 1 cup low-fat plain Greek yogurt
- 1 tablespoon white vinegar
- 1 teaspoon garlic powder
- 2 tablespoons minced fresh dill
- 2 tablespoons olive oil
- 2.5-ounces cucumber, seeded and grated (¼-whole)
- Salt and pepper to taste

Directions:

1. Make the sauce first: make sure to squeeze out all the excess liquid from the cucumber after grating. In a small bowl, mix all sauce ingredients thoroughly and refrigerate.
2. Prepare and slice all wrap ingredients.
3. On a flat surface, spread one collard green leaf. Spread 2 tablespoons of Tzatziki sauce on middle of the leaf.
4. Layer ¼ of each of the tomatoes, feta, olives, onion, pepper, and cucumber. Place them on the center of the leaf, like piling them high instead of spreading them.
5. Fold the leaf like you would a burrito. Repeat process for remaining ingredients.
6. Serve and enjoy.

Nutrition Facts Per Serving

Calories 463, Total Fat 31g, Saturated Fat 3g, Total Carbs 31g, Net Carbs 24g, Protein 20g, Sugar: 18g, Fiber 7g, Sodium 795mg, Potassium 960mg

414. ZUCCHINI GARLIC FRIES

Preparation Time: 10 minutes
Cooking Time: 20 minutes
Serving: 6

Ingredients:

- ¼ teaspoon garlic powder
- ½ cup almond flour
- 2 large egg whites, beaten
- 3 medium zucchinis, sliced into fry sticks
- Salt and pepper to taste

Directions:

1. Preheat oven to 400oF.
2. Mix all ingredients in a bowl until the zucchini fries are well coated.
3. Place fries on cookie sheet and spread evenly.
4. Put in oven and cook for 20 minutes.
5. Halfway through cooking time, stir fries.

Nutrition Facts Per Serving

Calories 11, Total Fat 0.1g, Saturated Fat 0g, Total Carbs 1g, Net Carbs 0.5g, Protein1.5 g, Sugar: 0.5g, Fiber 0.5g, Sodium 19mg, Potassium 71mg

415. MASHED CAULIFLOWER

Preparation Time: 10 minutes
Cooking Time: 10 minutes
Serving: 3

Ingredients:

- 1 cauliflower head
- 1 tablespoon olive oil
- ½ tsp salt
- ¼ tsp dill
- Pepper to taste
- 2 tbsp low fat milk

Directions:

1. Bring a small pot of water to a boil.
2. Chop cauliflower in florets.

3. Add florets to boiling water and boil uncovered for 5 minutes. Turn off fire and let it sit for 5 minutes more.
4. In a blender, add all ingredients except for cauliflower and blend to mix well.
5. Drain cauliflower well and add into blender. Puree until smooth and creamy.
6. Serve and enjoy.

Nutrition Facts Per Serving

Calories 78, Total Fat 5g, Saturated Fat 1g, Total Carbs 6g, Net Carbs 4g, Protein 2g, Sugar: 3g, Fiber 2g, Sodium 420mg, Potassium 327mg

416. STIR-FRIED EGGPLANT

Preparation Time: 10 minutes
Cooking Time: 10 minutes
Serving: 2

Ingredients:

- 1 tablespoon coconut oil
- 2 eggplants, sliced into 3-inch in length
- 4 cloves of garlic, minced
- 1 onion, chopped
- 1 teaspoon ginger, grated
- 1 teaspoon lemon juice, freshly squeezed
- ½ tsp salt
- ½ tsp pepper

Directions:

1. Heat oil in a nonstick saucepan.
2. Pan-fry the eggplants for 2 minutes on all sides.
3. Add the garlic and onions until fragrant, around 3 minutes.
4. Stir in the ginger, salt, pepper, and lemon juice.
5. Add a ½ cup of water and bring to a simmer. Cook until eggplant is tender.

Nutrition Facts Per Serving

Calories 232, Total Fat 8g, Saturated Fat 1g, Total Carbs 41g, Net Carbs 23g, Protein 7g, Sugar: 22g, Fiber 18g, Sodium 596mg, Potassium 1404mg

417. SAUTÉED GARLIC MUSHROOMS

Preparation Time: 10 minutes
Cooking Time: 10 minutes
Serving: 4

Ingredients:

- 1 tablespoon olive oil
- 3 cloves of garlic, minced
- 16 ounces fresh brown mushrooms, sliced
- 7 ounces fresh shiitake mushrooms, sliced
- ½ tsp salt
- ½ tsp pepper or more to taste

Directions:

1. Place a nonstick saucepan on medium high fire and heat pan for a minute.
2. Add oil and heat for 2 minutes.
3. Stir in garlic and sauté for a minute.
4. Add remaining ingredients and stir fry until soft and tender, around 5 minutes.
5. Turn off fire, let mushrooms rest while pan is covered for 5 minutes.
6. Serve and enjoy.

Nutrition Facts Per Serving

Calories 95, Total Fat 4g, Saturated Fat 0.5g, Total Carbs 14g, Net Carbs 10g, Protein 3g, Sugar: 5g, Fiber 4g, Sodium 296mg, Potassium 490mg

418. STIR FRIED ASPARAGUS AND BELL PEPPER

Preparation Time: 10 minutes
Cooking Time: 10 minutes
Serving: 6

Ingredients:

- 1 tablespoon olive oil
- 4 cloves of garlic, minced
- 1-pound fresh asparagus spears, trimmed
- 2 large red bell peppers, seeded and julienned
- ½ teaspoon thyme
- 5 tablespoons water
- ½ tsp salt
- ½ tsp pepper or more to taste

Directions:

1. Place a nonstick saucepan on high fire and heat pan for a minute.
2. Add oil and heat for 2 minutes.
3. Stir in garlic and sauté for a minute.
4. Add remaining ingredients and stir fry until soft and tender, around 6 minutes.
5. Turn off fire, let veggies rest while pan is

covered for 5 minutes.

6. Serve and enjoy.

Nutrition Facts Per Serving

Calories 45, Total Fat 2g, Saturated Fat 0.3g, Total Carbs 5g, Net Carbs 3g, Protein 2g, Sugar: 2g, Fiber 2g, Sodium 482mg, Potassium 219mg

419. STIR FRIED BRUSSELS SPROUTS AND PECANS

Preparation Time: 10 minutes
Cooking Time: 10 minutes
Serving: 7

Ingredients:

- 1 ½ pounds fresh Brussels sprouts, trimmed and halved
- 1 tablespoon olive oil
- 4 cloves of garlic, minced
- 3 tablespoons water
- ¼ tsp salt
- ½ tsp pepper or more to taste
- ½ cup chopped pecans

Directions:

1. Place a nonstick saucepan on high fire and heat pan for a minute.
2. Add oil and heat for 2 minutes.
3. Stir in garlic and sauté for a minute.
4. Add remaining ingredients and stir fry until soft and tender, around 6 minutes.
5. Turn off fire, let veggies rest while pan is covered for 5 minutes.
6. Serve and enjoy.

Nutrition Facts Per Serving

Calories 112, Total Fat 7g, Saturated Fat 0.8g, Total Carbs 11g, Net Carbs 8g, Protein 4g, Sugar: 4g, Fiber 3g, Sodium 108mg, Potassium 425mg

420. STIR FRIED KALE

Preparation Time: 10 minutes
Cooking Time: 10 minutes
Serving: 6

Ingredients:

- 1 tablespoon coconut oil
- 2 cloves of garlic, minced
- 1 onion, chopped
- 2 teaspoons crushed red pepper flakes
- 4 cups kale, chopped
- 2 tbsp water
- Salt and pepper to taste

Directions:

1. Place a nonstick saucepan on high fire and heat pan for a minute.
2. Add oil and heat for 2 minutes.
3. Stir in garlic and sauté for a minute. Add onions and stir fry for another minute.
4. Add remaining ingredients and stir fry until soft and tender, around 4 minutes.
5. Turn off fire, let veggies rest while pan is covered for 3 minutes.
6. Serve and enjoy.

Nutrition Facts Per Serving

Calories 37, Total Fat 2g, Saturated Fat 2g, Total Carbs 4g, Net Carbs 3g, Protein 1g, Sugar: 1g, Fiber 1g, Sodium 6mg, Potassium 111mg

421. STIR FRIED BOK CHOY

Preparation Time: 10 minutes
Cooking Time: 12 minutes
Serving: 1

Ingredients:

1. 1 tablespoon coconut oil
2. 4 cloves of garlic, minced
3. 1 onion, chopped
4. 2 heads bok choy, rinsed and chopped
5. ¼ tsp salt
6. ½ tsp pepper or more to taste
7. 1 tablespoons sesame seeds

Directions:

1. Place a nonstick saucepan on high fire and heat pan for a minute.
2. Add sesame seeds and toast for a minute. Transfer to a bowl.
3. In same pan, add oil and heat for 2 minutes.
4. Stir in garlic and sauté for a minute. Add onions and stir fry for another minute.
5. Add remaining ingredients and stir fry until soft and tender, around 4 minutes.
6. Turn off fire, let veggies rest while pan is covered for 3 minutes.
7. Serve and enjoy.

Nutrition Facts Per Serving

Calories 334, Total Fat 20g, Saturated Fat 5g, Total Carbs 36g, Net Carbs 22g, Protein 12g, Sugar: 6g, Fiber 14g, Sodium 731mg, Potassium 1043mg

422. VEGETABLE CURRY

Preparation Time: 10 minutes
Cooking Time: 20 minutes
Serving: 4

Ingredients:

- 1 tablespoon coconut oil
- 1 medium onion, chopped
- 1 teaspoon minced garlic
- 1 teaspoon minced ginger
- 2 cup broccoli florets
- 2 cups fresh spinach leaves
- 1 tablespoon garam masala
- ½ cup coconut milk
- ½ tsp salt
- ½ tsp pepper

Directions:

1. Place a nonstick pot on high fire and heat pot for a minute.
2. Add oil and heat for 2 minutes.
3. Stir in garlic and ginger, sauté for a minute. Add onions and garam masala and stir fry for another minute.
4. Add remaining ingredients, except for spinach leaves and simmer for 10 minutes.
5. Stir in spinach leaves, turn off fire, let veggies rest while pot is covered for 5 minutes.
6. Serve and enjoy.

Nutrition Facts Per Serving

Calories 121, Total Fat 11g, Saturated Fat 4g, Total Carbs 6g, Net Carbs 4g, Protein 2g, Sugar: 3g, Fiber 2g, Sodium 315mg, Potassium 266mg

423. BRAISED CARROTS 'N KALE

Preparation Time: 10 minutes
Cooking Time: 10 minutes
Serving: 2

Ingredients:

- 1 tablespoon coconut oil
- 1 onion, sliced thinly
- 5 cloves of garlic, minced
- 3 medium carrots, sliced thinly
- 10 ounces of kale, chopped
- ½ cup water
- Salt and pepper to taste
- A dash of red pepper flakes

Directions:

1. Heat oil in a skillet over medium flame and sauté the onion and garlic until fragrant.
2. Toss in the carrots and stir for 1 minute. Add the kale and water. Season with salt and pepper to taste.
3. Close the lid and allow to simmer for 5 minutes.
4. Sprinkle with red pepper flakes.
5. Serve and enjoy.

Nutrition Facts Per Serving

Calories 161, Total Fat 8g, Saturated Fat 1g, Total Carbs 20g, Net Carbs 14g, Protein 8g, Sugar: 6g, Fiber 6g, Sodium 63mg, Potassium 900mg

424. BUTTERNUT SQUASH HUMMUS

Preparation Time: 10 minutes
Cooking Time: 15 minutes
Serving: 8

Ingredients:

- 2 pounds butternut squash, seeded and peeled
- 1 tablespoon olive oil
- ¼ cup tahini
- 2 tablespoons lemon juice
- 2 cloves of garlic, minced
- Salt and pepper to taste

Directions:

1. Heat the oven to 3000F.
2. Coat the butternut squash with olive oil.
3. Place in a baking dish and bake for 15 minutes in the oven.
4. Once the squash is cooked, place in a food processor together with the rest of the ingredients.
5. Pulse until smooth.

6. Place in individual containers.
7. Put a label and store in the fridge.
8. Allow to warm at room temperature before heating in the microwave oven.
9. Serve with carrots or celery sticks.

Nutrition Facts Per Serving

Calories 109, Total Fat 6g, Saturated Fat 0.8g, Total Carbs 15g, Net Carbs 11g, Protein 2g, Sugar: 3g, Fiber 4g, Sodium 14mg, Potassium 379mg

425. STIR FRIED GINGERY VEGGIES

Preparation Time: 10 minutes
Cooking Time: 10 minutes
Serving: 4

Ingredients:

- 1 tablespoon oil
- 3 cloves of garlic, minced
- 1 onion, chopped
- 1 thumb-size ginger, sliced
- 1 tablespoon water
- 1 large carrots, peeled and julienned
- 1 large green bell pepper, seeded and julienned
- 1 large yellow bell pepper, seeded and julienned
- 1 large red bell pepper, seeded and julienned
- 1 zucchini, julienned
- Salt and pepper to taste

Directions:

- Heat oil in a nonstick saucepan over high flame and sauté the garlic, onion, and ginger until fragrant.
- Stir in the rest of the ingredients.
- Keep on stirring for at least 5 minutes until vegetables are tender.
- Serve and enjoy.

Nutrition Facts Per Serving

Calories 70, Total Fat 4g, Saturated Fat 1g, Total Carbs 9g, Net Carbs 7g, Protein 1g, Sugar: 4g, Fiber 2g, Sodium 273mg, Potassium 263mg

426. CAULIFLOWER FRITTERS

Preparation Time: 10 minutes
Cooking Time: 15 minutes
Serving: 6

Ingredients:

- 1 large cauliflower head, cut into florets
- 2 eggs, beaten
- ½ teaspoon turmeric
- ½ teaspoon salt
- ¼ teaspoon black pepper
- 1 tablespoon coconut oil

Directions:

1. Place the cauliflower florets in a pot with water and bring to a boil. Cook until tender, around 5 minutes of boiling. Drain well.
2. Place the cauliflower, eggs, turmeric, salt, and pepper into the food processor.
3. Pulse until the mixture becomes coarse.
4. Transfer into a bowl. Using your hands, form six small flattened balls and place in the fridge for at least 1 hour until the mixture hardens.
5. Heat the oil in a nonstick pan and fry the cauliflower patties for 3 minutes on each side.
6. Serve and enjoy.

Nutrition Facts Per Serving

Calories 53, Total Fat 6g, Saturated Fat 2g, Total Carbs 2g, Net Carbs 1g, Protein 3g, Sugar: 1g, Fiber 1g, Sodium 228mg, Potassium 159mg

427. STIR-FRIED SQUASH

Preparation Time: 10 minutes
Cooking Time: 10 minutes
Serving: 4

Ingredients:

- 1 tablespoon olive oil
- 3 cloves of garlic, minced
- 1 butternut squash, seeded and sliced
- 1 tablespoon coconut aminos
- 1 tablespoon lemon juice
- 1 tablespoon water
- Salt and pepper to taste

Directions:

1. Heat oil over medium flame and sauté the

garlic until fragrant.
2. Stir in the squash for another 3 minutes before adding the rest of the ingredients.
3. Close the lid and allow to simmer for 5 more minutes or until the squash is soft.
4. Serve and enjoy.

Nutrition Facts Per Serving

Calories 83, Total Fat 3g, Saturated Fat 0.5g, Total Carbs 14g, Net Carbs 12g, Protein 2g, Sugar: 1g, Fiber 2g, Sodium 8mg, Potassium 211mg

428. CAULIFLOWER HASH BROWN

Preparation Time: 10 minutes
Cooking Time: 20 minutes
Serving: 6

Ingredients:

- 4 eggs, beaten
- ½ cup coconut milk
- ½ teaspoon dry mustard
- Salt and pepper to taste
- 1 large head cauliflower, shredded

Directions:

1. Place all ingredients in a mixing bowl and mix until well combined.
2. Place a nonstick frypan and heat over medium flame.
3. Add a large dollop of cauliflower mixture in the skillet.
4. Fry one side for 3 minutes, flip and cook the other side for a minute, like a pancake. Repeat process to remaining ingredients.
5. Serve and enjoy.

Nutrition Facts Per Serving

Calories 102, Total Fat 8g, Saturated Fat 1g, Total Carbs 4g, Net Carbs 3g, Protein 5g, Sugar: 2g, Fiber 1g, Sodium 63mg, Potassium 251mg

429. SWEET POTATO PUREE

Preparation Time: 10 minutes
Cooking Time: 15 minutes
Serving: 6

Ingredients:

- 2 pounds sweet potatoes, peeled
- 1 ½ cups water
- 5 Medjool dates, pitted and chopped

Directions:

1. Place water and potatoes in a pot.
2. Close the lid and allow to boil for 15 minutes until the potatoes are soft.
3. Drain the potatoes and place in a food processor together with the dates.
4. Pulse until smooth.
5. Serve and enjoy.

Nutrition Facts Per Serving

Calories 172, Total Fat 0.2g, Saturated Fat 0g, Total Carbs 41g, Net Carbs 36g, Protein 3g, Sugar: 14g, Fiber 5g, Sodium 10mg, Potassium 776mg

430. CURRIED OKRA

Preparation Time: 10 minutes
Cooking Time: 12 minutes
Serving: 4

Ingredients:

- 1 lb. small to medium okra pods, trimmed
- ¼ tsp curry powder
- ½ tsp kosher salt
- 1 tsp finely chopped serrano chile
- 1 tsp ground coriander
- 1 tbsp canola oil
- ¾ tsp brown mustard seeds

Directions:

1. On medium high fire, place a large and heavy skillet and cook mustard seeds until fragrant, around 30 seconds.
2. Add canola oil. Add okra, curry powder, salt, chile, and coriander. Sauté for a minute while stirring every once in a while.
3. Cover and cook low fire for at least 8 minutes. Stir occasionally.
4. Uncover, increase fire to medium high and cook until okra is lightly browned, around 2 minutes more.
5. Serve and enjoy.

Nutrition Facts Per Serving

Calories 78, Total Fat 6g, Saturated Fat 0.7g, Total Carbs 6g, Net Carbs 3g, Protein 2g, Sugar: 3g, Fiber 3g, Sodium 553mg, Potassium 187mg

431. ZUCCHINI PASTA WITH MANGO-KIWI SAUCE

Preparation Time: 10 minutes
Cooking Time: 0 minutes
Serving: 2

Ingredients:

- 1 tsp dried herbs – optional
- ½ Cup Raw Kale leaves, shredded
- 2 small dried figs
- 3 medjool dates
- 4 medium kiwis
- 2 big mangos, peeled and seed discarded
- 2 cup zucchini, spiralized
- ¼ cup roasted cashew

Directions:

1. On a salad bowl, place kale then topped with zucchini noodles and sprinkle with dried herbs. Set aside.
2. In a food processor, grind to a powder the cashews. Add figs, dates, kiwis and mangoes then puree to a smooth consistency.
3. Pour over zucchini pasta, serve and enjoy.

Nutrition Facts Per Serving

Calories 370, Total Fat 9g, Saturated Fat 2g, Total Carbs 76g, Net Carbs 67g, Protein 6g, Sugar: 62g, Fiber 9g, Sodium 8mg, Potassium 868mg

432. RATATOUILLE

Preparation Time: 10 minutes
Cooking Time: 25 minutes
Serving: 4

Ingredients:

- freshly ground black pepper
- ½ cup shredded fresh basil leaves
- 1 tsp salt
- 4 plum tomatoes, coarsely chopped
- 1 red bell pepper, julienned
- 1 small zucchini, spiralized
- 1 small eggplant, spiralized
- 1 small bay leaf
- 4 garlic cloves, peeled and minced
- 1 onion, sliced thinly
- 1 tbsp olive oil

Directions:

1. Place a large nonstick saucepan on medium slow fire and heat oil.
2. Add bay leaf, garlic and onion. Sauté until onions are translucent and soft.
3. Add eggplant and cook for 7 minutes while occasionally stirring.
4. Add salt, tomatoes, red bell pepper and zucchini then increase fire to medium high. Continue cooking until veggies are tender around 5 to 7 minutes.
5. Turn off fire and add pepper and basil. Stir to mix.
6. Serve and enjoy.

Nutrition Facts Per Serving

Calories 116, Total Fat 4g, Saturated Fat 0.5g, Total Carbs 21g, Net Carbs 16g, Protein 2g, Sugar: 16g, Fiber 5g, Sodium 595mg, Potassium 421mg

433. ROASTED EGGPLANT WITH FETA DIP

Preparation Time: 10 minutes
Cooking Time: 30 minutes
Serving: 6

Ingredients:

- Pinch of sugar
- ¼ tsp salt
- ¼ tsp cayenne pepper or to taste
- 1 tbsp parsley, flat leaf and chopped finely
- 2 tbsp fresh basil, chopped
- 1 small chili pepper, seeded and minced, optional
- ½ cup red onion, finely chopped
- ½ cup Greek feta cheese, crumbled
- ¼ cup extra virgin olive oil
- 2 tbsp lemon juice
- 1 medium eggplant, around 1 lb.

Directions:

1. Preheat broiler and position rack 6 inches away from heat source.
2. Pierce the eggplant with a knife or fork. Then with a foil, line a baking pan and place the eggplant and broil. Make sure to turn eggplant every five minutes or until the skin is charred and eggplant is soft

which takes around 14 to 18 minutes of broiling. Once done, remove from heat and let cool.

3. In a medium bowl, add lemon. Then cut eggplant in half, lengthwise, and scrape the flesh and place in the bowl with lemon. Add oil and mix until well combined. Then add salt, cayenne, parsley, basil, chili pepper, bell pepper, onion and feta. Toss until well combined and add sugar to taste if wanted.

Nutrition Facts Per Serving

Calories 139, Total Fat 12g, Saturated Fat 3g, Total Carbs 7g, Net Carbs 4g, Protein 3g, Sugar: 4g, Fiber 3g, Sodium 178mg, Potassium 249mg

434. VEGETABLE POTPIE

Preparation Time: 10 minutes
Cooking Time: 10 minutes
Serving: 8

Ingredients:

- 1 recipe pastry for double crust pie
- 2 tbsp cornstarch
- 1 tsp ground black pepper
- 1 tsp kosher salt
- 3 cups vegetable broth
- 1 cup fresh green beans, trimmed and snapped into ½ inch pieces
- 2 cups cauliflower florets
- 2 stalks celery, sliced ¼ inch wide
- 2 potatoes, peeled and diced
- 2 large carrots, diced
- 1 clove garlic, minced
- 8 oz mushroom
- 1 onion, chopped
- 2 tbsp olive oil

Directions:

1. In a large saucepan, sauté garlic in oil until lightly browned, add onions and continue sautéing until soft and translucent.
2. Add celery, potatoes and carrots and sauté for 3 minutes.
3. Add vegetable broth, green beans and cauliflower and bring to a boil. Slow fire and simmer until vegetables are slightly tender. Season with pepper and salt.
4. Mix ¼ cup water and cornstarch in a small bowl. Stir until mixture is smooth and has no lumps. Then pour into the vegetable pot while mixing constantly.
5. Continue mixing until soup thickens, around 3 minutes. Remove from fire.
6. Meanwhile, roll out pastry dough and place on an oven safe 11x7 baking dish. Pour the vegetable filling and then cover with another pastry dough. Seal and flute thee edges of the dough and prick the top dough with fork on several places.
7. Bake the dish in a preheated oven of 425oF for 30 minutes or until crust has turned a golden brown.

Nutrition Facts Per Serving

Calories 202, Total Fat 10g, Saturated Fat 2g, Total Carbs 26g, Net Carbs 23g, Protein 4g, Sugar: 3g, Fiber 3g, Sodium 466mg, Potassium 483mg

435. MARSALA ROASTED CARROTS

Preparation Time: 10 minutes
Cooking Time: 40 minutes
Serving: 8

Ingredients:

- Chopped fresh parsley – optional
- Pepper and salt to taste
- 2 tbsp balsamic vinegar
- 2 tbsp extra virgin olive oil
- ½ cup marsala
- 2 lbs. julienned carrots

Directions:

1. Peel and julienne carrots.
2. Place carrots on baking sheet.
3. Add vinegar, olive oil and marsala. Toss to coat.
4. Roast carrots in oven for 30 minutes at 425oF, while occasionally stirring.
5. Carrots are cooked once tender and lightly browned. Remove from oven and season with pepper, salt and fresh parsley.

Nutrition Facts Per Serving

Calories 62, Total Fat 2g, Saturated Fat 0.2g, Total Carbs 11g, Net Carbs 7g, Protein 1g, Sugar: 5g,

Fiber 4g, Sodium 101mg, Potassium 333mg

436. CAJUN ASPARAGUS

Preparation Time: 10 minutes
Cooking Time: 10 minutes
Serving: 3

Ingredients:

- 1 teaspoon Cajun seasoning
- 1-pound asparagus
- 1 tsp Olive oil

Directions:

1. Snap the asparagus and make sure that you use the tender part of the vegetable.
2. Place a large skillet on stovetop and heat on high for a minute.
3. Then grease skillet with cooking spray and spread asparagus in one layer.
4. Cover skillet and continue cooking on high for 5 to eight minutes.
5. Halfway through cooking time, stir skillet and then cover and continue to cook.
6. Once done cooking, transfer to plates, serve, and enjoy!

Nutrition Facts Per Serving

Calories 47, Total Fat 2g, Saturated Fat 0.2g, Total Carbs 6g, Net Carbs 3g, Protein 3g, Sugar: 3g, Fiber 3g, Sodium 73mg, Potassium 315mg

437. BEEF STROGANOFF SOUP

Hands-on: 20 minutes
Cooking time: 40 minutes
Servings: 6

Ingredients:

- 2 large beef rump (sirloin) steaks (800 g/ 1.76 lbs.)
- 600 g brown or white mushrooms (1.3 lbs.)
- ¼ cup of ghee or lard (55 g/ 1.9 oz.)
- 2 cloves garlic, minced
- 1 medium white or brown onion, chopped (110 g/ 3.9 oz.)
- 5 cups bone broth or chicken stock or vegetable stock (1.2 l/ quart)
- 2 teaspoons of paprika
- 1 tablespoon of Dijon mustard you can make your own
- Juice from 1 lemon (~ 4 tbsp.)
- 1½ cup sour cream or heavy whipping cream (345 g/ 12.2 oz.) - you can use paleo-friendly coconut cream
- ¼ cup of freshly chopped parsley
- 1 teaspoon of salt
- ¼ teaspoon of freshly ground black pepper
- Optionally, you can use a thickener: 1 tablespoon of ground chia seeds (+ 0.1 g net carbs per serving) or arrowroot powder (+ 1.2 g net carbs per serving) mixed in ¼ cup of water or use cream & egg yolk mixture like I did in my Pork & Kohlrabi Stew.

Directions:

1. Lay the steaks in the freezer in a single layer for 30 to 45 minutes. This will make it easy to slice the steaks into thin strips. Meanwhile, clean and slice the mushrooms. When the steaks are ready, use a sharp knife and slice them as thin as you can. Season with some salt and pepper.Grease a large heavy bottom pan with half of the ghee and heat. Then, add the beef slices in a single layer. Do not overcrowd the pan. Fry over a medium-high heat until it's cooked through and browned from all sides. Remove the slices from the pan and place in a bowl. Set aside for later. Do the same for the remaining slices. Grease the pan with the remaining ghee. Add in the chopped onion and minced garlic in the pan and cook until lightly browned and fragrant.Add the sliced mushrooms and cook for 3 to 4 more minutes while stirring occasionally. Then add your Dijon mustard, paprika, and pour in the bone broth. Add lemon juice and boil for 2 to 3 minutes. Add the browned beef slices and sour cream. Remove from heat. If you are using a thickener, add it to the pot and stir well. Finally, add freshly chopped parsley. 1 Eat hot with a slice of toasted Keto Bread or let it cool down and store in the fridge for up to 5 days. Enjoy!

Nutrition:

Calories from carbs; 7%, protein; 27%, fat; 66%. Total carbs; 10.8 grams, Fibre 1.4 grams, Sugars 4.8 grams, Saturated fat; 18.4 grams, Sodium; 783 mg (34% RDA), Magnesium; 152 mg (38% RDA), Potassium; 1,398 mg (70% EMR).

438. BUFFALO RANCH CHICKEN SOUP

Preparation time: 20 minutes
Cooking time: 30 minutes

Ingredients:

- 4 cups of Boneless Skinless Chicken Breast
- 2 tablespoons of (I added more to mine, but made it very mild for the family)
- 4 tablespoons of Ranch Dressing
- 2 Celery Stalks (chopped of sliced)
- ¼ cup of Yellow Onion (chopped)
- 6 tablespoons of Butter (salted)
- 8 ounces of Cream Cheese

- 1 cup of Heavy Whipping Cream
- 8 cups of Chicken Broth
- 7 slices of Hearty Bacon

Directions:

1. First, cook and shred chicken by coating the bottom of a deep-frying pan with olive oil on medium heat. Then place the chicken in pan and cook for 5 minutes. Flip to the other side and add ¾ cup of water. Cover and cook for 7 to 10 minutes (add little drops of water occasionally). Shred after cooling.Cook and crumble bacon. I always precook bacon to make cooking a little easier.While waiting add all ingredients to a saucepan and cook on medium. When chicken and bacon are properly cooked add to the sauce pan and cover. Allow to cook for 5 to 10 minutes before serving. Enjoy.

Nutrition:

Calories: 444, Total Fat: 34g, Cholesterol: 133mg, Sodium: 1572mg, Potassium: 3mg, Carbohydrates: 4g, Dietary Fibre = 1g, Net Carbs= 3g, Dietary Fibre 1g, Sugars: 2g (all from natural sources), Protein: 28g

439. CHICKEN STEW

Preparation time: 5 minutes
Cooking time: 2 hours
Gross time: 2 hours 5 minutes
Servings: 4

Ingredients:

- 2 cups of chicken stock
- 2 medium carrots (½ cup), peeled and finely diced
- 2 celery sticks (1 cup), diced
- ½ onion (½ cup), diced
- 28 ounces skinless and deboned chicken thighs diced into 1" pieces
- 1 spring fresh rosemary or ½ teaspoon dried rosemary
- 3 garlic cloves, minced
- ¼ teaspoon of dried thyme
- ½ teaspoon of dried oregano
- 1 c. fresh spinach
- ½ cup of heavy cream
- salt and pepper, to taste
- xantham gum, to desired thickness starting at ⅛ teaspoon

Directions:

1. In a 3-quart crockpot, place the chicken stock, carrots, celery, onion, chicken thighs, rosemary, garlic, thyme, and oregano. Cook on low for 4 hours or on high for 2 hours. Add salt and pepper, to taste. Stir in spinach and the heavy cream.Sprinkle and thicken with xantham gum to desired thickness starting at ⅛ teaspoon. Continue to whisk until mix and cook for another 10 minutes.Serve and enjoy.

Nutrition:

Calories: 228 Fat: 11 Carbohydrates: 6 Protein: 23

440. CHICKEN FAJITA SOUP

Servings: 8 serves
Preparation time: 10 minutes
Cooking time: 6 hours 30 minutes
Total time: 6 hours 40 minutes

Ingredients:

- 2 pounds of boneless skinless chicken breasts
- 1 cup of chicken broth this is to pour over chicken in slow cooker
- 1 onion chopped
- 1 green pepper chopped
- 3 garlic cloves minced
- 1 tablespoon of butter
- 6 ounces of cream cheese
- 2 10 ounces of cans diced tomatoes with green chilis
- 2½ cups of chicken broth
- ½ cup of heavy whipping cream
- 2½ tablespoons of homemade taco seasoning recipe here or 1 packet of taco seasoning
- salt and pepper to taste

Directions:

1. Add boneless skinless chicken breasts to a slow cooker and cook for 3 hours on high or 6 hours on low in a cup of chicken

broth. Season with salt and pepper.When the chicken is done, remove from slow cooker and shred. (You can strain the leftover broth for the soup.)In a large saucepan fry green pepper, onion, and garlic in 1 tablespoon of butter until they are translucent (2 to 3 minutes).Mash the cream cheese into the veggies with a spoon so that it will combine smoothly as it melts.Add the canned tomatoes, chicken broth, heavy whipping cream, and taco seasoning.Cook on low uncovered for 20 minutes. Add chicken, cover and cook for 10 minutes.Add salt and pepper to taste. Serve and enjoy!

Nutrition:

Calories: 306kcal, Carbohydrates: 8.2g, Protein: 26g, Fat: 17g, Saturated Fat: 9g, Cholesterol: 120mg, Sodium: 880mg, Potassium: 757mg, Fibre: 1.6g, Sugar: 3g, Vitamin A: 12.7%, Vitamin C: 26.5%, Calcium: 4.9%, Iron: 4.4%.

441. ITALIAN WEDDING SOUP

Preparation time: 15 minutes
Cooking time: 25 minutes
Servings: 6 serves

Ingredients:

Meatballs:

- 1 pound of ground beef OR ground pork
- ½ cup of crushed pork rinds OR almond flour
- ½ cup of grated Parmesan cheese
- 1 teaspoon of Italian seasoning
- ¾ teaspoon of salt
- ½ teaspoon of pepper
- 1 large egg

Soup:

- 2 tablespoons of avocado oil
- ¼ cup of chopped onion
- 4 celery stalks chopped
- 1 teaspoon of salt
- ½ teaspoon of pepper
- 3 cloves garlic minced
- 1 teaspoon of dried oregano
- 6 cups of chicken broth
- 2 cups of riced cauliflower
- 2 cups of packed spinach leaves
- Additional salt and pepper
- Parmesan for sprinkling

Directions:

1. Mix together the ground meat, crushed pork rinds, cheese, Italian seasoning, salt, and pepper in a large mixing bowl. Add the egg and mix well using your hands. Form into ½ inch meatballs and place on a waxed paper-lined tray. Refrigerate until soup is ready.Heat the oil over medium heat until shimmering in a large saucepan or stock pot. Add the onion, celery, salt, and pepper and fry until vegetables are soft and tender (7 minutes). Add the garlic and cook for 1 minute.Stir in the chicken broth and oregano and simmer for 10 minutes. Add the cauliflower rice and the meatballs and cook for about 5 minutes.Add the spinach leaves and cook until wilted, 2 minutes more. Season to taste.Serve and enjoy.

Nutrition:

Food energy: 303kcal, Total fat: 20.16g, Calories from fat: 181, Cholesterol: 73mg, Carbohydrate: 5.73g, Total dietary fibre: 1.86g, Protein: 29.48g.

442. CREAM OF CHICKEN SOUP

Preparation time: 10 minutes
Cooking time: 20 minutes
Servings: 2

Ingredients:

- 2 cups (500 grams) of cauliflower florets
- 2/3 cup (157 mL) of unsweetened original almond milk
- 1 cup (250 mL) of chicken broth
- 1 teaspoon (5 mL) of onion powder
- ½ teaspoon (2.5 mL) of grey sea salt
- ¼ teaspoon (1.23 mL) of garlic powder
- ¼ teaspoon (1.23 mL) of freshly ground black pepper
- 1/8 teaspoon (0.61 mL) of celery seed (optional)
- 1/8 teaspoon (0.61 mL) of dried thyme
- ¼ cup (30 grams) of Beef Gelatin
- ¼ cup (54 grams) of finely diced cooked

chicken thighs

Directions:

1. Place all ingredients but cook chicken and gelatin in a small saucepan. Cover and bring to a boil over medium heat. Turn heat to low and cook for about 7 to 8 minutes, until cauliflower is softened. Remove from the heat. Add ½ cup or so of the hot liquid to a medium-sized bowl using a ladle. Add gelatin, one scoop at a time. Stir until dissolved, then add the next scoop.Transfer the cauliflower mixture and gelatin mixture to your food processor, immersion blender or high-powered blender. Blend until totally smooth.Add cauliflower and gelatin mixture back to saucepan. Add cooked chicken to cauliflower and gelatin mixture. Cover and heat on low for 2 to 5 minutes, until it thickens.Serve immediately. Enjoy friend.

Nutrition:

Calories: 198, Calories from Fat: 62.1, Total Fat: 6.9 g Saturated Fat: 1.1 g, Cholesterol: 24 mg, Sodium: 672 mg, Carbs: 9.4 g, Dietary Fibre: 3.8 g, Net Carbs: 5.6 g, Sugars: 3.3 g, Protein: 26.4 g,

443. COFFEE AND WINE BEEF STEW

Servings: 6
Preparation time: 20 minutes
Cooking time: 3 hours 20 minutes
Total time: 3 hours 40 minutes

Ingredients:

- Pounds Stew Meat
- 3 c. Coffee
- 1 c. Beef Stock
- 1½ c. Mushrooms (Baby Bella)
- 2/3 c. Red Wine (Merlot)
- 1 Medium Onion
- 3 tbsp. Coconut Oil
- 2 tbsp. Capers
- 2 tsp. Garlic
- 1 tsp. Salt
- 1 tsp. Pepper

Directions:

1. Cube all stew meat, then thinly slice onions and mushrooms. Bring 3 tablespoons of coconut oil and heat in a pan on the stove.Season beef with salt and pepper, then brown all of it in small batches. Ensure you don't overcrowd the pan.Once all meat is browned, cook onions, mushrooms, and garlic in the remaining fat in the pan. Do this until onions are translucent.Then mix together coffee, beef stock, red wine, and capers to the vegetables. Stir mixture well.Add beef into the mixture, bring to a boil then reduce heat to low.Cover and cook for 3 hours. Serve and enjoy.

Nutrition:

504 Calories, 32.2g Fats, 2.7g Net Carbs, and 42.5g Protein.

444. GREEN CHICKEN ENCHILADA SOUP

Servings: 4
Preparation time: 10 minutes
Cooking time: 5 minutes

Ingredients:

- ½ cup of salsa Verde (see example)
- 4 ounces of cream cheese, softened
- 1 cup of sharp cheddar cheese, shredded
- 2 cups of bone broth or chicken stock
- 2 cups of cooked chicken, shredded

Directions:

1. Add the salsa, cream cheese, cheddar cheese and chicken stock in a blender and blend until smooth. Pour into a medium saucepan and cook on medium until hot. Add the shredded chicken and cook an additional 3 to 5 minutes until heated through.Garnish with additional shredded cheddar and chopped cilantro if desired. Enjoy.

NUTRITION:

Serving Size: 1.5 cups, Calories: 346, Fat: 22gCarbohydrates: 3g net, Protein: 32g.

445. BEEF STEW

Preparation time: 10 minutes

Cooking time: 1 hour
Total time: 1 hour 10 minutes
Servings: 4

Ingredients:

- 1 pound of Beef Short Rib
- 2 cups of beef broth
- 4 cloves minced garlic
- 100-gram Onion
- 100-gram carrot
- 100-gram radishes
- ¼ teaspoon of Pink Himalayan Salt
- ¼ teaspoon of pepper
- ½ teaspoon of xanthan Gum
- 1 tablespoon of Butter
- 1 tablespoon of coconut oil

Directions:

1. Cut the short rib into bite sized chunks, salt and pepper and set aside.At medium-high heat, heat a large saucepan and add coconut oil. Then add short rib and brown on all side. Remove from saucepan and set aside.Chop onions, carrots and radishes into bite sized pieces and mince garlic. Add onions, garlic and butter and cook down for a couple minutes.Once the onions are soft, add the broth and combine. Add the xanthan gum and mix.Allow broth mixture to come to boil and then transfer the meat back in and cook covered for 30 minutes. Stir frequently scrapping the bottom as you stir,After 30 minutes add the carrots and radishes and cook for 30 minutes, stirring frequently until it thickens. If you feel the need you can add more broth or some water. Serve warm and enjoy!

NUTRITION:

Calories: 432.25kcal, Carbohydrates: 5.5g, Protein: 19.25g, Fat: 36.5g, Fibre: 1.5g.

446. BACON CHEESEBURGER SOUP

Cooking time: 40 minutes
Preparation time: 20 minutes

Ingredients:

- 5 slices Bacon
- 12 ounces of Ground Beef (80/20)
- 2 tablespoons of Butter
- 3 cups of Beef Broth
- ½ teaspoon of Garlic Powder
- ½ teaspoon of Onion Powder
- 2 teaspoons of Brown Mustard
- 1½ teaspoon of Kosher Salt
- ½ teaspoon of Black Pepper
- ½ teaspoon of Red Pepper Flakes
- 1 teaspoon of Cumin
- 1 teaspoon of Chili Powder
- 2½ tablespoons of Tomato Paste
- 1 medium Dill Pickle, diced
- 1 cup of Shredded Cheddar Cheese
- 3 ounces of Cream Cheese
- ½ cup of Heavy Cream

Directions:

1. Start with cooking the bacon in a pan until crispy, then set aside.Add ground beef in the bacon fat and cook until browned on one side, flip and cook other side until brown.Place beef in a pot, and move it to the sides. Add butter and spices to the pan and let the spices sweat for 30 to 45 seconds.Then add beef broth, tomato paste, mustard, cheese, and pickles to the pot and let cook for a few minutes until it melts.Cover pot and turn to low heat. Cook for another 20 to 30 minutes. Turn stove off, then finish with heavy cream and crumbled bacon. Stir well and serve. Enjoy.

Nutrition:

Calories, 48.6g Fats, 3.4g Net Carbs, and 23.4g Protein.

447. ROASTED GARLIC SOUP

Preparation time: 10 minutes
Cooking time: 55 minutes
Servings: 6

Ingredients:

- 2 bulbs of garlic
- 1 tablespoon extra-virgin olive oil, divided
- 3 shallots, chopped

- 1 large head of cauliflower, chopped (approximately 5 cups)
- 6 cups of gluten-free vegetable broth
- ¾ teaspoon of sea salt
- Freshly ground pepper, to taste

Directions:

1. First heat oven to 400F. Peel the outer layers of the garlic bulb. Cut off about ¼-inch from the top of the bulb. Place in on a square of aluminium foil and coat each with ½ teaspoon of olive oil. Heat in the oven for 35 minutes.Once complete, allow to cool slightly before removing from aluminium foil and squeezing out the garlic from each clove.Meanwhile, pour remaining olive oil in a medium-sized saucepan. Turn heat to medium-high and add chopped shallots. Fry until tender for about 6 minutes.In the saucepan, add the roasted garlic along with remaining ingredients. Cover and bring to a boil. Bring down the heat to low and cook for 15 to 20 minutes until the cauliflower is tender.Drop mixture into the bowl of your blender. Puree until smooth, about 30 seconds. Adjust with salt and pepper and serve. Enjoy.

448. FAT BOMB HAMBURGER SOUP

Preparation time: 30 minutes
Cooking time: 60 minutes
Total time: 1 hour 30 minutes
Servings: 6

Ingredients:

- 125-grams red onion, sliced (approx. ½ onion)
- 125-grams mushrooms, chopped (approx. 10 count)
- 200-grams yellow bell pepper, sliced (approx. 1 count)
- 200 grams Brussels sprouts, halved (approx. 20 count)
- ¼ cup of red palm oil, melted
- Himalayan rock salt, to taste
- Freshly ground pepper, to taste
- 1 pound of grass-fed regular ground beef
- 3 cloves garlic, minced
- 200-grams celery (approx. 6 sticks)
- 4 cups of homemade beef stock, with the fat
- 2 cups of organic whole tomatoes
- 1 tablespoon of organic tomato paste
- 1 bay leaf
- 1 teaspoon of dried oregano
- pinch cayenne pepper or ½ teaspoon chili powder
- 25-grams (¼ cup) fresh parsley, chopped

Cooking Instruction:

1. Preheat your oven to 350F. On a large baking sheet, place onions, mushrooms, bell pepper, Brussels sprouts, palm oil, salt and pepper. Place sheet to the oven and roast vegetables for 25 to 30 minutes. Once complete, remove and set aside.In a large soup pot, add ground beef and cook on medium-low heat until just cooked through. Then add garlic and celery, cook for another 3 minutes. Do not drain the fat, keep it in there.Add stock, tomatoes, paste and spices. Bring to a boil, reduce heat to low and simmer for 15 to 20 minutes.Stir in roasted vegetables and chopped parsley. Serve with a slice of Flax Focaccia. Enjoy.

449. MULLIGATAWNY

Preparation time: 10 minutes
Cooking time: 30 minutes
Servings: 10

Ingredients:

- 10 cups turkey or chicken broth
- 1½ tablespoon of curry powder
- 5 cups of chopped turkey or chicken, cooked
- 3 cups of celery root, riced or chopped finely
- ¼ cup of apple cider or juice
- 2 tablespoons of Swerve sweetener
- ½ cup of sour cream
- ¼ cup of fresh parsley, chopped
- Salt and pepper to taste

Directions:

1. In a large soup pot, add the broth, curry powder, turkey or chicken, celery root rice, and apple cider.Bring to a boil and simmer for about 25 to 30 minutes.Add the sweetener, sour cream, and fresh parsley and stir well.Taste and season with salt and pepper to taste.Serve hot. Enjoy friend.

Nutrition

Information per serving: 214 calories, 4g fat, 4g net carbs, 36g protein.

450. CHICKEN "NOODLE" SOUP

Preparation time: 10 minutes
Cooking time: 15 minutes
Total time: 25 minutes
Servings: 4 Serves

Ingredients:

- 2 tablespoons coconut oil
- 1 pound (453 grams) boneless, skinless chicken thighs
- 1 cup of diced celery* see note
- 1 cup diced carrots
- ¾ cup (approx. 6) chopped green onion, green part only
- 6 cups of chicken stock
- ½ teaspoon of dried basil
- ½ teaspoon of dried oregano
- 1 teaspoon of grey sea salt
- ⅛ teaspoon fresh ground pepper
- 2 cups (300 grams) of spiralized daikon noodles* see note

Directions:

1. To make on a stove top: In a large saucepan, add coconut oil and chicken thighs. Cook on medium for 15 minutes, until chicken is just about cooked through. Then shred with a fork. Add your celery, carrots and onions and cook for another 5 minutes. Add remaining ingredients. Cover and bring to a boil. Reduce heat and simmer for 20 to 25 minutes. Once complete, add daikon noodles and serve. Enjoy.

451. BROCCOLI CHEDDAR SOUP

Cooking Time: 20 minutes
Preparation time: 10 minutes
Servings: 4; ¾ Cup per Serving

Ingredients:

- 2 tbsp. Butter
- 1/ 8 c. White Onion
- ½ teaspoon Garlic, finely minced
- 2 c. Chicken Broth
- Salt and Pepper, to taste
- 1 c. Broccoli, chopped into bite size pieces
- 1 tbsp. Cream Cheese
- ¼ c. Heavy Whipping Cream
- 1 c. Cheddar Cheese; shredded
- 2 Slices Bacon; Cooked and Crumbled (Optional)
- ½ teaspoon xanthan gum (optional, for thickening)

Directions:

1. Sauté onion and garlic with butter in large pot over medium heat until onions are tender and translucent.Add broth and broccoli to pot. Cook broccoli until softened. Add salt, pepper and desired seasoning as necessary.In a small bowl, place cream cheese and heat in microwave for 30 seconds until soft and easily stirred.Stir heavy whipping cream and cream cheese into soup; bring to a boil.Remove from heat and quickly stir in cheddar cheese.Stir in xanthan gum, if desired. Allow to thicken.Serve hot with bacon crumbles. Enjoy.

452. FRENCH ONION SOUP

Preparation time: 10 minutes
Cooking time: 40 minutes
Servings: 6

Ingredients:

- 5 tablespoons of Butter
- 500 g Brown Onion Medium
- 2 teaspoons of Natvia (Or Erythritol) 4 drops stevia, or erythritol
- 4 tablespoons of olive oil
- 3 cups of Beef Stock

Directions:

2. Add butter and olive oil in a medium-large pot over medium low heat. Add onions and 1 teaspoon of Salt. Add chopped onions.Cook without lid, stirring often for 20 minutes or until onions are golden brown. Stir in the stevia and cook for another 5 minutes.Add the stock to the saucepan and cook. Turn to a low heat and simmer for 25 minutes.Ladle into soup bowls and serve. Enjoy

.Nutrition:

Keto French Onion Soup - Keto French Food Amount per Serving: Calories 212, Calories from Fat; 162% Daily Value*, Total Fat; 18g 14%, Total Carbohydrates; 5g 17%, Protein; 3g 3%.

453. CURRIED BEEF STEW

Preparation time: 10 minutes
Cooking time: 30 minutes
Servings: 4

Ingredients:

- pounds of stew beef meat
- 1 tablespoon of coconut oil
- ½ medium white onion, diced
- 3 teaspoons of minced garlic
- 2 teaspoons of curry powder
- 1 teaspoon of Cumin
- 1 teaspoon of Pink Himalayan Salt
- ½ teaspoon of chili powder
- 1 can coconut milk, refrigerated
- ½ cup of Water
- 4 ounces of cauliflower (optional)

Directions:

1. Freeze the can of coconut milk until ready to use in the recipe.Heat a large pan over medium-high heat and add ½ tablespoon of coconut oil. Once hot, add in the stew meat pieces and brown on all side.Remove from the pan and set aside in a bowl. Add the ½ tablespoon of coconut oil to hot pan and turn the heat to medium. Scrape up the bottom using a spatula. Add in the diced onion, and cook until translucent. Add in the garlic, curry powder, cumin, salt and chili powder. Mix using the spatula and cook until spices are fragrant.Place the stew meat back in and stir to combine. Remove the coconut milk from the freezer (should have been at least 10 minutes) and open can. Add the hardened coconut milk to the beef mixture and allow it to melt down. Add the water and stir until thoroughly combined. Cover the pan and allow to simmer for 20 minutes. If you are adding in the cauliflower, add it after 10 minutes have passed. Then replace with the lid and allow to cook remaining time. Remove the lid and either serve. Serve over cauliflower rice. Enjoy!

454. GREEN CHILE PORK STEW

Preparation time: 15 minutes
Cooking time: 1 hour 30 minutes
Total time: 1 hour 45 minutes
Servings: 8
Calories: 182kcal

Ingredients:

- 2 pounds of pork loin (cubed)
- 2 teaspoons ground cumin
- 2 teaspoons granulated garlic
- 1 teaspoon pure ground chili powder optional
- 2 ounces of onion (about ½ cup, chopped)
- 2 cloves garlic
- 1 can whole Hatch green chilies and liquid (27 ounces can)
- 3 tablespoons oil
- 2 cups water
- fried or poached eggs optional

Directions:

1. Heat oil in a big frying pan and brown the cubed pork loin.Chop the onion and garlic. Open the can of chilies and blend with the onion and garlic in a blender until the chilies resemble a thick chunky paste. Add the spices to the browned pork and give a nice stir until fragrant. Pour the pureed chilies, and their juice from the can, over the browned pork.Add the two cups of water, and the liquid from the can. Stir and reduce pan down from medium-

low to low heat.Cover the pan with the lid ajar and simmer for 1 to 1 ½. Add water occasionally. It will be very flavourful just by adding water.Adjust seasonings. Ladle into a bowl over cauliflower rice, over zoodles and top with a fried or poached egg (optional). Enjoy.

455. WONDERFUL MULTI-VEGGIE SOUP

Total time: 15 mins
Servings: 4

Ingredients:

- cups frozen mixed vegetables
- 1 cup chopped onion
- 2 tbsp minced ginger and garlic mixture
- 1 tsp oregano
- Salt and pepper

Directions:

1. Put all the ingredients in the instant pot and cover them with just enough water. Seal the pot and cook on Soup setting for 15 minutes.
2. When the cooking time is up, let the pressure release naturally and then open the lid. Stir the soup thoroughly and serve hot by adding some more seasoning.

456. HEALTHY KALE SOUP

Total time: 15 mins
Servings: 4

Ingredients:

  - cups frozen kale
- 1 cup chopped onion
- 2 tbsp minced ginger and garlic mixture
- 1 tsp oregano
- Salt and pepper

Directions:

1. Put all the ingredients in the instant pot and cover them with just enough water. Seal the pot and cook on Soup setting for 15 minutes.
2. When the cooking time is up, let the pressure release naturally and then open the lid. Use a hand blender to make the soup smooth and creamy. Stir the soup thoroughly once again and serve hot by adding some more seasoning.

457. DELICIOUS CARROT SOUP

Total time: 15 mins
Servings: 4

Ingredients:

- cups carrot cubes
- 1 tbsp minced ginger
- Salt and pepper

Directions:

1. Put all the ingredients in the instant pot and cover them with just enough water. Seal the pot and cook on Soup setting for 15 minutes.
2. When the cooking time is up, let the pressure release naturally and then open the lid. Use a hand blender to make the soup smooth and creamy. Stir the soup thoroughly once again and serve hot by adding some more seasoning.

458. MIND BLOWING PUMPKIN SOUP

Total time: 15 mins
Servings: 4

Ingredients:

- cups pumpkin cubes
- 1 tbsp minced ginger
- Salt and pepper

Directions:

1. Put all the ingredients in the instant pot and cover them with just enough water. Seal the pot and cook on Soup setting for 15 minutes.
2. When the cooking time is up, let the pressure release naturally and then open the lid. Use a hand blender to make the soup smooth and creamy. Stir the soup thoroughly once again and serve hot by adding some more seasoning.

459. HEALTHY CABBAGE SOUP

Total time: 15 mins
Servings: 4

Ingredients:

- cups shredded cabbage
- 1 tbsp minced ginger
- 1 tsp lemon juice
- ½ tsp hot sauce
- Salt and pepper

Directions:

1. Put all the ingredients in the instant pot and cover them with just enough water. Seal the pot and cook on Soup setting for 15 minutes.
2. When the cooking time is up, let the pressure release naturally and then open the lid. Use a hand blender to make the soup smooth and creamy. Stir the soup thoroughly once again and serve hot by adding some more seasoning.

460. BROCCOLI DELIGHT SOUP

Total time: 15 mins
Servings: 4

Ingredients:

- cups broccoli florets, cut into very small pieces
- 1 tbsp minced ginger
- 1 tsp lemon juice
- Salt and pepper

Directions:

1. Put all the ingredients in the instant pot and cover them with just enough water. Seal the pot and cook on Soup setting for 15 minutes.
2. When the cooking time is up, let the pressure release naturally and then open the lid. Stir the soup thoroughly once again and serve hot by adding some more seasoning.

461. CHICKEN & EGG DROP SOUP

Total time: 25 mins
Servings: 4

Ingredients:

- 1 large egg
- 1 cup chicken cubes
- 2 tbsp ginger and garlic, minced
- Salt and pepper
- 6 cups chicken broth

Directions:

1. Put all the ingredients in the instant pot cooker and lock the lid. Cook with Soup setting for 25 minutes and then let the pressure release naturally.
2. Beat the egg with one tablespoon water and season it with salt. Pour out one cup of soup from the instant pot into a bowl and add this beaten egg into the soup. Remember to stir the soup constantly. The egg will become set in a few minutes and will resemble water drops. Pour the egg-mixed soup into the instant pot and cook for another 5 minutes. The soup must be very runny.
3. Serve hot by seasoning with some more pepper and salt.

462.BEEF & EGG DROP DELIGHT

Total time: 25 mins
Servings: 4

Ingredients:

- 1 large egg
- 1 cup cooked beef, small cubes
- 2 tbsp ginger and garlic, minced
- Salt and pepper
- 5 cups beef broth

Directions:

1. Put all the ingredients in the instant pot cooker and lock the lid. Cook with Soup setting for 20 minutes and then let the pressure release naturally.
2. Beat the egg with one tablespoon water and season it with salt. Pour out one cup of soup from the instant pot into a bowl and add this beaten egg into the soup. Remember to stir the soup constantly. The egg will become set in a few minutes and will resemble water drops. Pour the egg-mixed soup into the instant pot and cook for another 5 minutes. The soup must be very runny.
3. Serve hot by seasoning with some more pepper and salt.

463. SUPER-CRAFTED EGG & VEGETABLE SOUP

Total time: 20 mins
Servings: 4

Ingredients:

- 1 large egg
- 1 cup mixed vegetables
- ½ cups chopped onion
- Salt and pepper
- 5 cups vegetable broth

Directions:

1. Put all the ingredients in the instant pot cooker and lock the lid. Cook with Soup setting for 10 minutes and then let the pressure release naturally.
2. Beat the egg with one tablespoon water and season it with salt. Pour out one cup of soup from the instant pot into a bowl and add this beaten egg into the soup. Remember to stir the soup constantly. The egg will become set in a few minutes and will resemble water drops. Pour the egg-mixed soup into the instant pot and cook for another 5 minutes. The soup must be very runny.
3. Serve hot by seasoning with some more pepper and salt.

464. BACON MASTER BLASTER

Total time: 25 mins
Servings: 4

Ingredients:

- 3 cups mixed vegetables
- 2 tbsp ginger and garlic, minced
- Salt and pepper
- 3 bacon slices
- 3 cups vegetable broth

Directions:

1. Put all the ingredients (except bacon) in the instant pot cooker and lock the lid. Cook with Soup setting for 20 minutes and then let the pressure release naturally.
2. Cook the bacon pieces in a skillet till they turn crispy. Let them cool down and then crumble them. Add the bacon into the soup and stir the soup thoroughly and cook for another 5 minutes without the lid to get the right consistency of the soup.
3. Serve hot by seasoning with some more pepper and salt.

465. BASIC QUINOA SOUP

Total time: 25 mins
Servings: 4

Ingredients:

- 1 cups mixed vegetables
- 1 cup quinoa
- Salt and pepper
- 3 cups vegetable broth

Directions:

1. Put all the ingredients in the instant pot cooker and lock the lid. Cook with Soup setting for 20 minutes and then let the pressure release naturally. Open the lid and let the soup simmer for another 5 minutes.
2. Serve hot by seasoning with some more pepper and salt.

466. MARVELLOUS BEANS SOUP

Total time: 25 mins
Servings: 4

Ingredients:

- 3 cups green beans, chopped
- 2 tbsp ginger, minced
- Salt and pepper
- 3 cups vegetable broth

Directions:

1. Put all the ingredients in the instant pot cooker and lock the lid. Cook with Soup setting for 20 minutes and then let the pressure release naturally.
2. Open the lid of the instant pot and simmer the soup for another 5 minutes without the lid to get the right consistency of the soup.
3. Serve hot by seasoning with some more pepper and salt.

467. TASTY SHRIMP SOUP

Total time: 25 mins

Servings: 4

Ingredients:

- 1 cup small shrimp, boiled
- 1 tbsp garlic, minced
- Salt and pepper
- 3 cups vegetable broth
- 1 tsp lemon juice

Directions:

1. Put all the ingredients in the instant pot cooker and lock the lid. Cook with Soup setting for 20 minutes and then let the pressure release naturally.
2. Open the lid of the instant pot and simmer the soup for another 5 minutes without the lid to get the right consistency of the soup.
3. Serve hot by seasoning with some more pepper and salt.

468. ROASTED PEPPER SOUP

Total time: 15 mins
Servings: 4

Ingredients:

- 2 roasted red bell pepper, chopped
- 1 tbsp ginger, minced
- Salt and pepper
- 3 cups vegetable broth
- 1 tsp hot sauce

Directions:

1. Put all the ingredients in the instant pot cooker and lock the lid. Cook with Soup setting for 10 minutes and then let the pressure release naturally.
2. Open the lid of the instant pot and simmer the soup for another 5 minutes. Use a hand blender to make smooth soup.
3. Serve hot by seasoning with some more pepper and salt.

469. HERB FLAVORED POTATO SOUP

Total time: 20 mins
Servings: 4

Ingredients:

- 3 medium potatoes
- 2 tbsp ginger, minced
- Salt and pepper
- 3 cups vegetable broth
- 2 tbsp rosemary, chopped

Directions:

1. Put all the ingredients in the instant pot cooker and lock the lid. Cook with Soup setting for 15 minutes and then let the pressure release naturally.
2. Open the lid of the instant pot and simmer the soup for another 5 minutes. Use a hand blender to make the soup smooth.
3. Serve hot by seasoning with some more pepper and salt.

470. CREAMY CARROT SOUP

Total time: 25 mins
Servings: 4

Ingredients:

- 3 diced carrots
- 2 tbsp ginger, minced
- Salt and pepper
- 3 cups vegetable broth
- ½ cup heavy cream

Directions:

1. Put all the ingredients (except heavy cream) in the instant pot cooker and lock the lid. Cook with Soup setting for 20 minutes and then let the pressure release naturally.
2. Open the lid of the instant pot and simmer the soup for another 5 minutes. Use a hand blender to make the soup smooth. Now, remove from heat and add the heavy cream.
3. Serve hot by seasoning with some more pepper and salt.

471. ROASTED PORK SOUP

Total time: 25 mins
Servings: 4

Ingredients:

- 3 cups mixed vegetables

- 2 tbsp ginger and garlic, minced
- Salt and pepper
- 1 cup roasted pork cubes
- 3 cups vegetable broth

Directions:

1. Put all the ingredients (except pork) in the instant pot cooker and lock the lid. Cook with Soup setting for 10 minutes and then let the pressure release naturally.
2. Now, add the roasted pork cubes and stir the soup thoroughly and cook for another 5 minutes without the lid to get the right consistency of the soup.
3. Serve hot by seasoning with some more pepper and salt.

SAUCE RECIPES

472. EASY GARLICKY CHERRY TOMATO SAUCE

Preparation Time: 5 minutes
Cooking Time: 25 minutes
Serving: 4

Ingredients:

- ¼ cup extra virgin olive oil
- ¼ thinly sliced garlic cloves
- 2 pounds organic cherry tomatoes
- ½ teaspoon dried oregano
- 1 teaspoon coconut sugar
- ¼ cup chopped fresh basil
- 1 teaspoon salt

Directions:

1. Heat oil in a large saucepan over medium heat.
2. Sauté the garlic for a minute until fragrant.
3. Add in the cherry tomatoes and season with salt, oregano, coconut sugar, and fresh basil.
4. Allow to simmer for 25 minutes until the tomatoes are soft and becomes a thick sauce.
5. Place in containers and store in the fridge until ready to use.

Nutrition Facts Per Serving

Calories 198, Total Fat 6g, Saturated Fat 0.8g, Total Carbs 37g, Net Carbs 32g, Protein 3g, Sugar: 30g, Fiber: 5g, Sodium: 116mg, Potassium 514mg

473. AVOCADO CILANTRO DETOX DRESSING

Preparation Time: 5 minutes
Cooking Time: 0 minutes
Serving: 3

Ingredients:

- 5 tablespoons lemon juice, freshly squeezed
- 1 clove of garlic, chopped
- 1 avocado, pitted and flesh scooped out
- 1 bunch cilantro, chopped
- ¼ teaspoon salt
- ¼ cup water

Directions:

1. Place all ingredients in a food processor and pulse until well combined.
2. Pulse until creamy.
3. Place in a lidded container and store in the fridge until ready to use.
4. Use on salads and sandwiches.

Nutrition Facts Per Serving

Calories 114, Total Fat 10g, Saturated Fat 1g, Total Carbs 8g, Net Carbs 3g, Protein 2g, Sugar: 2g, Fiber:5 g, Sodium: 5mg, Potassium 355mg

474. GOLDEN TURMERIC SAUCE

Prep time:10 minutes
Cooking Time: 15 minutes
Serving: 4

Ingredients:

- 2 tablespoons coconut oil
- 1 onion, chopped
- 2-inch piece ginger, peeled and minced
- 2 cloves of garlic, minced
- 2 cups white sweet potato, cubed
- 2 tablespoons turmeric powder
- ½ teaspoon ginger powder
- ¼ teaspoon cinnamon powder
- 2 cups coconut milk
- Juice from 1 lemon, freshly squeezed
- 1 cup water
- 1 ½ teaspoon salt

Directions:

1. Heat oil in a saucepan over medium flame.
2. Sauté the onion, ginger, and garlic until fragrant.
3. Add in the sweet potatoes, turmeric powder, ginger powder, and cinnamon powder.
4. Pour in water and season with salt.
5. Bring to a boil for 10 minutes.
6. Once the potatoes are soft, place in a

blender pulse until smooth.
7. Return the mixture into the saucepan. Turn on the stove.
8. Add in the coconut milk and lemon juice.
9. Allow to simmer for 5 minutes.
10. Store in lidded containers and put inside the fridge until ready to use.

Nutrition Facts Per Serving

Calories 172, Total Fat 11g, Saturated Fat 2g, Total Carbs 15g, Net Carbs 12g, Protein 5g, Sugar: 8g, Fiber: 3g, Sodium: 36mg, Potassium 408mg

475. CREAMY TURMERIC DRESSING

Preparation Time: 5 minutes
Cooking Time: 0 minutes
Serving: 6

Ingredients:

- ½ cup tahini
- ½ cup olive oil
- 2 tablespoons lemon juice
- 2 teaspoons honey
- Salt to taste
- a dash of black pepper

Directions:

1. Mix all ingredients in a bowl until the mixture becomes creamy and smooth.
2. Store in lidded containers.
3. Put in the fridge until ready to use.

Nutrition Facts Per Serving

Calories 286, Total Fat 29g, Saturated Fat 4g, Total Carbs 7g, Net Carbs 5g, Protein 4g, Sugar: 2g, Fiber:2 g, Sodium: 24mg, Potassium 89mg

476. DIJON MUSTARD VINAIGRETTE

Preparation Time: 5 minutes
Cooking Time: 0 minutes
Serving: 6

Ingredients:

- ¾ cup olive oil
- ¼ cup apple cider vinegar
- 3 tablespoons Dijon mustard
- 2 shallots, quartered
- 1 garlic clove, chopped
- A handful of parsley, chopped

Directions:

1. Place all ingredients in a food processor.
2. Pulse until smooth.
3. Place in containers and store in the fridge until ready to use.

Nutrition Facts Per Serving

Calories 252, Total Fat 27g, Saturated Fat 4g, Total Carbs 2g, Net Carbs 1.3g, Protein 0.6g, Sugar: 1g, Fiber: 0.7g, Sodium:80 mg, Potassium 93mg

477. ANTI-INFLAMMATORY CAESAR DRESSING

Preparation Time: 5 minutes
Cooking Time: 0 minutes
Serving: 6

Ingredients:

- ½ cup cashew nuts, soaked in water then drained
- 1/3 cup fresh lemon juice
- 1 clove of garlic, minced
- 1 tablespoon Dijon mustard
- 1 tablespoon anchovy paste
- 2 tablespoon extra-virgin olive oil
- ½ cup plain Greek yogurt

Directions:

1. Place all ingredients in a food processor.
2. Pulse until a smooth paste is formed.
3. Place in containers and store in the fridge until ready to use.

Nutrition Facts Per Serving

Calories 96, Total Fat 7g, Saturated Fat 1.2g, Total Carbs 5g, Net Carbs 4.5g, Protein 4g, Sugar: 1g, Fiber: 0.5g, Sodium: 113mg, Potassium 132mg

478. FRESH TOMATO VINAIGRETTE

Preparation Time: 5 minutes
Cooking Time: 0 minutes
Serving: 5

Ingredients:

- 1 fresh tomato, chopped
- ¾ cup olive oil
- ¼ cup apple cider vinegar
- 1 clove of garlic, chopped
- ½ teaspoon dried oregano
- Salt and pepper to taste

Directions:

1. Place all ingredients in a food processor.
2. Pulse until a smooth paste is formed.
3. Place in containers and store in the fridge until ready to use.

Nutrition Facts Per Serving

Calories 298, Total Fat 32g, Saturated Fat 5g, Total Carbs 2g, Net Carbs g, Protein 0.2g, Sugar: 2g, Fiber: 0.4g, Sodium: 3mg, Potassium 75mg

479. GINGER SESAME SAUCE

Preparation Time: 5 minutes
Cooking Time: 0 minutes
Serving: 6

Ingredients:

- ½ cup olive oil
- ¼ cup sesame oil
- 1/3 cup rice wine vinegar
- 1 tablespoon fresh ginger
- 1 tablespoon sesame seeds

Directions:

1. Place all ingredients in a food processor.
2. Pulse until a smooth paste is formed.
3. Place in containers and store in the fridge until ready to use.

Nutrition Facts Per Serving

Calories250, Total Fat 28g, Saturated Fat 4g, Total Carbs 0.2g, Net Carbs 0.1g, Protein 0.3g, Sugar: 0.01g, Fiber: 0.1g, Sodium: 2mg, Potassium 10 mg

480. GOLDEN TURMERIC TAHINI SAUCE

Preparation Time: 5 minutes
Cooking Time: 0 minutes
Serving: 6

Ingredients:

- ¼ cup tahini
- ¼ cup lemon juice
- 1 tablespoon olive oil
- 1 tablespoon nutritional yeast
- ½ tablespoon maple syrup
- ¼ teaspoon ground turmeric
- A pinch of cayenne pepper
- 2 tablespoons water
- ¼ teaspoon salt
- ¼ teaspoon black pepper

Directions:

1. Place all ingredients in a food processor.
2. Pulse until a smooth paste is formed.
3. Place in containers and store in the fridge until ready to use.

Nutrition Facts Per Serving

Calories 71, Total Fat 6g, Saturated Fat 1g, Total Carbs4 g, Net Carbs 3g, Protein 2g, Sugar: 1g, Fiber: 1g, Sodium: 56mg, Potassium 341mg

481. HEALTHY TERIYAKI SAUCE

Preparation Time: 5 minutes
Cooking Time: 8 minutes
Serving: 6

Ingredients:

- ½ cup reduced-sodium tamari
- ¼ cup pitted dates, pulsed until smooth
- 1 ½ teaspoons minced garlic
- 1 ½ teaspoons minced ginger
- 1 tablespoon blackstrap molasses
- 2 tablespoons sweet rice cooking wine
- 2 teaspoons arrowroot powder + 2 teaspoons water
- ¼ cup water

Directions:

1. Place all ingredients except for the arrowroot slurry in a saucepan.
2. Turn on the heat and bring to a simmer for 5 minutes over medium flame.
3. Add in the arrowroot slurry and continue cooking for another 3 minutes or until the sauce thickens.
4. Place in containers and store in the fridge.

Nutrition Facts Per Serving

Calories 236, Total Fat 11g, Saturated Fat 2g, Total Carbs 31g, Net Carbs 29g, Protein 7g,

Sugar: 11g, Fiber: 2g, Sodium: 245mg, Potassium 274mg

482. YOGURT GARLIC SAUCE

Preparation Time: 5 minutes
Cooking Time: 0 minutes
Serving: 4

Ingredients:

- 1 cup yogurt
- 1 clove of garlic, minced
- 1/3 cup parsley, finely chopped
- Juice from ½ lemon

Directions:

1. Place all ingredients in a bowl.
2. Whisk to combine everything.
3. Put in a container with lid and store in the fridge until ready to use.

Nutrition Facts Per Serving

Calories 42, Total Fat 2g, Saturated Fat 1g, Total Carbs 4g, Net Carbs 3.8g, Protein 2g, Sugar: 3g, Fiber:0.2 g, Sodium: 31mg, Potassium 132mg

483. CHUNKY TOMATO SAUCE

Preparation Time: 5 minutes
Cooking Time: 15 minutes
Serving: 6

Ingredients:

- ¼ cup extra virgin olive oil
- 2 onions, chopped
- 5 cloves of garlic, minced
- 2 red bell peppers, chopped
- ½ cup sliced Portobello mushrooms
- 3 cups diced tomatoes
- 1 teaspoon dried oregano
- 2 teaspoons honey
- 2 teaspoons balsamic vinegar
- 1 teaspoon dried basil
- ½ cup fresh spinach, chopped
- salt and pepper to taste

Directions:

1. In a heavy pan, heat oil over medium flame.
2. Stir in the onions, garlic, and bell pepper until fragrant.
3. Add in the mushrooms, tomatoes, oregano, honey, balsamic vinegar, and basil. Season with salt and pepper to taste.
4. Close the lid and bring to a simmer for 10 minutes until the tomatoes have wilted.
5. Add in the spinach last and cook for another 5 minutes.
6. Place in containers and store in the fridge until ready to use.

Nutrition Facts Per Serving

Calories 86, Total Fat 4g, Saturated Fat 0.6g, Total Carbs 11g, Net Carbs 9g, Protein 2g, Sugar: 7g, Fiber: 2g, Sodium: 88mg, Potassium 358mg

484. SWEET BALSAMIC DRESSING

Preparation Time: 5 minutes
Cooking Time: 0 minutes
Serving: 5

Ingredients:

- 1 cup olive oil
- ½ cup balsamic vinegar
- 2 teaspoons raw honey
- 2 teaspoons mustard
- 2 cloves of garlic, minced
- Salt and pepper to taste

Directions:

1. Combine all ingredients in a blender and combine until the mixture becomes smooth.
2. Place in contains until ready to use.

Nutrition Facts Per Serving

Calories 416, Total Fat 43g, Saturated Fat 6g, Total Carbs 7g, Net Carbs 6.9g, Protein 0.3g, Sugar:6 g, Fiber: 0.1g, Sodium: 29mg, Potassium 38mg

485. CITRUS SALAD SAUCE

Preparation Time: 5 minutes
Cooking Time: 0 minutes
Serving: 4

Ingredients:

- 1/3 cup fresh orange juice
- 2 tablespoons balsamic vinegar
- 1 tablespoon extra-virgin olive oil

- salt and pepper to taste

Directions:

1. Place all ingredients in a bowl.
2. Whisk until well-combined.
3. Place in a small jar and shake well before using.
4. Keep inside the fridge for two days.

Nutrition Facts Per Serving

Calories 43, Total Fat 4g, Saturated Fat 0.5g, Total Carbs 4g, Net Carbs 4g, Protein 0.1g, Sugar: 1g, Fiber: 0g, Sodium:73 mg, Potassium 103mg

486. ANTI-INFLAMMATORY APPLESAUCE

Prep time:10 minutes
Cooking Time: 15 minutes
Serving: 4

Ingredients:

- 12 organic apples, peeled, cored, and sliced
- 2 teaspoons cinnamon
- Water for steamer pot

Directions:

- Pour water in a deep pan and place a steamer basket on top.
- Place apples in the steamer and steam for 15 minutes until soft.
- Place the apples in a food processor and add in cinnamon.
- Pulse until smooth.
- Place in containers and store in the fridge until ready to consume.

Nutrition Facts Per Serving

Calories 287, Total Fat 0.9g, Saturated Fat 0.1g, Total Carbs 76g, Net Carbs 62g, Protein 2g, Sugar:56 g, Fiber: 14g, Sodium: 6mg, Potassium 590mg

487. HEALTHY PIZZA SAUCE

Preparation Time: 5 minutes
Cooking Time: 10 minutes
Serving: 8

Ingredients:

- 2 cups tomato, diced
- ½ teaspoon oregano
- ½ teaspoon garlic powder
- ¼ teaspoon dried thyme
- 1/8 teaspoon ground red pepper
- 1/8 teaspoon cinnamon
- ¼ teaspoon basil
- ¼ teaspoon black pepper
- ¼ teaspoon salt

Directions:

1. Place all ingredients in a saucepan.
2. Heat over medium flame and heat for 10 minutes.
3. Transfer to a food processor and pulse until smooth.
4. Transfer to a container and store inside the fridge until ready to use.

Nutrition Facts Per Serving

Calories 8, Total Fat 0.08g, Saturated Fat 0.01g, Total Carbs 2g, Net Carbs 1.5g, Protein 0.4g, Sugar:1 g, Fiber: 0.5g, Sodium: 2mg, Potassium 93mg

488. GREEN GODDESS SAUCE

Preparation Time: 5 minutes
Cooking Time: 0 minutes
Serving: 8

Ingredients:

- 1 cup basil, chopped
- 1 cup flat leaf parsley, chopped
- ¼ cup green onion
- 1 clove of garlic, minced
- 1 teaspoon apple cider vinegar
- 2 tablespoons lemon juice, freshly squeezed
- ¼ cup olive oil
- 1 cup plain non-fat Greek yogurt
- 1/8 teaspoon salt
- 1/8 teaspoon black pepper
- 1/8 teaspoon cayenne pepper

Directions:

1. Place all ingredients in a food processor and blend until smooth.
2. Place in containers and store in the fridge until ready to use.

Nutrition Facts Per Serving

Calories 78, Total Fat 7g, Saturated Fat 1g, Total Carbs 2g, Net Carbs 1.6g, Protein 3g, Sugar: 0.9g, Fiber: 0.4g, Sodium: 13mg, Potassium 90mg

489. CHIMICHURRI SAUCE

Preparation Time: 5 minutes
Cooking Time: 0 minutes
Serving: 5

Ingredients:

- ½ cup packed fresh parsley leaves
- ½ cup fresh cilantro leaves
- 4 cloves of garlic, minced
- ½ seeded and chopped jalapeno pepper
- 2 tablespoons chopped onion
- 2 tablespoons lemon juice
- 1 teaspoon dried oregano
- ¼ cup apple cider vinegar
- ¾ cup extra virgin olive oil
- Salt and pepper to taste

Directions:

1. Place all ingredients in a food processor until smooth.
2. Put in container and store in the fridge until ready to use.

Nutrition Facts Per Serving

Calories 149, Total Fat 16g, Saturated Fat 2g, Total Carbs 1g, Net Carbs 0.6g, Protein 2g, Sugar: 0g, Fiber: 0.4g, Sodium: 3 mg, Potassium 25mg

490. RASPBERRY VINAIGRETTE SAUCE

Preparation Time: 5 minutes
Cooking Time: 0 minutes
Serving: 5

Ingredients:

- ¾ cup olive oil
- ¼ cup apple cider vinegar
- 1 teaspoon dried basil
- ½ cup raspberries
- 1 teaspoon salt
- ¼ cup water

Directions:

1. Place all ingredients in a food processor until smooth.
2. Put in container and store in the fridge until ready to use.

Nutrition Facts Per Serving

Calories 316, Total Fat 32g, Saturated Fat 5g, Total Carbs 8g, Net Carbs 7g, Protein 0.3g, Sugar:6 g, Fiber: 1g, Sodium: 2mg, Potassium 41mg

491. CLEAN BBQ SAUCE

Preparation Time: 5 minutes
Cooking Time: 10 minutes
Serving: 5

Ingredients:

- 3 tablespoons extra virgin olive oil
- ½ onion, chopped
- 4 cloves of garlic, minced
- 1 cup tomatoes, chopped
- 2 teaspoons Dijon mustard
- 2 tablespoons apple cider vinegar
- 3 tablespoons raw honey
- 5 medjool dates, pitted
- 1 teaspoon chili powder
- 1 teaspoon chili powder
- a dash of salt

Directions:

1. Heat oil in a pan over medium flame and sauté the onion and garlic until fragrant.
2. Add in the rest of the ingredients and season with salt to taste.
3. Allow to simmer for 15 minutes until the tomatoes have wilted.
4. Place in containers and store in the fridge until ready to use.

Nutrition Facts Per Serving

Calories 156, Total Fat 4g, Saturated Fat 0.5g, Total Carbs 32g, Net Carbs 29g, Protein 1g, Sugar: 28g, Fiber: 3g, Sodium: 128mg, Potassium 301mg

EGGS AND DAIRY

492. CHEESE STUFFED PEPPERS

Preparation Time: 25 minutes
Servings: 4

Nutrition: 140 Calories; 9.8g Fat; 6.4g Carbs; 7.8g Protein; 0.9g Fiber

Ingredients

- 4 summer bell peppers, divined and halved
- 2 ounces mozzarella cheese, crumbled
- 2 tablespoons Greek-style yogurt
- 4 ounces cream cheese
- 1 clove garlic, minced

Directions

1. Boil the peppers until they are just tender.
2. Thoroughly combine the cheese, yogurt, and garlic. Stuff your peppers with this filling. Place the stuffed peppers in a foil-lined baking dish.
3. Bake in the preheated oven at 365 degrees F for about 10 minutes. Bon appétit!

493. ITALIAN ZUCCHINI SANDWICHES

Preparation Time: 10 minutes
Servings: 2

Nutrition: 352 Calories; 26.5g Fat; 6.6g Total Carbs; 22.1g Protein; 0.6g Fiber

Ingredients

- 4 thin zucchini slices, cut lengthwise
- 2 eggs
- 4 slices Sopressata
- 2 slices provolone cheese
- 1 red bell pepper, sliced thinly

Directions

1. Melt 1 tablespoon of butter in a frying pan over medium-high flame. Then, fry the eggs for about 5 minutes.
2. Place one zucchini slice on each plate. Add the cheese, Sopressata, and peppers on top; season with salt and black pepper to taste.
3. Add fried eggs and top with the remaining zucchini slices. Bon appétit!

494.CREAMY DILLED EGG SALAD

Preparation Time: 20 minutes + chilling time | 3

Nutrition: 212 Calories; 19.4g Fat; 0.9g Carbs; 7.6g Protein; 0.2g Fiber

Ingredients

- 4 eggs, peeled and chopped
- 1 scallion, chopped
- 1 tablespoon fresh dill minced
- 1 teaspoon Dijon mustard
- 4 tablespoons mayonnaise

Directions

1. Add the eggs and water to a saucepan and bring to a boil; remove from heat. Allow the eggs to sit, covered, for about 11 minutes.
2. Peel and rinse the eggs under running water. Then, chop the eggs and transfer them to a nice salad bowl; stir in the scallions, dill, mustard, and mayonnaise.
3. Taste and season with salt and pepper. Enjoy!

495. EGGS WITH GOAT CHEESE

Preparation Time: 10 minutes
Servings: 2

Nutrition: 287 Calories; 22.6g Fat; 1.3g Carbs19.8g Protein; 0g Fiber

Ingredients

- 4 eggs, whisked
- 2 teaspoons ghee, room temperature
- 1 teaspoon paprika
- Sea salt and ground black pepper, to taste
- 4 tablespoons goat cheese

Directions

1. In a frying pan, melt the ghee over a moderate heat. Then, cook the eggs, covered, for about 4 minutes.
2. Stir in goat cheese, paprika, salt, and black pepper; continue to cook for 2 to 3 minutes more or until cooked through.
3. Taste and adjust seasonings. Enjoy!

496. DUKKAH FRITTATA WITH CHEESE

Preparation Time: 30 minutes
Servings: 3

Nutrition: 354 Calories; 29.2g Fat; 3.5g Carbs; 19.1g Protein; 0.5g Fiber

Ingredients

- 3 tablespoons milk
- 1 tablespoon Dukkah spice mix
- 5 eggs
- 2 tablespoons olive oil
- 1 cup cheddar cheese, shredded

Directions

1. Preheat your oven to 360 degrees F.
2. Whisk the milk, spices mix and eggs until well mixed.
3. Grease the bottom of a small-sized baking pan with olive oil. Spoon the egg mixture into the pan and top with cheese.
4. Bake in the preheated oven for about 25 minutes until the eggs are set but the center jiggles just a bit. Bon appétit!

497. CLASSIC ITALIAN OMELET

Preparation Time: 15 minutes
Servings: 3

Nutrition: 481 Calories; 43.3g Fat; 4.8g Carbs; 17.2g Protein; 0.6g Fiber

Ingredients

- 3 ounces bacon, diced
- 1 Italian pepper, chopped
- 6 eggs, whisked
- 1 teaspoon Italian seasoning blend
- 1/2 cup goat cheese, shredded

Directions

1. Preheat a frying pan over a medium-high heat. Now, fry the bacon until crisp or 3 to 4 minutes; set aside.
2. Stir in Italian pepper and continue to sauté for 2 minutes more or until just tender and fragrant. Pour the eggs into the pan.
3. Sprinkle with the Italian seasoning blend; add the salt and black pepper to taste and cook until the eggs are ser. Top with the reserved bacon and goat cheese.
4. Slide your omelet onto serving plates and serve. Bon appétit!

498. EGG SALAD WITH ANCHOVIES

Preparation Time: 15 minutes + chilling time | 3

Nutrition: 329 Calories; 23.4g Fat; 2.6g Carbs; 25g Protein; 0.3g Fiber

Ingredients

- 3 ounces anchovies, flaked
- 5 eggs
- 2 tablespoons mayonnaise
- 1 teaspoon Dijon mustard
- 2 tablespoons Ricotta cheese

Directions

1. Add the eggs and water to a saucepan and bring to a boil; remove from heat. Allow the eggs to sit, covered, for about 11 minutes.
2. Then, peel the eggs and rinse them under running water. Then, transfer chopped eggs to a salad bowl.
3. Add in the remaining ingredients, gently stir to combine and enjoy!

499. CLASSIC KETO MUFFINS

Preparation Time: 20 minutes
Servings: 4

Nutrition: 292 Calories; 23.1g Fat; 5.4g Carbs; 16.4g Protein; 3.3g Fiber

Ingredients

- 4 ounces cheddar cheese, shredded
- 6 tablespoons almond flour
- 2 tablespoons flaxseed meal
- 4 eggs
- 1/4 teaspoon baking soda

Directions

1. Start by preheating an oven at 355 degrees F
2. Thoroughly combine all of the above ingredients until well mixed.
3. Coat a muffin pan with cupcake liners. Spoon the batter into the muffin pan.

Bake in the preheated oven for 16 minutes.

4. Place on a wire rack for 10 minutes before unmolding and serving. Enjoy!

500. AUTHENTIC SPANISH MIGAS

Preparation Time: 15 minutes
Servings: 3

Nutrition: 193 Calories; 12.3g Fat; 6g Carbs; 12g Protein; 1.7g Fiber

Ingredients

- 6 eggs
- 6 lettuce leaves
- 1 white onion, chopped
- 1 tomato, chopped
- 1 Spanish pepper, chopped

Directions

1. Melt 1 tablespoon of butter in a cast-iron skillet over medium-high flame. Sauté the onion for about 4 minutes, stirring continuously to ensure even cooking.
2. Stir in the peppers and continue to sauté an additional 3 to 4 minutes. Whisk in the eggs. Continue to cook until the eggs are set.
3. Divide the egg mixture between lettuce leaves; top with tomatoes. Season with salt and black pepper and serve. Devour!

501. DOUBLE CHEESE FONDUE

Preparation Time: 10 minutes
Servings: 8

Nutrition: 196 Calories; 15.7g Fat; 3.4g Carbs; 10.1g Protein; 0g Fiber

Ingredients

- 4 ounces Ricotta cheese
- 1 cup double cream
- Cayenne pepper, to taste
- 8 ounces Swiss cheese, shredded
- 4 tablespoons Greek-style yogurt

Directions

1. Warm Ricotta cheese and double cream and in a saucepan over medium-low flame.
2. Remove from the heat. Fold in cayenne pepper, Swiss cheese, and Greek-style yogurt. Stir until everything is well combined.
3. Bon appétit!

502. SAVORY ROLLS WITH BACON AND CHEESE

Preparation Time: 30 minutes
Servings: 8

Nutrition: 176 Calories; 15.8g Fat; 3g Carbs; 6g Protein; 0.6g Fiber

Ingredients

- 1/2 cup goat cheese, crumbled
- 1/2 cup cream cheese
- 8 eggs
- 6 ounces bacon, diced
- 1/2 cup marinara sauce

Directions

1. In a nonstick skillet, fry the bacon over the highest heat until crisp; set aside.
2. Whisk the crema cheese and eggs until foamy. Add in the fried bacon along with salt and black pepper; whisk to combine well.
3. Spoon the mixture into greased muffin cups. Top each muffin with goat cheese. Bake in the preheated oven at 355 degrees F for about 14 minutes or until golden on the top.
4. Serve with marinara sauce and enjoy!

503. BROCCOLI CHEESE PIE

Preparation Time: 30 minutes
Servings: 4

Nutrition: 308 Calories; 23.2g Fat; 5.3g Carbs; 19.2g Protein; 0.9g Fiber

Ingredients

- 6 eggs
- 1 red onion, sliced
- 6 tablespoons Greek yogurt
- 2 cups broccoli florets
- 1/2 cup cheddar cheese, shredded

Directions

1. Heat 2 teaspoon of olive oil in an oven-safe skillet over medium-high heat. Sweat red onion and broccoli until they have softened or about 4 minutes.
2. Season with salt and black pepper.
3. In a mixing bowl, whisk Greek yogurt and eggs until well mixed. Scrape the mixture into the pan.
4. Bake at 365 degrees F for 15 to 20 minutes or until a toothpick inserted into a muffin comes out dry and clean.
5. Top with cheddar cheese and bake for 5 to 6 minutes more. Bon appétit!

504. HERBED CHEESE BALL

Preparation Time: 10 minutes + chilling time | 10

Nutrition: 176 Calories; 15.7g Fat; 2g Carbs; 7.2g Protein; 0.9g Fiber

Ingredients

- 1/2 cup sour cream
- 8 ounces extra-sharp cheddar cheese, shredded
- 6 ounces cream cheese, softened
- 2 tablespoons mayonnaise
- 1 tablespoon Moroccan herb mix

Directions

1. Thoroughly combine sour cream, cheddar cheese, cream cheese, and mayonnaise.
2. Cover the mixture with a plastic wrap and place in your refrigerator for about 3 hours.
3. Roll the mixture over Moroccan herb mix until well coated. Serve with assorted keto veggies. Enjoy!

505. MEXICAN EGGS WITH VEGETABLES

Preparation Time: 15 minutes
Servings: 2

Nutrition: 287 Calories; 20.5g Fat; 7.2g Total Carbs; 17.4g Protein; 2.9g Fiber

Ingredients

- 1/2 cup cauliflower florets
- 2 ounces Cotija cheese, crumbled
- 2 scallion stalks, chopped
- 2 bell peppers, chopped
- 3 eggs

Directions

1. Warm 2 teaspoons of olive oil in a frying pan over medium-high heat.Sauté the cauliflower, scallions and peppers until tender and aromatic about 3 minutes.
2. In the meantime, beat the eggs with salt and black pepper. Add in Mexican oregano, if desired.
3. Pour the egg mixture over the vegetables in the frying pan. Continue to cook for about 5 minutes.
4. Top with Cotija cheese and cook for 2 minutes longer. Serve immediately.

506. MASALA EGGS WITH BROWN MUSHROOMS

Preparation Time: 15 minutes
Servings: 2

Nutrition: 217 Calories; 15.6g Fat; 5g Carbs; 14.4g Protein; 1.2g Fiber

Ingredients

- 4 eggs, whisked
- 1/2 brown onion, thinly sliced
- 1/2 pound brown mushrooms, sliced
- 1 garlic clove, thinly sliced
- 1/2 teaspoon garam masala

Directions

1. Heat 1 tablespoon of oil in a frying pan over medium-high heat. Sauté the onion, garlic, and mushrooms for 3 to 4 minutes until tender and aromatic. Set aside.
2. Add the eggs and garam masala to the pan. Give it a quick swirl and cook for about 3 minutes.
3. Turn the omelet over and cook for a further 2 minutes. Add the mushroom mixture, fold your omelet and serve. Enjoy!

507. EASY KETO QUESADILLAS

Preparation Time: 15 minutes
Servings: 2

Nutrition: 417 Calories; 34.5g Fat; 5.3g Carbs;

20.6g Protein; 1.1g Fiber

Ingredients

- 4 tablespoons sour cream
- 4 eggs
- 1 white onion, chopped
- 1/2 cup Monterey-Jack cheese, shredded
- 1 cup kale, torn into pieces

Directions

1. Heat 1 tablespoon of olive oil in an oven-proof skillet over medium-high heat. Cook the onion until tender and translucent about 3 minutes.
2. Fold in the kale leaves and stir for a minute or so.
3. Then, thoroughly combine the sour cream with eggs; season with the salt and black pepper to taste. Spoon the mixture into the skillet and tilt to distribute evenly.
4. Top with Monterey-Jack cheese.
5. Bake in the preheated oven at 380 degrees F for 10 minutes until the eggs are golden brown. Slice into wedges and serve.

508. HAM AND CHEESE MUFFINS

Preparation Time: 30 minutes
Servings: 2

Nutrition: 249 Calories; 15.3g Fat; 5.5g Carbs; 22.5g Protein; 1.4g Fiber

Ingredients

- 1/4 cup mozzarella cheese, shredded
- 4 eggs
- 1/4 cup double cream
- 2 ounces ham, chopped
- 1 cup broccoli florets

Directions

1. In a frying pan, melt 1 teaspoon of butter. Cook the broccoli until crisp tender about 3 minutes.
2. In a mixing bowl, combine the eggs and double cream. Stir in the sautéed broccoli and ham; divide the mixture between muffin cups.
3. Top with shredded mozzarella cheese.
4. Bake in the preheated oven at 365 degrees F for 12 minutes or until a knife inserted into a muffin comes out clean. Bon appétit!

509. ALEPPO PEPPER DEVILED EGGS

Preparation Time: 15 minutes
Servings: 4

Nutrition: 163 Calories; 12.7g Fat; 1.7g Carbs; 10.1g Protein; 0.3g Fiber

Ingredients

- 4 eggs
- 1 teaspoon Aleppo chili pepper
- 2 slices bacon, diced
- 1/3 cup Asiago cheese, grated
- 1 tablespoon Dijon mustard

Directions

1. Place the eggs and water in a saucepan and bring to a boil. Let them sit, covered, for 9 minutes; then, place the eggs in the ice bath.
2. Peel the eggs and cut them in half. Then, fry the bacon in the preheated skillet for about 4 minutes.
3. Mash the yolks with fried bacon, mustard, Aleppo chili pepper, and Asiago cheese; mix to combine well.
4. Stuff the egg whites with this filling and serve.

510. SKINNY EGGS WITH SPINACH

Preparation Time: 10 minutes
Servings: 2

Nutrition: 183 Calories; 13.1g Fat; 3.3g Carbs; 12.9g Protein; 1.4g Fiber

Ingredients

- 4 eggs, well whisked
- 2 teaspoons olive oil
- 1/2 teaspoon garlic powder
- Sea salt cayenne pepper, to taste, to taste
- 4 cups baby spinach

Directions

1. Heat the olive oil in a cast-iron skillet over

medium-high heat.

2. Add in the baby spinach and garlic powder; season with salt and cayenne pepper and cook for 1 to 2 minutes or until wilted.
3. Fold in the eggs, and continue to cook, stirring continuously with a spatula. Enjoy!

511. OVEN-BAKED EGGS WITH HAM

Preparation Time: 35 minutes
Servings: 5

Nutrition: 258 Calories; 17.3g Fat; 2.8g Carbs; 20.5g Protein; 0.2g Fiber

Ingredients

- 8 eggs
- 2 tablespoons bacon drippings
- 1 shallot, chopped
- 6 ounces cooked ham, diced
- 3 tablespoons cream of celery soup

Directions

1. In an oven-safe skillet, warm the bacon drippings over medium-high heat.
2. Sweat the shallot until tender and caramelized or about 10 minutes.
3. Mix the eggs with the celery soup. Stir in the cooked ham and pour the egg mixture into the skillet.
4. Bake in the preheated oven at 380 degrees F for 20 to 23 minutes. Bon appétit!

512. FAMOUS DOUBLE-CHEESE CHIPS

Preparation Time: 10 minutes
Servings: 6

Nutrition: 148 Calories; 11.7g Fat; 1.1g Carbs; 9.4g Protein; 0.2g Fiber

Ingredients

- 3/4 cup Romano cheese, shredded
- 1 tablespoon Italian seasoning blend
- 1 cup Asiago cheese, shredded

Directions

1. Start by preheating your oven to 360 degrees F.
2. Mix the ingredients together in a bowl. Spoon tablespoon-sized heaps of the mixture onto foil-lined baking sheets.
3. Bake in the preheated oven approximately 7 minutes until they are browned around the edges.
4. Transfer the cheese chips to paper towels and allow them to cool until crisp. Enjoy!

513. FAST AND SIMPLE SPICY EGGS

Preparation Time: 15 minutes
Servings: 3

Nutrition: 317 Calories; 24.3g Fat; 4.2g Carbs; 19g Protein; 0.4g Fiber

Ingredients

- 2 scallions, chopped
- 1 tablespoon olive oil
- 1/2 teaspoon chili powder
- 1/3 cup full-fat milk
- 6 eggs

Directions

1. Heat the olive oil in a frying pan over medium-high flame. Cook the scallions until tender and aromatic about 3 minutes.
2. In a mixing dish, whisk the milk, eggs, and chili powder. Season with the salt and black pepper to your liking.
3. Spoon the egg mixture into the pan; shake the pan to spread the mixture evenly.
4. Cook the eggs for about 5 minutes. Taste, adjust the seasonings, and serve immediately.

514. FAVORITE BREAKFAST TABBOULEH

Preparation Time: 20 minutes
Servings: 3

Nutrition: 204 Calories; 8.6g Fat; 8.6g Carbs; 13.7g Protein; 2.8g Fiber

Ingredients

- 6 eggs, beaten
- 1 shallot, sliced
- 2 cups cauliflower rice
- 1 bell pepper, deseeded and sliced

- 1/2 cup cherry tomatoes, halved

Directions

1. Melt 1 tablespoon of butter in an oven-safe skillet over medium-high heat.
2. Cook the cauliflower rice for 5 to 6 minutes or until it has softened. Stir in shallot and bell pepper and continue to cook for 4 minutes more.
3. Pour the beaten eggs over vegetables and cook until the eggs are set; do not overcook eggs.
4. Top with cherry tomatoes and place under the preheated broiler for 5 minutes. Taste and adjust seasonings. Bon appétit!

515. EGG CUPS WITH HAM

Preparation Time: 30 minutes
Servings: 6

Nutrition: 258 Calories; 19.1g Fat; 2.8g Carbs; 17.5g Protein; 0.2g Fiber

Ingredients

- 6 thin slices ham
- 6 eggs
- 4 ounces cream cheese
- 1 teaspoon mustard
- 6 ounces Colby cheese, shredded

Directions

1. Line muffin cups with cupcake liners. Add a ham slice to each muffin cup and gently press down.
2. In a mixing dish, whisk the eggs, cream cheese, and mustard; season with salt and pepper to taste.
3. Spoon the egg mixture into the cups. Top with the shredded cheese. Bake in the preheated oven at 355 degrees F approximately 27 minutes.
4. Garnish with 2 tablespoons of green onions just before serving and enjoy!

516. SEASONED EGG PORRIDGE FOR BREAKFAST.

Serving: 4
Prep + Cook Time:50 minutes

Ingredients:

- rinsed and drained white rice - 1/2 cup.
- Black pepper to taste
- water - 2 cups.
- Eggs - 4
- salt - 1/2 tsp.
- Sugar - 1 tbsp.
- olive oil - 1 tbsp.
- soy sauce - 2 tsp.
- chopped scallions - 4
- chicken broth - 2 cups.

Directions:

1. Add water, broth, sugar, salt, and rice to the Instant Pot before closing the lid
2. Press "Porridge" and leave it on "High" pressure for 30 minutes.
3. As that continues to cook, heat the oil in a saucepan.
4. When cracking the eggs, ensure to do so one at a time, this is so they won't touch each other
5. Keep cooking till the whites become crispy on the edges, while the yolks remain runny. Add a pinch of salt and pepper to taste.
6. Immediately the Instant Pot timer goes off, you are to press the "Cancel" button and allow the pressure to go down by itself.
7. Now, if the porridge isn't thick enough, press the "Sauté" button and cook uncovered for about 5 to 10 minutes.
8. Finally, you can serve with scallions, soy sauce, and an egg for each bowl

517. SAVORY FETA SPINACH EGG CUPS.

Serving: 4
Prep + Cook Time:22 minutes

Ingredients:

- feta cheese - 1/4 cup.
- chopped tomato – 1
- eggs - 6
- salt - 1/2 tsp.
- water - 1 cup.
- black pepper - 1 tsp.
- 1/2 cup.mozzarella cheese

- chopped baby spinach - 1 cup.

Directions:

1. Add water to the Instant Pot and lower in trivet
2. Place silicone ramekins with spinach.
3. Mix the remaining ingredients in a bowl and transfer to cups, allowing 1/4-inch head room
4. Introduce to the instant pot pressure cooker; note that you may have to cook in batches before adjusting time to 8 minutes on "High" pressure
5. Turn off the instant pot and quick-release immediately the time is up.

518. TASTY AND SOFT-BOILED EGG.

Serving: 2
Prep + Cook Time:6 minutes

Ingredients:

- water - 1 cup.
- eggs - 4
- toasted English muffins – 2
- Salt and pepper to taste

Directions:

1. Add the 1 cup of water to the Instant Pot and insert the steamer basket. Transfer four canning lids to the basket, then place the eggs on top of them, in order to ensure they are separated
2. Ensure the lid is secured.
3. Hit the STEAM setting and select a time of 4 minutes
4. Quick-release the steam valve once you are ready.
5. Remove the eggs using tongs and move them to a bowl containing cold water.
6. Wait for about one or two minutes.
7. Then peel and serve with one egg for each half of a toasted English muffin
8. Add salt and pepper as seasoning.

519. POACHED TOMATOES WITH EGGS.

Serving: 4
Prep + Cook Time:15 minutes

Ingredients:

- eggs – 4
- salt - 1 tsp.
- paprika - 1/2 tsp
- olive oil - 1 tbsp.
- white pepper - 1/2 tsp.
- red onion – 1
- medium tomatoes - 3
- fresh dill - 1 tbsp.

Directions:

1. Add the olive oil inside to the ramekins by spraying.
2. Then, make sure to beat the eggs into every ramekin.
3. Mix the paprika, white pepper, fresh dill, and salt together in the mixing bowl. Ensure to stir the mixture gently as you mix.
4. Follow this by cutting the red onion into the mix.
5. Cut the tomatoes into the small pieces and then mix the pieces with the onion. Once again, stir the mixture gently and well.
6. Then sprinkle tomato mixture on the eggs.
7. Add spice mixture and move the eggs to the Instant Pot.
8. Close the lid and set the Instant Pot to STEAM mode
9. Cook the dish for about 5 minutes before removing the dish from the Instant Pot and let it chill for a while.
10. Serve the dish immediately and enjoy your meal!

520. TASTY AND SIMPLE FRENCH TOAST.

Serving: 4
Prep + Cook Time:35 minutes

Ingredients:

- butter - 1 tsp.
- stale cinnamon-raisin bread - 3 cups; cut into cubes
- water - 1 ½ cups.
- whole milk - 1 cup.
- pure vanilla extract - 1 tsp
- maple syrup - 2 tbsp.

- sugar - 1 tsp.
- Big and beaten eggs – 3

Directions:

1. Add water to your Instant Pot and lower in the steam rack
2. Grease a 6 to 7-inch soufflé pan.
3. Mix milk, vanilla, maple syrup, and eggs in a clean bowl.
4. Add the bread cubes and let them soak for 5 minutes.
5. Pour the soaked bread cubes to the pan; ensure that the bread is totally submerged.
6. Make sure the instant pot pressure cooker is set.
7. Then select "Manual" and adjust the time settings to 15 minutes on "High" pressure
8. Quick-release the pressure immediately the time is out.
9. Top with sugar by sprinkling, then broil in the oven for about 3 minutes

521. HARD BOILED LARGE EGGS RECIPE.

Serving: 6
Prep + Cook Time:10 minutes

Ingredients:

- water - 1 cup.
- large white eggs - 12

Directions:

1. Pour about 1 cup of water into the bowl in the Instant Pot.
2. Insert the stainless steamer basket inside the pot
3. Place the eggs in the steamer basket
4. Boil on manual "High" pressure for about 7 minutes.
5. Then quick release valve to ensure that the pressure is released
6. Open the lid and remove the eggs using tongs and move them into a bowl containing cold water.

522. SPINACH, SLICED BACON WITH EGGS.

Serving: 4
Prep + Cook Time:15 minutes

Ingredients:

- Bacon - 7 oz.
- cream - 3 tbsp.
- spinach - 1/2 cup.
- eggs - 4, boiled
- ground white pepper - 1/2 tsp.
- cilantro - 1 tsp.
- butter - 2 tsp.

Directions:

1. Slice the bacon neatly and sprinkle the ground white pepper on it as well as cilantro. Stir the mixture gently.
2. Remove the egg shells, then wrap them in the spinach leaves
3. Follow this by wrapping the eggs with the sliced bacon
4. Select the Instant Pot MEAT/STEW mode and move the wrapped eggs
5. Then add butter and cook the dish for about 10 minutes.
6. Remove the eggs from the Instant Pot and sprinkle the cream on them, immediately the time is up.
7. Ensure to serve the dish while it is still hot.

523. BREAKFAST JAR WITH BACON.

Serving: 3
Prep + Cook Time:25 minutes

Ingredients:

- eggs – 6
- Tater tots
- sharp cheese or shredded cheese - 9 slices; divided
- mason jars -- 3 pieces; that can hold about 2-cup worth ingredients
- bacon - 6 pieces; cooked of your preferred breakfast meat, such as sausage
- peach-mango salsa - 6 tbsp.; divided

Directions:

1. Add about 1 ¼ cups of water to the Instant Pot. Then add enough tater tots to ensure the bottom of the mason jars is covered.
2. Break 2 eggs into each Mason jar you

have. Then poke the egg yolks with a fork; you can also use the tip of a long knife.
3. Place a couple of your preferred meat to the mason jars. Then add 2 slices of cheese to each Mason jar; this should cover the ingredients.
4. Pour 2 tablespoon of salsa into each jar, right on top of the cheese. Also, add a couple more tater tots right on top of the salsa.
5. Then top the mix with 1 slice of cheese. Ensure to cover each jar using foil, make sure the cover is tight enough to prevent moisture from escaping into the jars.
6. Place the jars into the water in the Instant Pot. Close the lid of the instant pot.
7. Select "High" pressure and set the timer to clock out at 5 minutes; ensure the valve of the Instant Pot is also in pressure cooker mode.
8. Turn the steam valve to release pressure immediately the timer beeps; make sure to quick release the pressure.
9. Open the Instant Pot and gently remove the jar.

524. TASTY SCRAMBLED EGGS & BACON.

Serving: 4
Prep + Cook Time:15 minutes

Ingredients:

- fresh parsley - 1/4 cup.
- cilantro - 1 tbsp.
- butter - 1 tbsp.
- Eggs – 7
- basil - 1 tsp.
- milk - 1/2 cup.
- salt - 1 tsp.
- paprika - 1 tsp.
- bacon - 4 oz.

Directions:

1. Beat the eggs in a clean mixing bowl and whisk them well.
2. Also, add milk, basil, salt, paprika, and cilantro and stir the mixture gently. Chop the bacon and parsley.
3. Choose the Instant Pot "Sauté" mode and move the chopped bacon. Cook it for about 3 minutes
4. Also, add whisked egg mixture and cook the dish for another 5 minutes.
5. Follow that by mixing up the eggs gently using a wooden spoon
6. Then sprinkle some chopped parsley on the dish and cook it for another 4 minutes.
7. Remove them from the Instant Pot when the eggs are done.
8. Serve the dish immediately while the dish is still hot. Enjoy!

525. TOMATO SPINACH QUICHE WITH PARMESAN CHEESE.

Serving: 6
Prep + Cook Time:30 minutes

Ingredients:

- fresh ground black pepper - 1/4 tsp.
- large green onions - 3, sliced
- tomato slices – 4; for topping the quiche
- milk - 1/2 cup.
- large eggs - 12
- Tomato - 1 cup; seeded, diced
- salt - 1/2 tsp.
- Water - 1 ½ cup; for the pot
- Parmesan cheese - 1/4 cup; shredded.
- fresh baby spinach - 3 cups; roughly chopped

Directions:

1. Add water to the Instant Pot container. Whisk the eggs with the milk, pepper, and salt in a large-sized bowl.
2. Then add the tomato, spinach, and the green onions into a 1 ½ quart-sized baking dish; stir the mix well.
3. Add the egg mix on the vegetables; stir until properly mixed. Put the tomato slices gently on top
4. Sprinkle the shredded parmesan cheese on the mix. Place the baking dish into the rack using a handle.
5. Place the rack into the Instant Pot and ensure the lid is locked. Put the pressure on "High" and set the timer to 20 minutes.

6. Immediately the timer clocks out, wait for about 1o minutes, then turn the steamer valve to "Venting" in order to release the rest of the pressure. Open the lid of the pot gently.
7. Hold the rack handles carefully and remove the dish out from the pot
8. Broil till the top of the quiche turns to light brown color, if you like.
9. TIP: You can cover the baking dish with foil to prevent moisture from gathering on the quiche top. You can cook uncovered; just soak the moisture using a paper towel

526. SEASONED CHEESY HASH BROWN.

Serving: 8
Prep + Cook Time:10 minutes

Ingredients:

- Eggs - 8
- chopped bacon - 6 slices
- frozen hash browns - 2 cups.
- salt - 1 tsp.
- black pepper - 1/2 tsp.
- shredded cheddar cheese - 1 cup.
- milk - 1/4 cup.

Directions:

1. Set your Instant Pot to "Sauté" and cook the bacon until it gets crispy.
2. Add hash browns and stir for about 2 minutes, or until they start to thaw
3. Whisk the eggs, milk, cheese, and seasonings in a bowl.
4. Transfer the hash browns to the pot, then lock and seal lid
5. Hit "Manual" button and adjust time to 5 minutes.
6. Select "Cancel" and quick-release the pressure when the time is up
7. Ensue to serve in slices.

527. SEASONED CREAMY SAUSAGE FRITTATA.

Serving: 4
Prep + Cook Time:40 minutes

Ingredients:

- 1/2 cup.cooked ground sausage
- water - 1 ½ cups.
- grated sharp cheddar - 1/4 cup.
- beaten eggs - 4
- sour cream - 2 tbsp.
- butter - 1 tbsp.
- Black pepper to taste
- Salt to taste

Directions:

1. Pour water into the Instant Pot and lower in the steamer rack.
2. Grease a 6 to 7-inch soufflé dish
3. Whisk the eggs and sour cream together in a bowl.
4. Add cheese, sausage, salt, and pepper. Stir
5. Pour the mix into the dish and wrap with foil all over; ensure to wrap tightly.
6. Lower right into the steam rack and close the lid of the pot.
7. Press "Manual" and then put it on "Low" pressure for 17 minutes.
8. Quick-release the pressure when the time is up. Serve the dish while still hot!

528. SEASONED EGG SIDE DISH RECIPE.

Serving: 6
Prep + Cook Time:20 minutes

Ingredients:

- eggs - 8
- ground white pepper - 1 tsp.
- mustard - 1 tbsp.
- minced garlic - 1 tsp.
- mayo sauce - 1 tsp.
- dill - 1/4 cup.
- cream - 1/4 cup.
- salt - 1 tsp.

Directions:

1. Introduce the eggs in the Instant Pot, then add water to the pot.
2. Cook the eggs at high pressure for about 5 minutes
3. Then take out the eggs from the Instant Pot and chill
4. Remove the egg shells and cut them into 2

parts

5. Remove and do away with the egg yolks and mash them together.
6. Then add the mustard, cream, salt, mayo sauce, ground white pepper, and minced garlic in the mashed egg yolks
7. Cut the dill and sprinkle the chopped dill on the egg yolk mixture.
8. Mix it up gently until you get a smooth and homogenous mass
9. Then move the egg yolk mixture into a pastry bag.
10. Fill up the egg whites with the yolk mixture
11. Serve the dish as soon as possible. Enjoy your meal!

529. BACON AND EGG WITH CHEESE MUFFINS.

Serving: 8
Prep + Cook Time:25 minutes

Ingredients:

- green onion - 1, diced.
- lemon pepper seasoning - 1/4 tsp.
- cheddar or pepper jack cheese - 4 tbsp., shredded.
- Bacon - 4 slices; cooked and crumbled.
- water - 1 ½ cup; for the pot
- eggs - 4

Directions:

1. Add water to the Instant Pot container and then place a steamer basket to the pot. Break the eggs in a large measuring bowl using a pour pout.
2. Add the lemon pepper and beat properly. Cut the bacon, cheese, and green onion between 4 silicone muffin cups.
3. Pour the egg mix into each muffin cups; using a fork, stir using a fork to mix well. Place the muffin cups into the steamer basket, and make sure to close the lid.
4. Set the pressure on "High" pressure and the timer to 8 minutes
5. Immediately the timer beeps, turn off the pot. Then wait for about 2 minutes before turning the steam valve in order to quick release the pressure.
6. Open the pot lid gently, and lift the steamer basket right from the container, and then do away with the muffin cups.
7. Serve warm and enjoy your meal!
8. Tips: These muffins can be stored in the refrigerator for more than 1 week. When ready to serve, just microwave for 30 seconds on "High" to reheat

SNACKS

530. CHEESY SPICY SAUSAGE STUFFED MUSHROOMS

Preparation time: 20 minutes
Cooking time: 30 minutes
Servings: 12 People
Calories: 164 kcal

Ingredients:

- 24 ounces Baby Bella mushrooms stems removed
- 12 ounces of pork sausage
- 1 teaspoon garlic powder
- 1 teaspoon dried basil
- 1 teaspoon dried parsley
- 2 to 3 teaspoons chili pepper
- 8 ounces of cream cheese softened
- Optional: Gourmet Garden Slightly Dried Chili Pepper Flakes and Parsley
- Get Ingredients Powered by Chicory

Directions:

1. Start by heating the oven to 350 degrees F. Then scoop the inside of each mushroom to make room for the stuffing.Add each mushroom into a 9 by 13 baking dish. In a skillet over medium heat, brown the sausage.Once browned add stir in pastes and stir to combine. Taste and adjust seasonings to your taste.Place the cream cheese in a stand mixer then add in your sausage. Blend until fully mixed.Stuff each mushroom with mixture. Bake for about 25 to 30 minutes.Remove from oven, sprinkle on chili pepper and parsley if desired.Remove mushrooms to a serving platter. Enjoy.

531. BUFFALO CAULIFLOWER BITES WITH DAIRY FREE RANCH DRESSING

Preparation time: 15 minutes
Cooking time: 30 minutes
Servings: 8 Serves
Calories: 268 kcal

Ingredients:

- 4 cups of cauliflower florets
- 2 tablespoons of extra virgin olive oil
- ¼ teaspoon of salt
- ¼ teaspoon of smoked paprika
- ¼ teaspoon of garlic powder
- ½ cup of sugar free hot sauce I used Archie Moore's brand
- Dairy Free Ranch Dressing
- 1 cup organic mayonnaise
- ½ cup of Silk unsweetened coconut milk
- 1 teaspoon of garlic powder
- 1 teaspoon of onion powder
- ¼ teaspoon of pepper
- 1 tablespoon of fresh lemon juice
- ¼ cup fresh chopped parsley
- Get Ingredients Powered by Chicory

Directions:

1. First heat oven to 400 degrees F. Spray baking sheet with non-stick olive oil cooking spray.Place florets in a large bowl and toss with olive oil. In a small bowl mix the salt, paprika and garlic powder together with hot sauce.Add the hot sauce into cauliflower bowl and stir well until well coated. Spread cauliflower out evenly on baking sheet and bake for 30 minutes.Whisk ingredients together and pour into a mason jar. Cover and refrigerate until ready to serve with cauli bites.

532. MINI ZUCCHINI PIZZA BITES

Preparation time: 15 minutes
Cooking time: 15 minutes
Servings: 6
Calories: 230 kcal

Ingredients:

- 2 cups shredded zucchini
- 1 egg
- 1 teaspoon of Italian Seasonings
- ½ teaspoon of salt

- ¼ teaspoon of pepper
- ½ cup of grated provolone cheese
- 1 cup shredded mozzarella cheese
- ¼ cup of mini pepperoni slices
- Get Ingredients Powered by Chicory

Directions:

1. First heat oven to 400 degrees. Grease a mini muffin pan with natural olive oil cooking spray.Place the zucchini in a clean towel and squeeze as much liquid out as you can. Mix the zucchini, egg, Italian seasoning, salt, pepper and provolone cheese and cilantro in a bowl.Equally divide the mixture into the mini muffin pan, packed down in each cup. Then sprinkle mozzarella onto zucchini then top with mini pepperoni slices.Bake for about 15 to 18 minutes until golden brown around the edges. Allow to cool about 10 minutes before removing. Let cool.Use a knife to cut around edges to loosen from muffin pan. Serve and enjoy.

533. SUGAR FREE SWEET & SPICY BACON CHICKEN BITES

Preparation time: 20 minutes
Cooking time: 30 minutes
Total time 50 minutes
Servings: 8 people

Ingredients:

- 2 pounds of chicken tenderloin boneless, cut into 1 inch cubes
- 16 ounces of bacon cut into fourths (I used Applegate)
- ½ cup of Swerve sweetener
- 1 teaspoon of chili powder
- ½ teaspoon of pepper
- Get Ingredients Powered by Chicory

Directions:

1. First heat oven to 400 degrees F and then wrap the bacon over each piece of chicken.Prepare two baking sheets with aluminium foil or you can use a cooling rack over the baking pan.In a bowl whisk the last 3 ingredients together and roll each chicken bite into the mixture.Place chicken bites on baking pans or cooling rack over pans and bake for about 25 to 30 minutes.Serve immediately. Enjoy.

534. BAKED CREAM CHEESE CRAB DIP

Preparation time: 5 minutes
Cooking time: 30 minutes
Servings: 12 people
Calories: 142kcal

Ingredients:

- 8 oz. lump crab meat
- 8 oz. cream cheese softened
- ½ cup avocado mayonnaise
- 1 tablespoon lemon juice
- 1 teaspoon Worcestershire sauce
- ½ teaspoon of garlic powder
- ½ teaspoon of onion powder
- ½ teaspoon of salt
- ¼ teaspoon of dry mustard
- ¼ teaspoon of black pepper

Directions:

1. Add all ingredients into small baking dish and spread out evenly. Bake at 375°F for about 25 to 30 minutes.Serve with low carb crackers or vegetables. Enjoy.

535. PHILLY CHEESESTEAK STUFFED MUSHROOMS

Preparation time: 15 minutes
Cooking time: 15 minutes

Ingredients:

- 24 oz. baby bella mushrooms
- 1 cup chopped red pepper
- 1 cup chopped onion
- 2 tablespoons butter
- 1 teaspoon salt divided
- ½ teaspoon of pepper divided
- 1 pound of beef sirloin shaved or thinly sliced against the grain
- 4 ounces of provolone cheese
- Get Ingredients Powered by Chicory

Directions:

1. First heat oven to 350 degrees. Remove

stems from mushrooms and place mushrooms on a greased baby sheet.Sprinkle with ½ teaspoon of salt and ¼ teaspoon of pepper on both sides and bake for 15 minutes. Set aside.Melt 1 tablespoon butter in a large skillet and cook pepper and onions until soft. Then season with ½ teaspoon of salt and ¼ teaspoon of pepper.Remove from the skillet and set aside. In the same skillet, melt the remaining tablespoon of butter and cook the meat to your preference.Add the provolone cheese and stir until completely melted. Return back the veggies.Add mixture into the mushrooms, top with more cheese if you like and bake for 5 minutes.Serve and enjoy.

536. CHEDDAR CHEESE STRAWS AND THE CABOT FIT TEAM

Servings: 24 straws
Preparation time: 5 minutes
Cooking time: 35 minutes

Ingredients:

- 1 & ¼ cup of almond flour
- 2 tablespoons of coconut flour I used Bob's Red Mill
- 2 tablespoon of arrowroot starch I used Bob's Red Mill
- 1 teaspoon of xanthan gum
- ½ teaspoon of garlic powder
- ¼ teaspoon of salt
- 5 tablespoons of butter well chilled and cut into small pieces
- 2 to 4 tablespoons of ice water
- 4 ounces of finely shredded sharp cheddar

Directions:

1. Combine almond flour, coconut flour, arrowroot starch, xanthan gum, garlic powder and salt in the bowl of a food processor. Pulse a few times to mix.Evenly sprinkle butter over almond flour mixture and pulse until it resembles fine crumbs.Add water through feeding tube 1 tablespoon at a time until dough clumps together (Turn processor to low).Form into a flat disc and cover with plastic wrap. Chill 30 minutes. Meanwhile preheat oven to 300F and line a large baking sheet with parchment paper.Take about 1 tablespoon of dough and roll it between your palms. Continue to roll gently on a piece of parchment.Sprinkle evenly a few teaspoons of grated cheddar and gently press the cheese into the stick to adhere. Transfer to prepared baking sheet.Do the same for remaining dough and cheese. Bake for 25 to 30 minutes, until firm and cheese is lightly browned. Remove from oven and let cool completely. Enjoy.

537. CRISPY PARMESAN TOMATO CHIPS

Servings: 6 People
Preparation time: 10 minutes
Cooking time: 5 hours
Total time: 5 hours 10 minutes
Calories: 88 kcal

Ingredients:

- 6 cups thinly sliced beefsteak tomatoes
- 2 tablespoons extra virgin olive oil
- 2 tsp. sea salt
- 1 tsp. garlic powder
- 2 tablespoons fresh chopped parsley
- 2 tablespoons grated Parmesan cheese

Directions:

1. Gently drizzle and toss the sliced tomatoes in the olive oil to coat slices and place slices without overlapping in a baking pan.Preheat oven to 200 degrees F. Combine and whisk the remaining ingredients together in a small bowl whisk.Sprinkle mixture over each slice. Depending on how thick the slices of tomato are check every 30 minutes until edges show some charring, could take 4 to 5 hours.Serve and enjoy.

538. PARMESAN ZUCCHINI ROUNDS

Preparation time: 10 minutes
Cooking time: 20 minutes
Servings: 12 People

Ingredients:

- 3 large zucchinis, sliced (6 cups sliced rounds)
- 1 whole egg
- 1 egg white
- 1½ cups Parmesan cheese, grated
- ¼ cup of fresh parsley, chopped
- ½ teaspoon of garlic powder
- olive oil cooking spray

Directions:

1. Preheat oven to 425 degrees and spray baking sheets with cooking spray.Beat the egg and white in a shallow bowl, set aside. Meanwhile combine the Parmesan, garlic powder and parsley in another bowl and mix well.Dip zucchini rounds in egg mixture then in Parmesan and place on baking sheet. Bake for 10 minutes on both sides. Do not overlap zucchini on the baking sheet. Serve and enjoy.

539. CHEDDAR CAULIFLOWER BACON BITES

Preparation time: 10 minutes
Cooking time: 15 minutes
Servings: 6 Serves
Calories: 172 kcal

Ingredients:

- 4 cups cauliflower florets
- 6 ounces of uncured nitrate free bacon cooked till crisp
- 1 egg
- 1 teaspoon baking powder
- ¼ teaspoon salt
- 1/3 cup scallions chopped
- ½ cup coconut flour
- 1 cup shredded cheddar cheese
- Get Ingredients Powered by Chicory

Directions:

1. Start by heating the oven to 400 degrees. Steam cauliflower until tender. Allow to cool then add to food processor.Pulse until fine crumbs, then place in a large bowl and add the rest of the ingredients.Stir until combined. Oil a mini muffin tin. Fill mini muffin cups by adding a heaping tablespoon of batter and pressing into each cup, about 30 cups.Bake for 15 minutes and allow to cool about for 10 minutes then remove from pan.Enjoy immediately!

540. JALAPENO POPPER DIP

Preparation time: 10 minutes
Cooking time: 30 minutes

Ingredients:

- 1 pound of bacon, fried, drained, and chopped
- 2 8 ounces of packages reduced fat cream cheese, softened
- ½ cup mayonnaise
- ½ cup Greek yogurt
- 2 tablespoons of sriracha chili sauce
- 4 to 6 jalapenos, deseeded and chopped
- 1½ cups shredded cheese of choice (I used a Mexican blend)
- ½ teaspoon of each onion powder and dill weed

Topping:

- ¼ cup salted butter, melted
- ½ cup grated parmesan cheese (the kind from the green shake container)
- 6 Light Rye Wasa crackers, crushed (¾ cup crushed pork rinds or Joseph's pita crumbs might work as well)

Directions:

1. Set a small amount of chopped bacon aside for topping. Throw all the dip ingredients in a blender and blend until mostly smooth.Spread the dip into a 10-inch round baking. Combine the topping ingredients and sprinkle evenly on top of the dip. Then top with reserved bacon bits.Bake at 350 degrees F for 20 to 30 minutes. Serve with veggies. Enjoy.

541. CREAM CHEESE STUFFED MEATBALLS

Preparation time: 15 minutes
Cooking time: 15 minutes

Ingredients

Meatballs:

- 1 spring onion finely sliced
- 1 clove garlic crushed
- 750 g ground/mincemeat. I used pork
- salt and pepper to taste
- 1 egg slightly beaten
- 2 slices bacon finely chopped
- 3 tablespoons of sun-dried tomatoes finely diced
- 2 tablespoon of favourite herbs - I use rosemary, thyme, oregano and sage

Filling:

- 110 g cream cheese diced into squares

Instructions:

1. In a large mixing bowl combine all the meatball ingredients. Mix thoroughly with your hands.Scoop up a golf ball size of meatball mixture (Use a dessert spoon). Squeeze the mixture into a ball then flatten into a circle.In the centre of the meatball circle, place a cube of cream cheese then fold the meatball mixture around the cream cheese. Place the cream cheese stuffed meatball on a greased baking tray. Do the same for the remaining mixture. Spray them all with olive oil spray so they will crisp and brown beautifully. Place in the oven and bake at 180C/350F for 15 to 20minutes. Serve and enjoy.

542. CUCUMBER CREAM CHEESE SANDWICHES

Preparation time: 5 minutes
Cooking time: 15 minutes
Servings: Serves 20
Calories: 47kcal

Ingredients:

- 3 oz. of cream cheese
- 1 medium cucumber
- 1 tbsp. sour cream
- dash salt
- dash pepper
- dash celery salt
- dash garlic powder
- Flaxseed Bread or other low carb bread
- Low Carb Sweeteners | Keto Sweetener Conversion Chart

Directions:

1. Grate cucumber and let drain until most of the liquid is gone. Then mix the cream cheese, medium cucumber, sour cream until smooth. Season with salt, pepper, celery salt and garlic powder. Cut the low carb flax bread squares in half through the middle height of the slice to make them thinner. Spread cucumber mixture on bottom slice and cover with top slice. Cut in half to make finger size.Serve immediately, enjoy.

543. SALT AND VINEGAR ZUCCHINI CHIPS

Preparation time: 15 minutes
Cooking time: 12 hours
Total time: 12 hours 15 minutes
Servings: Serves 8

Ingredients:

- 4 cups thinly sliced zucchini about 2-3 medium
- 2 tablespoons extra virgin olive oil avocado oil or sunflower oil
- 2 tablespoons white balsamic vinegar
- 2 teaspoons coarse sea salt

Directions:

1. Use a mandolin or slice zucchini as thin as possible. Then whisk olive oil and vinegar together in a small bowl.Place zucchini in a large bowl and toss with oil and vinegar. Place zucchini in even layers to dehydrator then sprinkle evenly with coarse sea salt.Depending on how thin you sliced the zucchini and, on your dehydrator, the drying time will vary, about 8 to 14 hours. To make in the oven: Line a cookie sheet with parchment paper. Place zucchini evenly and bake at 200 degrees F for 2 to 3 hours. Rotate half way during cooking time. Store chips in an airtight container. Enjoy.

544. CHICKEN SALAD

CUCUMBER BITES

Servings: 8 people
Preparation time: 5 minutes
Cooking time: 20 minutes
Calories: 74 kcal

Ingredients:

- 1 English cucumber
- 7 oz. cooked chicken breast
- 2 tablespoons of mayonnaise
- 2 scallions chopped
- 2 tablespoons of fresh cilantro
- ¼ teaspoon of ground cumin
- salt and pepper to taste
- Kalamata, black or green olives for topping optional

Directions:

1. Slice the cucumber in squares. Shred your chicken with a food processor if you have one or you can use a fork.In a bowl thoroughly mix the chicken, mayo, cilantro, scallions and cumin and salt and pepper.Lay a slice of cucumber on the plate you will serve the appetizer on. Add a heaping tablespoon of the chicken salad on the cucumber, lay another piece on top.Use toothpick to hold it together. Place Kalamata, black or green olives through the top of the toothpick to pretty it up!Keep refrigerated until ready to serve. Enjoy.

545. HAM AND DILL PICKLE BITES

Preparation time: 5 minutes
Cooking time: 45 minutes

Ingredients:

- Dill pickles
- Thin deli ham slices
- Cream cheese (or use whipped cream cheese if you prefer)

Directions:

1. Let the cream cheese sit for at least 30 minutes at room temperature before you make these.Cut dill pickles lengthwise into sixths, depending on how thick the pickles are. You need as many cut pickle spears as you have ham slices.Spread each slice of ham with a very thin layer of cream cheese. Place a dill pickle on the edge of each ham slice. Then roll up the ham around the dill pickle, and place toothpicks where you want each piece to be cut. Arrange on plate and serve. Enjoy.

546. SMOKED SALMON & CUCUMBER

Preparation time: 5 minutes
Cooking time: 15 minutes
Gross time: 20 minutes
Servings: 24
Calories: 20.7kcal

- **Ingredients:**
- ½ cup non-fat plain Greek yogurt
- 1 tablespoon capers chopped
- 1 tablespoon chopped dill
- 24¼ -inch thick English cucumber slices
- 4 ounces smoked salmon cut into 24 pieces
- Dill for garnish

Directions:

1. Mix together the Greek yogurt, capers and chopped dill in a small bowl.Place 1 teaspoon of yogurt sauce onto each cucumber slice. Then top each with a piece of smoked salmon and a small sprig of dill. Serve and enjoy.

547. ALMONDS & BLUEBERRIES SMOOTHIE

Servings: 2
Preparation Time: 5 minutes

Ingredients

- 1/4 cup ground almonds, unsalted
- 1 cup fresh blueberries
- Fresh juice of a 1 lemon
- 1 cup fresh Kale leaves
- 1/2 cup coconut water
- 1 cup water
- 2 Tbsp plain yogurt (optional)

Directions:

1. Dump all Ingredients in your high-speed blender, and blend until your smoothie is smooth.
2. Pour the mixture in a chilled glass.
3. Serve and enjoy!

Nutrition:

Calories: 110 Carbohydrates: 8g Proteins: 2g Fat: 7g Fiber: 2g

548. ALMONDS AND ZUCCHINI SMOOTHIE

Servings: 2
Preparation Time: 5 minutes

Ingredients

- 1 cup zucchini, cooked and mashed - unsalted
- 1 1/2 cups almond milk
- 1 Tbsp almond butter (plain, unsalted)
- 1 tsp pure almond extract
- 2 Tbsp ground almonds or Macadamia almonds
- 1/2 cup water
- 1 cup Ice cubes crushed (optional, For serving)

Directions:

1. Dump all Ingredients from the list above in your fast-speed blender; blend for 45 - 60 seconds or to taste.
2. Serve with crushed ice.

Nutrition:

Calories: 322 Carbohydrates: 6g Proteins: 6g Fat: 30g Fiber: 3.5g

549. AVOCADO WITH WALNUT BUTTER SMOOTHIE

Servings: 2
Preparation Time: 5 minutes

Ingredients

- 1 avocado (diced)
- 1 cup baby spinach
- 1 cup coconut milk (canned)
- 1 Tbsp walnut butter, unsalted
- 2 Tbsp natural sweetener such as Stevia, Erythritol, Truvia...etc.

Directions:

1. Place all Ingredients into food processor or a blender; blend until smooth or to taste.
2. Add more or less walnut butter.
3. Drink and enjoy!

Nutrition:

Calories: 364 Carbohydrates: 7g Proteins: 8g Fat: 35g Fiber: 5.5g

550. BABY SPINACH AND DILL SMOOTHIE

Servings: 2
Preparation Time: 5 minutes

Ingredients

- 1 cup of fresh baby spinach leaves
- 2 Tbsp of fresh dill, chopped
- 1 1/2 cup of water
- 1/2 avocado, chopped into cubes
- 1 Tbsp chia seeds (optional)
- 2 Tbsp of natural sweetener Stevia or Erythritol (optional)

Directions:

1. Place all Ingredients into fast-speed blender. Beat until smooth and all Ingredients united well.
2. Serve and enjoy!

Nutrition:

Calories: 136 Carbohydrates: 8g Proteins: 7g Fat: 10g Fiber: 9g

551. BLUEBERRIES AND COCONUT SMOOTHIE

Servings: 5
Preparation Time: 5 minutes

Ingredients

1. 1 cup of frozen blueberries, unsweetened
2. 1 cup Stevia or Erythritol sweetener
3. 2 cups coconut milk (canned)
4. 1 cup of fresh spinach leaves
5. 2 Tbsp shredded coconut (unsweetened)
6. 3/4 cup water

Directions:

1. Place all Ingredients from the list in food-processor or in your strong blender.
2. Blend for 45 - 60 seconds or to taste.
3. Ready for drink! Serve!

Nutrition:

Calories: 190 Carbohydrates: 8g Proteins: 3g Fat: 18g Fiber: 2g

552. COLLARD GREENS AND CUCUMBER SMOOTHIE

Servings: 2
Preparation Time: 15 minutes

Ingredients

- 1 cup Collard greens
- A few fresh pepper mint leaves
- 1 big cucumber
- 1 lime, freshly juiced
- 1/2 cups avocado sliced
- 1 1/2 cup water
- 1 cup crushed ice
- 1/4 cup of natural sweetener Erythritol or Stevia (optional)

Directions:

1. Rinse and clean your Collard greens from any dirt.
2. Place all Ingredients in a food processor or blender,
3. Blend until all Ingredients in your smoothie is combined well.
4. Pour in a glass and drink. Enjoy!

Nutrition:

Calories: 123 Carbohydrates: 8g Proteins: 4g Fat: 11g Fiber: 6g

553. CREAMY DANDELION GREENS AND CELERY SMOOTHIE

Servings: 2
Preparation Time: 10 minutes

Ingredients

- 1 handful of raw dandelion greens
- 2 celery sticks
- 2 Tbsp chia seeds
- 1 small piece of ginger, minced
- 1/2 cup almond milk
- 1/2 cup of water
- 1/2 cup plain yogurt

Directions:

1. Rinse and clean dandelion leaves from any dirt; add in a high-speed blender.
2. Clean the ginger; keep only inner part and cut in small slices; add in a blender.
3. Add all remaining Ingredients and blend until smooth.
4. Serve and enjoy!

Nutrition:

Calories: 58 Carbohydrates: 5g Proteins: 3g Fat: 6g Fiber: 3g

554. DARK TURNIP GREENS SMOOTHIE

Servings: 2
Preparation Time: 10 minutes

Ingredients

- 1 cup of raw turnip greens
- 1 1/2 cup of almond milk
- 1 Tbsp of almond butter
- 1/2 cup of water

- 1/2 tsp of cocoa powder, unsweetened
- 1 Tbsp of dark chocolate chips
- 1/4 tsp of cinnamon
- A pinch of salt
- 1/2 cup of crushed ice

Directions:

1. Rinse and clean turnip greens from any dirt.
2. Place the turnip greens in your blender along with all other Ingredients.
3. Blend it for 45 - 60 seconds or until done; smooth and creamy.
4. Serve with or without crushed ice.

Nutrition:

Calories: 131 Carbohydrates: 6g Proteins: 4g Fat: 10g Fiber: 2.5g

555. BUTTER PECAN AND COCONUT SMOOTHIE

Servings: 2
Preparation Time: 5 minutes

Ingredients

- 1 cup coconut milk, canned
- 1 scoop Butter Pecan powdered creamer
- 2 cups fresh spinach leaves, chopped
- 1/2 banana frozen or fresh
- 2 Tbsp stevia granulated sweetener to taste
- 1/2 cup water
- 1 cup ice cubes crushed

Directions:

1. Place Ingredients from the list above in your high-speed blender.
2. Blend for 35 - 50 seconds or until all Ingredients combined well.
3. Add less or more crushed ice.
4. Drink and enjoy!

Nutrition:

Calories: 268 Carbohydrates: 7g Proteins: 6g Fat: 26g Fiber: 1.5g

556. FRESH CUCUMBER, KALE AND RASPBERRY SMOOTHIE

Servings: 3
Preparation Time: 10 minutes

Ingredients

- 1 1/2 cups of cucumber, peeled
- 1/2 cup raw kale leaves
- 1 1/2 cups fresh raspberries
- 1 cup of almond milk
- 1 cup of water
- Ice cubes crushed (optional)
- 2 Tbsp natural sweetener (Stevia, Erythritol...etc.)

Directions:

1. Place all Ingredients from the list in a food processor or high-speed blender; blend for 35 - 40 seconds.
2. Serve into chilled glasses.
3. Add more natural sweeter if you like. Enjoy!

Nutrition:

Calories: 70 Carbohydrates: 8g Proteins: 3g Fat: 6g Fiber: 5g

557. FRESH LETTUCE AND CUCUMBER-LEMON SMOOTHIE

Servings: 2
Preparation Time: 10 minutes

Ingredients

- 2 cups fresh lettuce leaves, chopped (any kind)
- 1 cup of cucumber
- 1 lemon, washed and sliced.
- 1/2 avocado
- 2 Tbsp chia seeds
- 1 1/2 cup water or coconut water
- 1/4 cup stevia granulate sweetener (or to taste)

Directions:

1. Add all Ingredients from the list above in the high-speed blender; blend until completely smooth.
2. Pour your smoothie into chilled glasses and enjoy!

Nutrition:

Calories: 51 Carbohydrates: 4g Proteins: 2g Fat: 4g Fiber: 3.5g

558. GREEN COCONUT SMOOTHIE

Servings: 2
Preparation Time: 10 minutes

Ingredients

- 1 1/4 cup coconut milk (canned)
- 2 Tbsp chia seeds
- 1 cup of fresh kale leaves
- 1 cup of spinach leaves
- 1 scoop vanilla protein powder
- 1 cup ice cubes
- Granulated stevia sweetener (to taste; optional)
- 1/2 cup water

Directions:

1. Rinse and clean kale and the spinach leaves from any dirt.
2. Add all Ingredients in your blender.
3. Blend until you get a nice smoothie.
4. Serve into chilled glass.

Nutrition:

Calories: 179 Carbohydrates: 5g Proteins: 4g Fat: 18g Fiber: 2.5g

559. INSTANT COFFEE SMOOTHIE

Servings: 2
Preparation Time: 20 minutes

Ingredients

- 2 cups of instant coffee
- 1 cup almond milk (or coconut milk)
- 1/4 cup heavy cream
- 2 Tbsp cocoa powder (unsweetened)
- 1 - 2 Handful of fresh spinach leaves
- 10 drops liquid stevia

Directions:

1. Make a coffee; set aside.
2. Place all remaining Ingredients in your fast-speed blender; blend for 45 - 60 seconds or until done.
3. Pour your instant coffee in a blender and continue to blend for further 30 - 45 seconds.
4. Serve immediately.

Nutrition:

Calories: 142 Carbohydrates: 6g Proteins: 5g Fat: 14g Fiber: 3g

560. KETO BLOOD SUGAR ADJUSTER SMOOTHIE

Servings: 2
Preparation Time: 10 minutes

Ingredients

- 2 cups of green cabbage
- 1/2 avocado
- 1 Tbsp Apple cider vinegar
- Juice of 1 small lemon
- 1 cup of water
- 1 cup of crushed ice cubes For serving

Directions:

1. Place all Ingredients in your high-speed blender or in a food processor and blend until smooth and soft.
2. Serve in chilled glasses with crushed ice.
3. Enjoy!

Nutrition:

Calories: 74 Carbohydrates: 7g Proteins: 2g Fat: 6g Fiber: 4g

561. LIME SPINACH SMOOTHIE

Servings: 2
Preparation Time: 5 minutes

Ingredients

- 1 cup water
- 1 lime juice (2 limes)
- 1 green apple cut into chunks; core discarded
- 2 cups fresh spinach, roughly chopped
- 1/2 cup fresh chopped fresh mint
- 1/2 avocado
- Ice crushed
- 1/4 tsp ground cinnamon
- 1 Tbsp natural sweetener of your choice (optional)

Directions:

1. Place all Ingredients in your high-speed

blender.
2. Blend for 45 - 60 seconds or until your smoothie is smooth and creamy.
3. Serve in a chilled glass.
4. Adjust sweetener to taste.

Nutrition:

Calories: 112 Carbohydrates: 8g Proteins: 4g Fat: 10g Fiber: 5.5g

562. PROTEIN COCONUT SMOOTHIE

Servings: 2
Preparation Time: 15 minutes

Ingredients

- 1 1/2 cup of coconut milk canned
- 1 cup of fresh spinach finely chopped
- 1 scoop vanilla protein powder
- 2 Tbsp chia seeds
- 1 cup of ice cubes crushed
- 2 - 3 Tbsp Stevia granulated natural sweetener (optional)

Directions:

1. Rinse and clean your spinach leaves from any dirt.
2. Place all Ingredients from the list above in a blender.
3. Blend until you get a smoothie like consistently.
4. Serve into chilled glass and it is ready to drink.

Nutrition:

Calories: 377 Carbohydrates: 7g Proteins: 10g Fat: 38g Fiber: 2g

563. STRONG SPINACH AND HEMP SMOOTHIE

Servings: 3
Preparation Time: 10 minutes

Ingredients

- 1 cup almond milk
- 1 small ripe banana
- 2 Tbsp hemp seeds
- 2 handful fresh spinach leaves
- 1 tsp pure vanilla extract
- 1 cup of water
- 2 Tbsp of natural sweetener such Stevia, Truvia...etc.

Directions:

1. First, rinse and clean your spinach leaves from any dirt.
2. Place the spinach in a blender or food processor along with remaining Ingredients.
3. Blend for 45 - 60 seconds or until done.
4. Add more or less sweetener.
5. Serve.

Nutrition:

Calories: 75 Carbohydrates: 7g Proteins: 4g Fat: 6g Fiber: 3g

564. TOTAL ALMOND SMOOTHIE

Servings: 2
Preparation Time: 15 minutes

Ingredients

- 1 1/2 cups of almond milk
- 2 Tbsp of almond butter
- 2 Tbsp ground almonds
- 1 cup of fresh kale leaves (or to taste)
- 1/2 tsp of cocoa powder
- 1 Tbsp chia seeds
- 1/2 cup of water

Directions:

1. Rinse and carefully clean kale leaves from any dirt.
2. Add almond milk, almond butter and ground almonds in your blender; blend for 45 - 60 seconds.
3. Add kale leaves, cocoa powder and chia seeds; blend for further 45 seconds.
4. If your smoothie is too thick, pour more almond milk or water.
5. Serve.

Nutrition:

Calories: 228 Carbohydrates: 7g Proteins: 8g Fat: 11g Fiber: 6g

565. ULTIMATE GREEN MIX SMOOTHIE

Servings: 2

Preparation Time: 15 minutes

Ingredients

- Handful of spinach leaves
- Handful of collard greens
- Handful of lettuce, any kind
- 1 1/2 cup of almond milk
- 1/2 cup of water
- 1/4 cup of stevia granulated sweetener
- 1 tsp pure vanilla extract
- 1 cup crushed ice cubes (optional)

Directions:

1. Rinse and carefully clean your greens from any dirt.
2. Place all Ingredients from the list above in your blender or food processor.
3. Blend until done or 45 - 30 seconds.
4. Serve with or without crushed ice.

Nutrition:

Calories: 73 Carbohydrates: 4g Proteins: 5g Fat: 7g Fiber: 1g

566. FRUIT TRIFLE

Preparation Time: 35 minutes
Cooking time: 5 minutes
Servings:10

Ingredients:

- 8 oz biscuits, chopped
- ¼ cup strawberries, chopped
- 1 banana, chopped
- 1 peach, chopped
- ½ mango, chopped
- 1 cup grapes, chopped
- 1 tablespoon liquid honey
- 1 cup of orange juice
- ½ cup Plain yogurt
- ¼ cup cream cheese
- 1 teaspoon coconut flakes

Directions:

1. Bring the orange juice to boil and remove it from the heat.
2. Add liquid honey and stir until it is dissolved.
3. Cool the liquid to the room temperature.
4. Add chopped banana, peach, mango, grapes, and strawberries. Shake the fruits gently and leave to soak the orange juice for 15 minutes.
5. Meanwhile, with the help of the hand mixer mix up together Plain yogurt and cream cheese.
6. Then separate the chopped biscuits, yogurt mixture, and fruits on 4 parts.
7. Place the first part of biscuits in the big serving glass in one layer.
8. Spread it with yogurt mixture and add fruits.
9. Repeat the same steps till you use all ingredients.
10. Top the trifle with coconut flakes.

Nutrition: calories 164, fat 6.2, fiber 1.3, carbs 24.8, protein 3.2

567. BERRY CRUMBLE

Preparation Time: 20 minutes
Cooking time: 35 minutes
Servings:6

Ingredients:

- 1 cup wheat flour, whole grain
- 1 cup blackberries
- 1/3 cup Erythritol
- ½ teaspoon ground clove
- ½ cup rolled oats
- 1/3 cup butter, softened

Directions:

1. In the mixing bowl combine together blackberries, Erythritol, and ground clove.
2. Then take another bowl and put rolled oats, butter, and wheat flour inside.
3. Mix up the ingredients until it is crumbly.
4. Line the round springform pan with baking paper.
5. Put the blackberry mixture inside the springform pan and flatten it with the help of the spoon.
6. After this, top the berries with all crumbly mixture.
7. Bake the crumble for 35 minutes at 365F.
8. Cook the crumble for 15 minutes before serving.

Nutrition: calories 203, fat 11, fiber 2.6, carbs 36.3, protein 3.5

568. GREEK CHEESECAKE

Preparation Time: 40 minutes
Cooking time: 10 minutes
Servings:6

Ingredients:

½ cup pistachio, chopped
4 teaspoons butter, softened
4 teaspoon Erythritol
2 cups cream cheese
½ cup cream, whipped

Directions:

1. Mix up together pistachios, butter, and Erythritol.

2. Put the mixture in the baking mold and bake for 10 minutes at 355F.
3. Meanwhile, whisk together cream cheese and whipped cream.
4. When the pistachio mixture is baked, chill it well.
5. After this, transfer the pistachio mixture in the round cake mold and flatten in one layer.
6. Then put the cream cheese mixture over the pistachio mixture, flatten the surface until smooth.
7. Cool the cheesecake in the fridge for 1 hour before serving.

Nutrition: calories 332, fat 33, fiber 0.5, carbs 7.4, protein 7

569. LEMON PIE

Preparation Time: 35 minutes
Cooking time: 30 minutes
Servings:6

Ingredients:

- ¼ cup lemon juice
- 1 cup cream
- 4 egg yolks
- 4 tablespoons Erythritol
- 1 tablespoon cornstarch
- 1 teaspoon vanilla extract
- 3 tablespoons butter
- 6 oz wheat flour, whole grain

Directions:

1. Mix up together wheat flour and butter and knead the soft dough.
2. Put the dough in the round cake mold and flatten it in the shape of pie crust.
3. Bake it for 15 minutes at 365F.
4. Meanwhile, make the lemon filling: Mix up together cream, egg yolks, and lemon juice. When the liquid is smooth, start to heat it up over the medium heat. Stir it constantly.
5. When the liquid is hot, add vanilla extract, cornstarch, and Erythritol. Whisk well until smooth.
6. Brin the lemon filling to boil and remove it from the heat.
7. Cool it to the room temperature.
8. Cook the pie crust to the room temperature.
9. Pour the lemon filling over the pie crust, flatten it well and leave to cool in the fridge for 25 minutes.

Nutrition: calories 225, fat 11.4, fiber 0.8, carbs 34.8, protein 5.2

570. GALAKTOBOUREKO

Preparation Time: 20 minutes
Cooking time: 1 hour
Servings:6

Ingredients:

- ½ cup milk
- 3 tablespoons semolina
- ½ cup butter, softened
- 8 Phyllo sheets
- 2 eggs, beaten
- 3 tablespoons Erythritol
- 1 teaspoon lemon rind
- 1 tablespoon lemon juice
- 1 teaspoon vanilla extract
- 2tablespoons liquid honey
- 1 teaspoon ground cinnamon
- ¼ cup of water

Directions:

1. Melt ½ part of all butter.
2. Then brush the casserole glass mold with the butter and place 1 Phyllo sheet inside.
3. Brush the Phyllo sheet with butter and cover it with second Phyllo sheet.
4. Make the dessert filling: heat up milk, and add semolina.
5. Stir it carefully.
6. After this, add remaining softened butter, Erythritol, and vanilla extract.
7. Bring the mixture to boil and simmer it for 2 minutes.
8. Remove it from the heat and cool to the room temperature.
9. Then add beaten eggs and mix up well.
10. Pour the semolina mixture in the mold over the Phyllo sheets, flatten it if needed.
11. Then cover the semolina mixture with remaining Phyllo sheets and brush with remaining melted butter.
12. Cut the dessert on the bars.

13. Bake galaktoboureko for 1 hour at 365F.
14. Then make the syrup: bring to boil lemon juice, honey, and water and remove the liquid from the heat.
15. Pour the syrup over the hot dessert and let it chill well.

Nutrition: calories 304, fat 18, fiber 1.1, carbs 39.4, protein 6.1

571. HONEY CAKE

Preparation Time: 15 minutes
Cooking time: 30 minutes
Servings: 6

Ingredients:

- ½ cup wheat flour, whole grain
- ½ cup semolina
- 1 teaspoon baking powder
- ½ cup Plain yogurt
- 1 teaspoon vanilla extract
- 4 tablespoons Erythritol
- 1 teaspoon lemon rind
- 2 tablespoons olive oil
- 1 tablespoon almond flakes
- 4 teaspoons liquid honey
- ½ cup of orange juice

Directions:

1. Mix up together wheat flour, semolina, baking powder, Plain yogurt, vanilla extract, Erythritol, and olive oil.
2. Then add lemon rind and mix up the ingredients until smooth.
3. Transfer the mixture in the non-sticky cake mold, sprinkle with almond flakes, and bake for 30 minutes at 365F.
4. Meanwhile, bring the orange juice to boil.
5. Add liquid honey and stir until dissolved.
6. When the cake is cooked, pour the hot orange juice mixture over it and let it rest for at least 10 minutes.
7. Cut the cake into the.

Nutrition: calories 179, fat 6.1, fiber 1.1, carbs 36.3, protein 4.5

572. PORTOKALOPITA

Preparation Time: 20 minutes
Cooking time: 60 minutes
Servings:8

Ingredients:

- 4 oranges
- 1/3 cup water
- ½ cup Erythritol
- ½ teaspoon ground cinnamon
- 4 eggs, beaten
- 3 tablespoons stevia powder
- 10 oz Phyllo pastry
- ½ teaspoon baking powder
- ½ cup Plain yogurt
- 3 tablespoons olive oil

Directions:

1. Squeeze the juice from 1 orange and pour it in the saucepan.
2. Add water, squeezed oranges, water, ground cinnamon, and Erythritol.
3. Bring the liquid to boil.
4. Simmer the liquid for 5 minutes over the medium heat. When the time is over, cool it.
5. Grease the baking mold with 1 tablespoon of olive oil.
6. Chop the phyllo dough and place it in the baking mold.
7. Slice ½ of orange for decorating the cake. Slice it.
8. Squeeze juice from remaining oranges.
9. Then mix up together, squeeze orange juice, Plain yogurt, baking powder, stevia powder, and eggs. Add remaining olive oil.
10. Mix up the mixture with the help of the hand mixer.
11. Pour the liquid over the chopped Phyllo dough.
12. Stir to evenly distribute.
13. Top the cake with sliced orange (that one which you leave for decorating).
14. Bake the dessert for 50 minutes at 370F.
15. Pour the baked cake with cooled orange juice syrup.
16. Leave it for 10 minutes to let the cake soaks the syrup.
17. Cut it into the.

Nutrition: calories 237, fat 9.9, fiber 3, carbs 46, protein 7

573. FINIKIA

Preparation Time: 15 minutes
Cooking time: 20 minutes
Servings:6

Ingredients:

- ½ teaspoon lemon zest, grated
- 4 tablespoons Erythritol
- 4 tablespoons semolina
- 2 tablespoons olive oil
- 8 tablespoons wheat flour, whole grain
- 1 teaspoon vanilla extract
- ½ teaspoon ground clove
- 3 tablespoons coconut oil
- ¼ teaspoon baking powder
- ¼ cup of water

Directions:

1. Make the dough: in the mixing bowl combine together lemon zest, semolina, olive oil, wheat flour, vanilla extract, ground clove, coconut oil, and baking powder.
2. Knead the soft dough.
3. Make the small cookies in the shape of walnuts and press them gently with the help of the fork.
4. Line the baking tray with the baking paper.
5. Place the cookies in the tray and bake them for 20 minutes at 375F.
6. Meanwhile, bring the water to boil.
7. Add Erythritol and simmer the liquid for 2 minutes over the medium heat. Cool it.
8. Pour the cooled sweet water over the hot baked cookies and leave them for 10 minutes.
9. When the cookies soak all liquid, transfer them in the serving plates.

Nutrition: calories 165, fat 11.7, fiber 0.6, carbs 23.7, protein 2

574. VASILOPITA

Preparation Time: 20 minutes
Cooking time: 40 minutes
Servings:4

Ingredients:

- 1 egg
- 3 tablespoons butter, softened
- 1 teaspoon baking powder
- 1/3 cup Erythritol
- 1 teaspoon vanilla extract
- ½ cup almond meal
- ½ cup wheat flour, whole grain
- 1 teaspoon orange zest, grated
- ¼ cup milk
- 1 tablespoon almond flakes

Directions:

1. Mix up together butter and Erythritol and start to mix it with the help of the cooking machine for 4 minutes over the medium speed.
2. Meanwhile, crack the egg and separate it into the egg yolk and egg white.
3. Add egg yolk in the butter mixture and keep mixing it for 2 minutes more,
4. After this, whisk the egg white till the strong peaks.
5. Add egg white in the butter mixture.
6. Then add vanilla extract and orange zest.
7. When the mixture is homogenous, switch off the cooking machine.
8. Add almond meal, wheat meal, and milk.
9. Mix up the dough until smooth and transfer it in the non-sticky round cake mold.
10. Flatten the surface of the cake with the help of the spatula and sprinkle with almond flakes.
11. Bake vasilopita for 40 minutes at 345F.
12. Chill the cooked pie well and cut on the.

Nutrition: calories 245, fat 17.4, fiber 2.3, carbs 36.4, protein 6.6

575. VANILLA BISCUITS

Preparation Time: 15 minutes
Cooking time: 40 minutes
Servings:6

Ingredients:

- 5 eggs
- ½ cup coconut flour
- ½ cup wheat flour
- 1/3 cup Erythritol

- 1 teaspoon vanilla extract
- Cooking spray

Directions:

1. Crack the eggs in the mixing bowl and mix it up with the help of the hand mixer.
2. Then add Erythritol and keep mixing the egg mixture until it will be changed into the lemon color.
3. Then add wheat flour, coconut flour, and vanilla extract.
4. Mix it up for 30 seconds more.
5. Spray the baking tray with cooking spray.
6. Pour the biscuit mixture in the tray and flatten it.
7. Bake it for 40 minutes at 350F.
8. When the biscuit is cooked, cut it on the serving squares.

Nutrition: calories 132, fat 4.7, fiber 4.3, carbs 28.3, protein 7

576. SEMOLINA PUDDING

Preparation Time: 15 minutes
Cooking time: 7 minutes
Servings:3

Ingredients:

- ½ cup organic almond milk
- ½ cup milk
- 1/3 cup semolina
- 1 tablespoon butter
- ¼ teaspoon cornstarch
- ½ teaspoon almond extract

Directions:

1. Pour almond milk and milk in the saucepan.
2. Bring it to boil and add semolina and cornstarch.
3. Mix up the ingredients until homogenous and simmer them for 1 minute.
4. After this, add almond extract and butter. Stir well and close the lid.
5. Remove the pudding from the heat and leave for 10 minutes.
6. Then mix it up again and transfer in the serving ramekins.

Nutrition: calories 201, fat 7.9, fiber 1.1, carbs 25.7, protein 5.8

577. WATERMELON JELLY

Preparation Time: 30 minutes
Cooking time: 5 minutes
Servings:2

Ingredients:

- 8 oz watermelon
- 1 tabelspoon gelatin powder

Directions:

1. Make the juice from the watermelon with the help of the fruit juicer.
2. Combine together 5 tablespoons of watermelon juice and 1 tablespoon of gelatin powder. Stir it and leave for 5 minutes.
3. Then preheat the watermelon juice until warm, add gelatin mixture and heat it up over the medium heat until gelatin is dissolved.
4. Then remove the liquid from the heat and pout it in the silicone molds.
5. Freeze the jelly for 30 minutes in the freezer or for 4 hours in the fridge.

Nutrition: calories 46, fat 0.2, fiber 0.4, carbs 8.5, protein 3.7

578. GREEK COOKIES

Preparation Time: 20 minutes
Cooking time: 725 minutes
Servings:6

Ingredients:

- ½ cup Plain yogurt
- ½ teaspoon baking powder
- 2 tablespoons Erythritol
- 1 teaspoon almond extract
- ½ teaspoon ground clove
- ½ teaspoon orange zest, grated
- 3 tablespoons walnuts, chopped
- 1 cup wheat flour
- 1 teaspoon butter, softened
- 1 tablespoon honey
- 3 tablespoons water

Directions:

1. In the mixing bowl mix up together Plain yogurt, baking powder, Erythritol, almond

extract, ground cloves orange zest, flour, and butter.

2. Knead the non-sticky dough. Add olive oil if the dough is very sticky and knead it well.
3. Then make the log from the dough and cut it into small pieces.
4. Roll every piece of dough into the balls and transfer in the lined with baking paper tray.
5. Press the balls gently and bake for 25 minutes at 350F.
6. Meanwhile, heat up together honey and water. Simmer the liquid for 1 minute and remove from the heat.
7. When the cookies are cooked, remove them from the oven and let them cool for 5 minutes.
8. Then pour the cookies with sweet honey water and sprinkle with walnuts.
9. Cool the cookies.

Nutrition: calories 134, fat 3.4, fiber 0.9, carbs 26.1, protein 4.3

579. BAKED FIGS WITH HONEY

Preparation Time: 10 minutes
Cooking time: 15 minutes
Servings:4

Ingredients:

- 4 figs
- 4 teaspoons honey
- 1 oz Blue cheese, chopped

Directions:

1. Make the cross cuts in the figs and fill them with chopped Blue cheese.
2. Then sprinkle the figs with honey and wrap in the foil.
3. Bake the figs for 15 minutes at 355F.
4. Remove the figs from the foil and transfer in the serving plates.

Nutrition: calories 94, fat 2.2, fiber 1.9, carbs 18.1, protein 2.2

580. CREAM STRAWBERRY PIES

Preparation Time: 20 minutes
Cooking time: 15 minutes
Servings:6

Ingredients:

- 1 cup strawberries
- 7 oz puff pastry
- 3 teaspoons butter, softened
- 3 teaspoons Erythritol
- ¼ teaspoon ground nutmeg
- 4 teaspoons cream

Directions:

1. Roll up the puff pastry and cut it on 6 squares.
2. Slice the strawberries.
3. Grease every puff pastry square with butter and then place the sliced strawberries on it.
4. Sprinkle every strawberry square with cream, ground nutmeg, and Erythritol.
5. Secure the edges of every puff pastry square in the shape of a pie.
6. Line the baking tray with baking paper.
7. Transfer the pies in the tray and place the tray in the oven.
8. Bake the pies for 15 minutes at 375F.

Nutrition: calories 209, fat 14.8, fiber 1, carbs 19.4, protein 2.6

581. BANANA MUFFINS

Preparation Time: 10 minutes
Cooking time: 12 minutes
Servings:4

Ingredients:

- 4 tablespoons wheat flour
- 2 bananas, peeled
- 1 tablespoon Plain yogurt
- ½ teaspoon baking powder
- ¼ teaspoon lemon juice
- 1 teaspoon vanilla extract

Directions:

1. Mash the bananas with the help of the fork.
2. Then combine mashed bananas with flour, yogurt, baking powder, and lemon juice.
3. Add vanilla extract and stir the batter until smooth.
4. Fill ½ part of every muffin mold with banana batter and bake them for 12 minutes at 365F.

5. Chill the muffins and remove them from the muffin molds.

Nutrition: calories 87, fat 0.3, fiber 1.8, carbs 20.2, protein 1.7

582. GRILLED PINEAPPLE

Preparation Time: 7 minutes
Cooking time: 5 minutes
Servings:4

Ingredients:

- 10 oz fresh pineapple
- ½ teaspoon ground ginger
- 1 tablespoon almond butter, softened

Directions:

1. Slice the pineapple into the serving pieces and brush with almond butter.
2. After this, sprinkle every pineapple piece with ground ginger.
3. Preheat the grill to 400F.
4. Grill the pineapple for 2 minutes from each side.
5. The cooked fruit should have a light brown surface of both sides.

Nutrition: calories 61, fat 2.4, fiber 1.4, carbs 10.2, proteinb 1.3

583. COCONUT-MINT BARS

Preparation Time: 35 minutes
Cooking time: 1 minute
Servings:6

Ingredients:

- 3 tablespoons coconut butter
- ½ cup coconut flakes
- 1 egg, beaten
- 1 tablespoon cocoa powder
- 3 oz graham crackers, crushed
- 2 tablespoons Erythritol
- 3 tablespoons butter
- 1 teaspoon mint extract
- 1 teaspoon stevia powder
- 1 teaspoon of cocoa powder
- 1 tablespoon almond butter, melted

Directions:

1. Churn together coconut butter, coconut flakes, and 1 tablespoon of cocoa powder.
2. Then microwave the mixture for 1 minute or until it is melted.
3. Chill the liquid for 1 minute and fast add egg. Whisk it until homogenous and smooth.
4. Stir the liquid in the graham crackers and transfer in the mold. Flatten it well with the help of the spoon.
5. After this, blend together Erythritol, butter, mint extract, and stevia powder.
6. When the mixture is fluffy, place it over the graham crackers layer.
7. Then mix up together 1 teaspoon of cocoa powder and almond butter.
8. Sprinkle the cooked mixture with cocoa liquid and flatten it.
9. Refrigerate the dessert for 30 minutes.
10. Then cut it into the bars.

Nutrition: calories 213, fat 16.3, fiber 2.9, carbs 20, protein 3.5

584. HUMMINGBIRD CAKE

Preparation Time: 20 minutes
Cooking time: 30 minutes
Servings:10

Ingredients:

- 1 cup of rice flour
- 1 cup coconut flour
- ½ cup wheat flour
- ½ cup Erythritol
- ½ teaspoon baking powder
- ¾ teaspoon salt
- 1/3 teaspoon ground cinnamon
- ½ cup olive oil
- 2 eggs, beaten
- 3 oz pineapple, chopped
- 1 banana, chopped
- 3 tablespoons walnuts, chopped
- 6 tablespoons cream cheese

Directions:

1. In the mixing bowl combine together 9 first ingredients from the list above.
2. When the mixture is smooth and add pineapple and bananas.
3. Add walnuts and mix up the dough well.

4. Put the dough into the baking pans and bake for 30 minutes at 355F.
5. Then remove the cooked cakes from the oven and chill well.
6. Spread every cake with cream cheese and form them into 1 big cake.

Nutrition: calories 278, fat 16, fiber 6, carbs 41.9, protein 5.5

585. COOL MANGO MOUSSE

Preparation Time: 8 minutes
Cooking time: 30 minutes
Servings:6

Ingredients:

- 2 cups coconut cream, chipped
- 6 teaspoons honey
- 2 mango, chopped

Directions:

1. Blend together honey and mango.
2. When the mixture is smooth, combine it with whipped cream and stir carefully.
3. Put the mango-cream mixture in the serving glasses and refrigerate for 30 minutes.

Nutrition: calories 272, fat 19.5, fiber 3.6, carbs 27, protein 2.8

586. SWEET POTATO BROWNIES

Preparation Time: 5 minutes
Cooking time: 30 minutes
Servings:6

Ingredients:

- 1 tablespoon cocoa powder
- 1 sweet potato, peeled, boiled
- ½ cup wheat flour
- 1 teaspoon baking powder
- 1 tablespoon butter
- 1 tablespoon olive oil
- 2 tablespoons Erythritol

Directions:

1. In the mixing bowl combine together all ingredients.
2. Mix them well until you get a smooth batter.
3. After this, pour the brownie batter in the brownie mold and flatten it.
4. Bake it for 30 minutes at 365F.
5. After this, cut the brownies into the serving bars.

Nutrition: calories 95, fat 4.5, fiber 1.2, carbs 17.8, protein 1.6

587. PUMPKIN COOKIES

Preparation Time: 10 minutes
Cooking time: 30 minutes
Servings:6

Ingredients:

- 1 egg, beaten
- 1 teaspoon vanilla extract
- ½ teaspoon ground cinnamon
- 1 teaspoon ground turmeric
- 1 tablespoon butter, softened
- 1 cup wheat flour
- 1 teaspoon baking powder
- 4 tablespoons pumpkin puree
- 1 tablespoon Erythritol

Directions:

1. Put all ingredients in the mixing bowl and knead the soft and non-sticky dough.
2. After this, line the baking tray with baking paper.
3. Make 6 balls from the dough and press them gently with the help of the spoon.
4. Arrange the dough balls in the tray.
5. Bake the cookies for 30 minutes at 355F.
6. Chill the cooked cookies well and store them in the glass jar.

Nutrition: calories 111, fat 2.9, fiber 1.1, carbs 20.2, protein 3.2

588. BAKED PLUMS

Preparation Time: 8 minutes
Cooking time: 20 minutes
Servings:4

Ingredients:

- 4 plums, pitted, halved, not soft
- 1 tablespoon peanuts, chopped
- 1 tablespoon honey
- ½ teaspoon lemon juice
- 1 teaspoon coconut oil

Directions:

1. Make the packet from the foil and place the plum halves in it.
2. Then sprinkle the plums with honey, lemon juice, coconut oil, and peanuts.
3. Bake the plums for 20 minutes at 350F.

Nutrition: calories 69, fat 2.5, fiber 1.1, carbs 12.7, protein1.1

589. CLASSIC PARFAIT

Preparation Time: 10 minutes
Cooking time: 20 minutes
Servings:4

Ingredients:

- 1 cup Plain yogurt
- 1 tablespoon coconut flakes
- 1 tablespoon liquid honey
- 4 teaspoons peanuts, chopped
- 1 cup blackberries
- 1 tablespoon pomegranate seeds

Directions:

1. Mix up together plain yogurt and coconut flakes.
2. Put the mixture in the freezer.
3. Meanwhile, combine together liquid honey and blackberries.
4. Place ½ part of blackberry mixture in the serving glasses.
5. Then add ¼ part of the cooled yogurt mixture.
6. Sprinkle the yogurt mixture with all peanuts and cover with ½ part of remaining yogurt mixture.
7. Then add remaining blackberries and top the dessert with yogurt.
8. Garnish the parfait with pomegranate seeds and cool in the fridge for 20 minutes.

Nutrition: calories 115, fat 3.1, fiber 3, carbs 13, protein 5.1

590. MELON POPSICLES

Preparation Time: 10 minutes
Cooking time: 2 hours
Servings:4

Ingredients:

- 9 oz melon, peeled, chopped
- 1 tablespoon Erythritol
- ½ cup of orange juice

Directions:

1. Blend the melon until smooth and combine it with Erythritol and orange juice.
2. Mix up the liquid until Erythritol is dissolved.
3. Then pour the liquid into the popsicles molds.
4. Freeze the popsicles for 2 hours in the freezer.

Nutrition: calories 36, fat 0.2, fiber 0.6, carbs 12.2, protein 0.8

591. WATERMELON SALAD WITH SHAVED CHOCOLATE

Preparation Time: 10 minutes
Cooking time: 0 minutes
Servings:6

Ingredients:

- 14 oz watermelon
- 1 oz dark chocolate
- 3 tablespoons coconut cream
- 1 teaspoon Erythritol
- 2 kiwi, chopped
- 1 oz Feta cheese, crumbled

Directions:

1. Peel the watermelon and remove the seeds from it.
2. Chop the fruit and place in the salad bowl.
3. Add chopped kiwi and crumbled Feta. Stir the salad well.
4. Then mix up together coconut cream and Erythritol.
5. Pour the cream mixture over the salad.
6. Then shave the chocolate over the salad with the help of the potato peeler.
7. The salad should be served immediately.

Nutrition: calories 90, fat 4.4, fiber 1.4, carbs 12.9, protein 1.9

592. NO-BAKE STRAWBERRY CHEESECAKE

Servings: 8
Preparation Time: 20 minutes
Cooking Time: 5 minutes

Ingredients:

For Crust:

- 1 cup almonds
- 1 cup pecans
- 2 tablespoons unsweetened coconut flakes
- 6 Medjool dates, pitted, soaked for 10 minutes and drained
- Pinch of salt

For Filling:

- 3 cups cashews, soaked and drained
- ¼ cup organic honey
- ¼ cup fresh lemon juice
- 1/3 cup coconut oil, melted
- 1 teaspoon organic vanilla flavor
- ¼ teaspoon salt
- 1 cup fresh strawberries, hulled and sliced

For Topping:

- 1/3 cup maple syrup
- 1/3 cup water
- Drop of vanilla flavor
- 5 cups fresh strawberries, hulled, sliced and divided

Directions:

1. Grease a 9-inch spring foam pan.
2. For crust in the small mixer, add almonds and pecans and pulse till finely grounded.
3. Add remaining all ingredients and pulse till smooth.
4. Transfer the crust mixture into prepared pan, pressing gently downwards. Freeze to create completely.
5. In a large blender, add all filling ingredients and pulse till creamy and smooth.
6. Place filling mixture over crust evenly.
7. Freeze for at least couple of hours or till set completely.
8. In a pan, add maple syrup, water, vanilla and 1 cup of strawberries on medium-low heat.
9. Bring to a gentle simmer. Simmer for around 4-5 minutes or till thickens.
10. Strain the sauce and allow it to go cool completely.
11. Top the chilled cheesecake with strawberry slices. Drizzle with sauce and serve.

Nutrition:

Calories: 294 Fat: 12g, Carbohydrates: 32g, Fiber: 2g, Protein: 5.2g

593. RAW LIME, AVOCADO & COCONUT PIE

Servings: 8
Preparation Time: 20 minutes

Ingredients:

For Crust:

- ¾ cup unsweetened coconut flakes
- 1 cup dates, pitted and chopped roughly

For Filing:

- ¾ cup young coconut meat
- 1½ avocados, peeled, pitted and chopped
- 2 tablespoons fresh lime juice
- ¼ cup raw agave nectar

Directions:

1. Lightly, grease an 8-inch pie pan.
2. In a sizable food processor, add all crust ingredients and pulse till smooth.
3. Transfer the crust mixture into prepared pan, pressing gently downwards.
4. With a paper towel, wipe out your blender completely.
5. In the same processor, add all filling ingredients and pulse till smooth.
6. Place filling mixture over crust evenly.
7. Freeze not less than 120 minutes or till set completely.

Nutrition:

Calories: 290 Fat: 14g, Carbohydrates: 31g, Fiber: 6g, Protein: 7g

594. BLACKBERRY & APPLE SKILLET CAKE

Servings: 4
Preparation Time: 20 minutes
Cooking Time: 25 minutes

Ingredients:

For Filling:

- 2 tablespoons coconut oil

- 1 tablespoon coconut sugar
- 3 sweet apples, cored and cut into bite sized pieces
- ½ teaspoon ground cinnamon
- ¼ teaspoon ground cardamom
- 1/8 teaspoon ground cloves
- 1/8 teaspoon ground ginger
- 1 cup frozen blackberries

For Cake Mixture:

- ¾ cup ground almonds
- ½ teaspoon baking powder
- 2 tablespoons coconut sugar
- Pinch of salt
- ¼ cup full- Fat coconut milk
- 1 tablespoon coconut oil, melted
- 1 organic egg, beaten
- ½ teaspoon organic vanilla extract

Directions:

1. Preheat the oven to 40 degrees F.
2. In an ovenproof skillet, add butter and coconut sugar on high heat.
3. Cook, stirring for approximately 2-3 minutes.
4. Stir in apples and spices and cook, stirring approximately 5 minutes.
5. Remove from heat and stir in blackberries.
6. Meanwhile in a bowl, mix together ground almonds, baking powder, coconut sugar and salt.
7. In another bowl, add remaining ingredients and beat till well combined.
8. Add egg mixture into ground almond mixture and mix till well combined.
9. Place a combination over fruit mixture evenly.
10. Transfer the skillet into oven.
11. Bake approximately 15-20 min. Serve warm.

Nutritional Information:

Calories: 294 Fat: 9g, Carbohydrates: 22g, Fiber: 44g, Protein: 6g

595. PUDDING MUFFINS

Servings: 5
Preparation Time: 15 minutes
Cooking Time: 26 minutes

Ingredients:

For Muffins:

- 12 dates, pitted and chopped
- 10 tablespoons water
- 2½-3 tablespoons coconut flour
- ½ teaspoon baking powder
- 2 organic eggs
- 1½ bananas, peeled and sliced
- 1 teaspoon organic honey
- 1 tablespoon organic vanilla flavoring

For Topping:

- 5-6, pitted and chopped
- 3 tablespoons almond milk
- Fresh juice of ½ orange
- 1 teaspoon organic honey
- 1 teaspoon organic vanilla flavoring

For Garnishing:

- Fresh raspberries, as required

Directions:

1. Preheat the oven to 365 degrees F. Grease 5 cups of an large muffin tin.
2. For muffins in a very small pan, mix together dates and water on low heat.
3. Cook for approximately 3-4 minutes or till the dates break down and be thick.
4. Remove from heat and having a fork, mash the dates completely.
5. In a bowl, add remaining ingredients and beat till well combined.
6. Add mashed dates and stir to combine.
7. Transfer the mix in prepared muffin cups evenly.
8. Bake for about 20-22 minutes.
9. Meanwhile in a pan, add all topping ingredients on low heat.
10. Cook for about 3-4 minutes or till the dates break up and turn into thick.
11. Remove from heat and having a fork, mash the dates completely. Keep aside.
12. Remove muffins from oven and keep aside to cool for approximately 5 minutes.
13. Carefully, take away the muffins from cups. Top with date mixture evenly.
14. Garnish with raspberries and serve

Nutrition:

Calories: 287 Fat: 7g, Carbohydrates: 27g, Fiber: 6g, Protein: 9 g

596. BLACK FOREST PUDDING

Servings: 2
Preparation Time: 15 minutes
Cooking Time: 2 minutes

Ingredients:

- 1 teaspoon coconut cream
- 1 teaspoon coconut oil
- 3-4 squares 70% chocolate bars, chopped
- 1 cup coconut cream, whipped till thick and divided
- 2 cups fresh cherries, pitted and quartered
- 70% chocolate bars shaving, for garnishing
- Shredded coconut, for garnishing

Directions:

1. In a smaller pan, add 1 teaspoon coconut cream, coconut oil and chopped chocolate on low heat.
2. Cook, stirring continuously for about 2 minutes or till thick and glossy. Immediately, remove from heat.
3. In 2 serving glasses, divide chocolate sauce evenly.
4. Now, place ½ cup of cream over chocolate sauce in the glasses.
5. Divide cherries in glasses evenly.
6. Top with remaining coconut cream.
7. Garnish with chocolate shaving and shredded coconut.

Nutrition:

Calories: 302 Fat: 10g, Carbohydrates: 30g, Fiber: 3g, Protein: 4g

597. PINEAPPLE STICKS

Servings: 8
Preparation Time: 10 minutes

Ingredients:

- ¼ cup fresh orange juice
- ¾ cup coconut, shredded and toasted
- 8 (3x1-inch) fresh pineapple pieces

Directions:

1. Line a baking sheet with wax paper.
2. In a shallow dish, place pineapple juice.
3. In another shallow dish, squeeze pineapple.
4. Insert 1 wooden skewer in each pineapple piece through the narrow end.
5. Dip each pineapple piece in juice and then coat with coconut evenly.
6. Arrange the pineapple sticks onto prepared baking sheet inside a single layer.
7. Cover and freeze for around 1-2 hours.

Nutrition:

Calories: 65, Fat: 3g, Carbohydrates: 10g, Fiber: 1g, Protein: 0g

598. FRIED PINEAPPLE SLICES

Servings: 6-8
Preparation Time: 15 minutes
Cooking Time: 6 minutes

Ingredients:

- 1 fresh pineapple, peeled and cut into large slices
- ¼ cup coconut oil
- ¼ cup coconut palm sugar
- ¼ teaspoon ground cinnamon

Directions:

1. Heat a large surefire skillet on medium heat.
2. Stir in oil and sugar till coconut oil is very melted.
3. Add pineapple slices in batches and cook for approximately 1-2 minutes.
4. Carefully flip the side and cook for around 1 minute.
5. Cook for approximately 1 minute more.
6. Repeat with remaining slices.
7. Sprinkle with cinnamon and serve.

Nutrition:

Calories: 97 Fat: 1g, Carbohydrates: 12g, Fiber: 2g, Protein: 1g

599. GRILLED PEACHES

Servings: 6
Preparation Time: 15 minutes
Cooking Time: 10 min

Ingredients:

- 3 medium peaches, halved and pitted
- ½ cup coconut cream

- 1 teaspoon vanilla flavoring
- ¼ cup walnuts, chopped
- Ground cinnamon, as required

Directions:

1. Preheat the grill to medium-low heat. Grease the grill grate.
2. Arrange the peach slices onto grill, cut-side down.
3. Grill for approximately 3-5 minutes per side or till desired doneness.
4. Meanwhile inside a bowl, add coconut cream and vanilla extract and beat till smooth.
5. Spoon the whipped cream over each peach half.
6. Top with walnuts and sprinkle with cinnamon and serve.

Nutrition:

Calories: 286 Fat: 7g, Carbohydrates: 22g, Fiber: 4g, Protein: 8g

600. BAKED APPLES

Servings: 4
Preparation Time: 15 minutes
Cooking Time: 18 minutes

Ingredients:

- 4 tart apples, cored
- ¼ cup coconut oil, softened
- 4 teaspoons ground cinnamon
- 1/8 teaspoon ground ginger
- 1/8 teaspoon ground nutmeg

Directions:

1. Preheat the oven to 350 degrees F.
2. Fill each apple with 1 tablespoon of coconut oil.
3. Sprinkle with spices evenly.
4. Arrange the apples onto a baking sheet.
5. Bake for around 12-18 minutes.

Nutrition:

Calories: 285 Fat: 8g, Carbohydrates: 17g, Fiber: 3g, Protein: 52g

601. STUFFED APPLES

Servings: 4
Preparation Time: 15 minutes
Cooking Time: 35 minutes

Ingredients:

- 4 large apples, peeled and cored
- 2 teaspoons fresh lemon juice
- 1 cup fresh blueberries
- ½ cup fresh apple juice
- ½ teaspoon ground cinnamon
- ¼ cup almond meal
- ¼ cup coconut flakes

Directions:

1. Preheat the oven to 375 degrees F.
2. Coat the apples with lemon juice evenly.
3. Arrange the apples inside a baking dish.
4. Stuff each apple with blueberries.
5. Scatter the rest of the blueberries around the apples.
6. Drizzle with apple juice.
7. Sprinkle each apple with cinnamon evenly.
8. Top with almond meal and coconut flakes evenly.
9. Bake approximately 30-35 minutes.

Nutrition:

Calories: 200, Fat: 2g, Carbohydrates: 15g, Fiber: 1g, Protein: 4g

602. RHUBARB & BLUEBERRY GRANITA

Servings: 8
Preparation Time: 15 minutes
Cooking Time: 10 minutes

Ingredients:

- 1 cup fresh blueberries
- 3cups rhubarb, sliced
- ½ cup raw honey
- 2½ cups water
- Fresh mint leaves, for garnishing

Directions:

1. In a pan, add all ingredients on medium heat.
2. Cook, stirring occasionally for around 10 minutes.
3. Strain the mix through a strainer by pressing a combination.
4. Discard the pulp of fruit.
5. Transfer the strained mixture right into a

13x9-inch glass baking dish.
6. Freeze for around 20-a half-hour.
7. Remove from freezer and with a fork scrap the mix.
8. Cover and freeze for approximately 60 minutes, scraping after every half an hour.

Nutrition:

Calories: 122, Fat: 2g, Carbohydrates: 16g, Fiber: 2g, Protein: 6.1g

603. CITRUS STRAWBERRY GRANITA

Servings: 4
Preparation Time: 15 minutes
Cooking Time: 5 minutes

Ingredients:

- 12-ounce fresh strawberries.hulled
- 1 grapefruit, peeled, seeded and sectioned
- 2 oranges, peeled, seeded and sectioned
- ¼ of a lemon
- ¼ cup raw honey

Directions:

1. In a juicer add strawberries, grapefruit, oranges and lemon and process based on manufacturer's directions.
2. In a pan, add 1½ cups from the fruit juice and honey on medium heat.
3. Cook, stirring approximately 5 minutes.
4. Remove from heat and stir within the remaining juice.
5. Keep aside to cool for approximately a half-hour.
6. Transfer the juice mixture into an 8x8-inch glass baking dish.
7. Freeze for approximately 4 hours, scraping after every 30 minutes.

Nutrition:

Calories: 211, Fat: 2g, Carbohydrates: 19g, Fiber: 3g, Protein: 2g

604. PUMPKIN ICE-CREAM

Servings: 6-8
Preparation Time: 15 minutes

Ingredients:

- 1 (15-ounce) can pumpkin puree
- ½ cup dates, pitted and chopped
- 2 (14-ounce) cans coconut milk
- ½ teaspoon vanilla extract
- 1½ teaspoons pumpkin pie spice
- ½ teaspoon ground cinnamon
- Pinch of salt

Directions:

1. In an increased speed blender, add all ingredients and pulse till smooth.
2. Transfer into an airtight container and freeze for approximately 1-couple of hours.
3. Now, transfer into an ice-cream maker and process based on manufacturer's directions.
4. Return the ice-cream into airtight container and freeze for approximately 1-couple of hours.

Nutrition:

Calories: 103, Fat: 6g, Carbohydrates: 16g, Fiber: 5g, Protein: 7g

605. CHOCOLATY CHERRY ICE-CREAM

Servings: 2
Preparation Time: 10 minutes

Ingredients:

- 1 cup raw cashews
- 1 cup frozen cherries
- ¼ cup coconut, shredded
- 1 tablespoon raw honey
- ¼ cup chocolate bars, chopped

Directions:

1. In a higher speed blender, add cashews and pulse till a flour like texture forms.
2. Add remaining ingredients except chocolate and pulse till smooth.
3. Add chocolate and pulse till just combined.
4. Transfer the ice-cream into airtight container and freeze for about 1-120 minutes or till set.

Nutrition:

Calories: 135, Fat: 9g, Carbohydrates: 23g, Fiber: 4g, Protein: 12g

606. PINEAPPLE & BANANA ICE-CREAM

Servings: 6
Preparation Time: 15 minutes
Cooking Time: 20 minutes

Ingredients:

- 1(14-ounce) can coconut milk
- 1 cup frozen pineapple chunks, thawed
- 4 cups frozen banana slices, thawed
- 2 tablespoons fresh lime juice
- Pinch of salt

Directions:

1. Line a glass baking dish with plastic wrap.
2. In a higher speed blender, add all ingredients and pulse till smooth.
3. Transfer the amalgamation into prepared baking dish evenly.
4. Freeze approximately 35-40 minutes.

Nutrition:

Calories: 129, Fat: 14.3g, Carbohydrates: 32.5g, Fiber: 4g, Protein: 2.7g

607. CHOCOLATE SORBET

Servings: 4-6
Preparation Time: 15 minutes
Cooking Time: 3-4 minutes

Ingredients:

- 1/3 cup chocolate bars, chopped
- ½ cup unsweetened cocoa powder
- ½ cup coconut sugar
- Pinch of salt
- 2¼ cups water
- 1 tablespoon plus 1 teaspoon extra-virgin olive oil

Directions:

1. Freeze ice-cream maker tub for around a day before making sorbet.
2. In a pan, add all ingredients except oil on medium heat.
3. Bring with a boil, beating continuously.
4. Reduce heat to low and simmer for approximately thirty seconds.
5. Remove from heat and transfer in a heat-proof bowl.
6. Refrigerate for about 2-8 hours.
7. Now, transfer into an ice-cream maker and process according to manufacturer's directions.
8. While motor is running, add 1 tablespoon of oil.
9. Return the ice-cream into airtight container and freeze for around couple of hours.
10. Serve using the drizzling of remaining oil.

Nutrition:

Calories: 153, Fat: 13g, Carbohydrates: 25g, Fiber: 2g, Protein: 17g

608. LEMON SORBET

Servings: 2
Preparation Time: 10 minutes

Ingredients:

- 2 tablespoons fresh lemon zest, grated
- ½ cup raw honey
- 2 cups water
- 1½ cups freshly squeezed lemon juice

Directions:

1. Freeze ice-cream maker tub for about one day prior to sorbet.
2. In a pan, add all ingredients except fresh lemon juice on medium heat.
3. Simmer, stirring for approximately 1 minute or till sugar dissolves.
4. Remove from heat and stir in fresh lemon juice.
5. Transfer into an airtight container.
6. Refrigerate approximately 2 hours.
7. Now, transfer into an ice-cream maker and process according to manufacturer's directions.
8. While motor is running, add 1 tablespoon of oil.
9. Return the ice-cream into airtight container and freeze approximately 120 minutes.

Nutrition:

Calories: 134, Fat: 5g, Carbohydrates: 17.5g, Fiber: 2g, Protein: 7g

609. ZESTY MOUSSE

Servings: 4
Preparation Time: 15 minutes

Ingredients:

- 2 cups bananas, peeled and chopped
- 2 ripe avocados, peeled, pitted and chopped
- 1 teaspoon fresh lime zest, grated finely
- 1 teaspoon fresh lemon zest, grated finely
- ½ cup fresh lime juice
- ½ cup fresh lemon juice
- 1/3 cup raw honey

Directions:

1. In a blender, add all ingredients and pulse till smooth.
2. Transfer the mousse in 4 serving glasses.
3. Refrigerate to relax approximately 3 hours.

Nutrition:

Calories: 121, Fat: 8g, Carbohydrates: 25g, Fiber: 3g, Protein: 7g

610. CHOCOLATE & COFFEE MOUSSE

Servings: 4
Preparation Time: 15 minutes
Cooking Time: 20 minutes

Ingredients:

- ¼ cup chocolate brown chips
- ½ cup coconut milk
- ¼ cup boiling water
- 1 tablespoon ground coffees
- Raw honey, to taste
- ¼ teaspoon almond extract
- 1 tablespoon vanilla flavor

Directions:

1. In a nonstick pan, add chocolate chips on medium-low heat.
2. Cook, stirring continuously for around 2-3 minutes or till chocolate chips are melted.
3. Add coconut milk and beat till well combined.
4. Cook, stirring continuously for around 1-2 minutes.
5. Meanwhile in a small bowl, mix together hot water and coffee beans.
6. In a sizable bowl, add chocolate mixture, coffee mixture, honey and both extracts and mix till well combined.
7. Transfer the mousse in 4 serving glasses.
8. Refrigerate to relax for approximately 2-3 hours.

Nutrition:

Calories: 112, Fat: 3g, Carbohydrates: 12g, Fiber: 1g, Protein: 2g

611. CHOCOLATY AVOCADO MOUSSE

Servings: 4-6
Preparation Time: 10 minutes

Ingredients:

- 2 ripe avocados, peeled, pitted and chopped
- ½ cup coconut milk
- ½ cup cacao powder
- 1 teaspoon ground cinnamon
- ¼ teaspoon ground ancho Chile
- 1/3 cup raw honey
- 2 teaspoons vanilla extract

Directions:

1. In a blender, add all ingredients and pulse till smooth.
2. Transfer the mousse in serving glasses.
3. Refrigerate to relax completely.

Nutrition:

Calories: 132, Fat: 5g, Carbohydrates: 26g, Fiber: 6g, Protein: 34g

612. CHOCOLATY CHIA PUDDING

Servings: 4
Preparation Time: 10 minutes

Ingredients:

- 6-9 dates, pitted and chopped
- 1½ cups unsweetened almond milk
- 1/3 cup chia seeds
- ¼ cup unsweetened cocoa powder
- ½ teaspoon ground cinnamon
- Salt, to taste
- ½ teaspoon vanilla flavor

Directions:

1. In a mixer, add all ingredients and pulse till smooth.
2. Transfer the mixture into serving bowls.
3. Refrigerate to chill completely before serving.

Nutrition:

Calories: 166, Fat: 7g, Carbohydrates: 21g, Fiber: 7g, Protein: 17g

613. CARROT CHIA PUDDING

Servings: 1 serving
Preparation Time: 15 minutes
Cooking Time: 7 minutes

Ingredients:

- ¾ cup carrot, peeled and chopped roughly
- 2-3 tablespoons walnuts, chopped
- ½ teaspoon ground cinnamon
- ¼ teaspoon ground ginger
- Pinch of ground nutmeg
- Pinch of ground cloves
- 1-2 tablespoons raw honey
- 1 cup unsweetened almond milk
- ½ cup water
- ½ teaspoon vanilla flavoring
- 2 tablespoons chia seeds

Directions:

1. In a mixer, add carrot and walnuts and pulse till chopped finely.
2. Transfer the carrot mixture in the nonstick pan on medium heat.
3. Add spices and honey and cook, stirring occasionally for about 5-7 minutes.
4. Stir in almond milk, water and vanilla extract.
5. Transfer a combination into a serving bowl.
6. Add chia seeds and stir to blend well.
7. Cover and refrigerate for overnight.

Nutrition:

Calories: 137, Fat: 2g, Carbohydrates: 24g, Fiber: 9g, Protein: 6g

614. APPLE CHIA PUDDING

Servings: 1 serving
Preparation Time: 15 minutes
Cooking Time: 20 minutes

Ingredients:

- ½ cup unsweetened almond milk
- 2 tablespoons chia seeds
- ½ teaspoon ground cinnamon, divided
- 1/8 teaspoon vanilla extract
- 1 apple, cored and chopped finely
- ½ teaspoon raw honey
- 1½ teaspoons water
- 2 tablespoons golden raisins

Directions:

1. In a bowl, mix together almond milk, chia seeds, ¼ teaspoon of cinnamon and vanilla flavoring.
2. Refrigerate for around 1-120 minutes.
3. In a microwave safe bowl, mix together apple, honey, water and remaining cinnamon and microwave on high for around 1-2 minutes, stirring once.
4. Remove from microwave and stir in raisins.
5. Add 50 % of apple mixture in chia seeds mixture and stir to blend.
6. Refrigerate before serving.
7. Top with remaining apple mixture and serve.

Nutrition:

Calories: 123, Fat: 3g, Carbohydrates: 15g, Fiber: 4g, Protein: 6g

28 DAY MEAL PLAN

DAY	BREAKFAST	MAINS	DESSERT
1.	Berry Chia with Yogurt	Dolmas Wrap	Semolina Pudding
2.	Arugula Eggs with Chili Peppers	Salad al Tonno	Fruit Trifle
3.	Breakfast Skillet	Arlecchino Rice Salad	Berry Crumble
4.	Eggs in Tomato Rings	Greek Salad	Greek Cheesecake
5.	Eggplant Chicken Sandwich	Sauteed Chickpea and Lentil Mix	Lemon Pie
6.	Eggplant Caprese	Baked Vegetables Soup	Galaktoboureko
7.	Chorizo Bowl with Corn	Pesto Chicken Salad	Honey Cake
8.	Panzanella Salad	Falafel	Portokalopita
9.	Shrimp Bruschetta	Israeli Pasta Salad	Finikia
10.	Strawberry Muesli	Artichoke Matzo Mina	Vasilopita
11.	Rhubarb Muffins	Stuffed Zucchini Boats with Goat Cheese	No-Bake Strawberry Cheesecake
12.	Apple Muesli		Chocolaty Chia Pudding
13.	Gingerbread Oatmeal		Chocolaty Avocado Mousse
14.	Breakfast Crepes		Zesty Mousse
15.			Carrot Chia Pudding
16.	Buckwheat Granola		Lemon Sorbet
17.	Mushroom Frittata		Chocolate Sorbet
18.	Millet Muffins	Light Paprika Moussaka	Grilled Peaches
19.	Kale Smoothie	Creamy Penne	Baked Apples
20.	Olive Bread	Greek Style Quesadillas	Stuffed Apples
21.	Chia Pudding	Cucumber Bowl with Spices and Greek Yogurt	Rhubarb & Blueberry Granita
22.	Yogurt Bulgur	Stuffed Meatballs with Eggs	Citrus Strawberry Granita
23.	Goat Cheese Omelet	Stuffed Tomatoes with Cheese and Meat	Semolina Pudding
24.	Vanilla Scones	Garlic Chicken Balls	Hummingbird Cake
25.	Yufka Pies	Prosciutto Wrapped Mozzarella Balls	Grilled Pineapple
26.	Breakfast Potato Latkes with Spinach	Sweet Potato Bacon Mash	Cream Strawberry Pies
27.	Cherry Tomatoes and Feta Fritatta	Stuffed Bell Peppers with Quinoa	Coconut-Mint Bars
28.	Egg White Scramble	Mediterranean Burrito	Banana Muffins

5 TIPS

You can do a lot of things if you want to keep your kidneys healthy and have them functioning properly. Here are certain tips that you can keep in mind for ensuring proper functioning of your kidneys.

Keep yourself hydrated:

You should always make sure that you are sufficiently hydrated, but you shouldn't overdo this. No studies have shown that over-hydration is good for enhancing the performance of your kidneys. It is definitely good to drink sufficient water and you can drink around four to six glasses of water per day. Consuming more water than this wouldn't definitely help your kidneys perform better. In fact, it would just increase the stress on your kidneys.

Consume healthy foods:

Your kidneys are capable of tolerating a wide variety of dietary habits and usually most of the kidney problems crop up from other existing medical conditions, like high blood pressure or diabetes. Because of this, it would be advisable if you were consuming foods that will help you in regulating your weight and blood pressure. If you were able to prevent diabetes and even high blood pressure, then your kidneys would be healthy as well.

Exercise regularly:

If you were already consuming foods that are healthy then it would also make sense if you were exercising regularly. Because regular physical activity will prevent weight gain and also regulate your blood pressure. But you should be careful about the amount of time you exercise or how much you exercise, especially if you aren't acclimatized to exercising. Don't overexert yourself if you are just getting started, because this would just increase the pressure on your kidneys and can also result in the breaking down of your muscles.

Be careful when making use of supplements:

If you are consuming any supplements or any other herbal remedies, then you should be mindful of the amount you are consuming. Consuming excessive amount of vitamin supplements as well as any herbal extracts can prove to be harmful to the functioning of your kidneys. You should talk to your doctor before you start taking any supplements.

Quit smoking:

Smoking causes damage to your blood vessels and this in turn would reduce the flow of blood to and in your kidneys. When the kidneys don't receive sufficient blood, they won't function like they are supposed to. Smoking also tends to increase your blood pressure and can also cause kidney cancer, apart from damaging your lungs.

CONCLUSION

With that recipe, we have come to the end of this book. I want to thank you for choosing this book.

I hope this book helped you understand what renal failure diet is all about. You would have understood by now that it isn't just about following a diet for ensuring the health of your kidneys. But you should also make certain lifestyle changes and make the renal failure diet a part of your daily life if you want to maintain the health of your kidneys in the long run.

Since kidneys are vital for the proper functioning of the human body, you need to take good care of them. The first step for having healthy kidneys would be to incorporate all that you have read about in this book. You should also make sure that these practices become a habit for you and you will definitely start to notice a positive change in your overall health!

Thank you and all the best!

Made in the USA
Columbia, SC
28 October 2020